Low-Intensity Control of Nerve Tissue Activity

Online at: https://doi.org/10.1088/978-0-7503-6034-0

About the Series

The series in Physics and Engineering in Medicine and Biology will allow the Institute of Physics and Engineering in Medicine (IPEM) to enhance its mission to 'advance physics and engineering applied to medicine and biology for the public good'.

It is focused on key areas including, but not limited to:

- clinical engineering
- diagnostic radiology
- informatics and computing
- magnetic resonance imaging
- nuclear medicine
- physiological measurement
- radiation protection
- radiotherapy
- rehabilitation engineering
- ultrasound and non-ionising radiation.

A number of IPEM–IOP titles are being published as part of the EUTEMPE Network Series for Medical Physics Experts.

A full list of titles published in this series can be found here: https://iopscience.iop.org/bookListInfo/physics-engineering-medicine-biology-series.

Low-Intensity Control of Nerve Tissue Activity

Mikhail N Shneider
Princeton University, Princeton, NJ, USA

Mikhail Pekker
Retired, Princeton, NJ, USA

IOP Publishing, Bristol, UK

ISBN 978-0-7503-6034-0 (ebook)
ISBN 978-0-7503-6032-6 (print)
ISBN 978-0-7503-6035-7 (myPrint)
ISBN 978-0-7503-6033-3 (mobi)

DOI 10.1088/978-0-7503-6034-0

Version: 20241201

IOP ebooks

British Library Cataloguing-in-Publication Data: A catalogue record for this book is available from the British Library.

Published by IOP Publishing, wholly owned by The Institute of Physics, London

IOP Publishing, No.2 The Distillery, Glassfields, Avon Street, Bristol, BS2 0GR, UK

US Office: IOP Publishing, Inc., 190 North Independence Mall West, Suite 601, Philadelphia, PA 19106, USA

To our grandchildren

Contents

Preface

Wonder is the seed of knowledge.

—Francis Bacon

This book is written in a way that is unusual for the scientific tradition. It not only presents the results of research on nonthermal stimulation of nervous tissue by low-intensity microwave radiation and pulsed weak currents (in which the authors actively participated) but also traces the process of determining the underlying ideas of each research discovery. It is the latter that can transform science into a fascinating journey for the reader rather than an unconnected collection of questions and answers.

Our book is written primarily for biologists and physicians, but also for physicists, engineers, students, and curious readers interested in science who want to understand the basics of stimulation and propagation of signals in nervous tissue and the mechanisms that cause them. We did not set out to provide an exhaustive introduction to modern neuroscience, which is the subject of a number of excellent textbooks and monographs, some of which we referred to in writing our book. Moreover, we have not attempted to summarize or comment on the numerous journal articles on the subject. Our goal is to describe the phenomena and the biophysical mechanisms that explain them. For this reason, the book does not provide a detailed review of the literature but instead is based on works that allow the reader to understand the essence of the phenomena in the most understandable and simple way.

In our presentation, we first sketch the history of the science of signal propagation along nerves from Galvani's 'animal electricity' to Hodgkin and Huxley's phenomenological model of unmyelinated fibers, which is based on experiments with the giant squid axon. We also briefly review the evolution of experimental methods for observing the nervous system and its processes, which have been refined over time, up to the most recent, such as optogenetics, thermogenetics, and those based on the use of green fluorescent proteins.

We have considered in detail the phenomenon of ephaptic coupling, which consists of the transmission of excitation by currents in the intercellular medium from an active neuron to an inactive neuron in its vicinity. This phenomenon plays an important role in the functioning of the nervous system and, in particular, is the key to understanding the processes of stimulation of nerve tissue activity by weak current pulses initiated by an external source.

In the 1960s, experiments showed that low-intensity microwave electromagnetic fields can have a strong effect on living organisms and that the effect is selective to the frequency of microwave radiation. In 2010, experiments were conducted on the direct effect of microwave irradiation on nerve tissue. In these experiments, it was found that at very low intensities, the excitability of nerve tissue increases and that action potentials can be self-initiated. However, these and other experiments did not elucidate the mechanism of microwave effects on the excitation thresholds of action potentials in neurons. Surprisingly, until recently, the question of the mechanism of the experimentally observed effect of low-intensity microwave electromagnetic fields on the excitation of action potentials in nerve tissue has remained unanswered. This issue is important because of the widespread electromagnetic noise associated with, for example, the development of mobile communications and wireless Wi-Fi technologies. We have shown that the electric field of an electromagnetic wave directed along the axon surface leads to longitudinal acoustic oscillations of the membrane, which in turn lead to the displacement of unbound ion channels that are subject to lateral diffusion. This interaction and the resulting redistribution of transmembrane ion channels have a pronounced resonant character and lead to an increase in the density of sodium channels in a region of the initial segment of the axon, resulting in a lower threshold for action potential excitation.

In this book, we consider nonthermal effects that stimulate the activity of nervous tissue, but microwave radiation is inevitably partially absorbed in nervous tissue, which leads to its heating. It is known that when a membrane is heated by an external source above a certain phase transition threshold, irreversible conformation of proteins embedded in the membrane occurs. This allows us to determine the temperature at which the effects of stimulating the activity of nerve tissue can be considered thermal.

To date, the medical community has gained extensive experience in the treatment of paralyzed patients with spinal cord injuries using external electrodes to initiate relatively low currents to stimulate muscle activity and anesthesia. However, there is no understanding of how weak currents introduced into the body can lower the excitation thresholds of action potentials and have a therapeutic effect on paralyzed patients, while also raising the excitation thresholds of action potentials, thus blocking the sensation of pain. This book presents a theory that answers these questions.

In recent decades, plasma medicine, which studies the interaction between weakly ionized low-temperature plasma and cell ensembles in physiological solutions in Petri dishes, has attracted great interest. In such an interaction, ions from the plasma enter the solution, changing the ionic composition of the solution and thus the osmotic pressure in the cells. We have found in our research that osmotic pressure offers an explanation for the experimentally observed change in cell morphology under the influence of low-temperature plasma on the surface of the solution in the cuvette where the cells are located. Furthermore, changes in osmotic pressure and associated changes in cell shape lead to changes in the water content of lipid membranes and thus to changes in their effective dielectric constant. In the case of neurons in solution interacting with the plasma source, this may lead to changes in the resting potential at the axon membranes and in the thresholds of action potential excitation. A separate chapter of this book is devoted to these issues, which require further in-depth research.

One of the main goals of our book is to provide a clear understanding of the biophysical phenomena underlying the stimulation and propagation of action potentials along nerve fibers. We hope that our book will attract physicians, students, and researchers of various specialties to theoretical and experimental studies in the field of neurostimulation and anesthesia of nerve fibers by weak electromagnetic fields and the study of the corresponding mechanisms of influence on the excitation thresholds of action potentials.

Acknowledgements

We are thankful to our colleagues and friends E Cohen, Yu Gerasimenko, R Gimatdinov, V R Edgerton, A Filippov, M Keidar, L Lurya, E Nikolsky, P Porazik, M Possover, S Reuter, V Semak, A Shashurin, A Starikovskiy, S Starikovskaia, S Talyansky, and A Zheltikov for their encouragement, stimulating discussions, and interest in the issues we address in this book.

We are also grateful to Lora Shneider and Rita Polishchuk for their understanding and support of our work.

Author biographies

Mikhail N Shneider

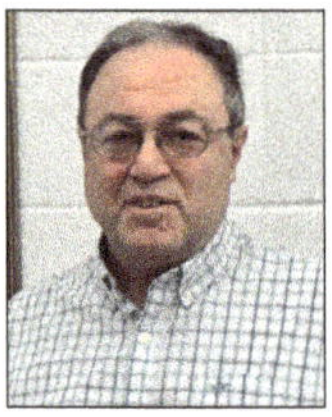

Dr Mikhail N Shneider received a master's degree in theoretical physics (with honors) from Kazan State University, Russia, a PhD in plasma physics and chemistry from the All-Union Electrotechnical Institute, Moscow, and a Doctor of Sciences (the highest scientific degree in Russia) in plasma physics and chemistry from the Institute of High Temperatures, Russian Academy of Sciences, Moscow. Since 1998, Dr Shneider has worked at the Department of Mechanical and Aerospace Engineering, Princeton University, where he is currently a senior research scholar. His research interests include the theoretical study of gas-discharge physics, physical gas dynamics, biophysics, atmospheric electrical phenomena, nonlinear optics, and laser–matter interaction. He has published about 250 papers in refereed journals (including 11 review papers), three U.S. patents, and two books. Dr Shneider has been a visiting professor at universities in Austria, China, France, Germany, Great Britain, Israel, and Russia. He is the recipient of the 2020 AIAA Plasma Dynamics and Lasers Award and Medal.

Mikhail Pekker

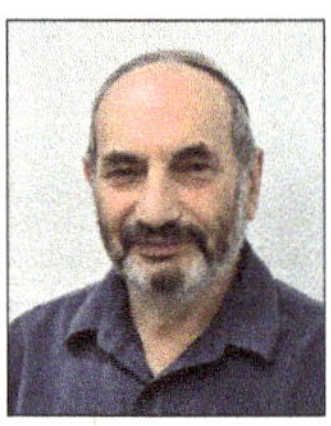

Dr Mikhail Pekker received his master's degree in physics and applied mathematics from Novosibirsk State University, Russia, and his PhD in physics and mathematics from the Institute of Theoretical and Applied Mechanics, Novosibirsk, Russia. From 1993 until 2007, he worked at the Institute for Fusion Studies at the University of Texas, Austin; from 2010 to 2014, he worked at the Drexel Plasma Institute, Drexel University, as an Assistant Research Professor; and from 2015 to 2017, he worked at the Department of Mechanical and Aerospace Engineering at George Washington University. At present, he is retired. His research interests include the theoretical study of gas discharge physics, biophysics, and the general theory of relativity. Dr Mikhail Pekker has authored about 100 papers (three review papers), one U.S. patent, and one book. He is the author of several fiction books and the winner of the Literary Prize of Writers of Russia for 2006 and the 2018 'Golden Pen of Russia.'

Nomenclature

A_s	Sound wave amplitude
$A_\parallel$, $A_\perp$	Amplitudes of longitudinal and transverse membranes
C_m	Displacement membrane capacitance per unit area of skin
C_{skin}	Capacitance per unit area
C_M	Capacitance per unit length of myelin segment
D_L	Lateral diffusion coefficient
$\overline{E}$	Electric field of an electromagnetic wave
$E_\parallel$	Electric field of an electromagnetic wave directed along the axon
$E_\perp$	Electric field of an electromagnetic wave perpendicular to the axon
$\overline{E}_s$	Energy density of the sound wave
$\vec{F}$	Force acting on the ion channel in the acoustic field in the membrane
$F_\parallel$, F_x	Longitudinal force acting per unit area of charged membrane
$F_\perp$, F_z	Transverse force acting per unit area of charged membrane
$F_{n,\,z}$	Amplitude of the Fourier component of the external force perpendicular to the membrane
$F_{n,\,x}$	Amplitude of the Fourier component of the external force along the membrane
F_{tr}	Force acting on a particle in the field of a traveling sound wave
F_{st}	Force acting on a particle in a standing sound wave field
$G_{\text{Na}} \sim g_{\text{Na}}, G_{\text{K}} \sim g_{\text{K}}, G_L = g_L$	Membrane conductances per unit area for sodium, potassium and leakage in the Hodgkin–Huxley equations.
I_{Na}	Current density of sodium ions through a unit area of membrane
I_{K}	Current density of potassium ions through a unit area of membrane
I_L	Leakage current density per unit area of membrane
$I_\parallel$	Current density per unit area of axon cross section
$I_\perp$	Current density normal to the membrane surface
I_r, I_z	Radial and longitudinal current densities outside the axon ($r > a$)
I_{MW}	Microwave radiation intensity
J	Total current
$J_\parallel = \pi a^2 I_\parallel$	Longitudinal current through the axon cross-section
$J_\perp = 2\pi a I_\perp \, dz$	Transverse current through the membrane
L_{IS}	Length of the initial segment
L_R	Length of the node of Ranvier
L_M	Length of the myelin sheath
N_{A}	Avogadro's number (in SI: $6.023 \cdot 10^{23}\ \text{mol}^{-1}$)
$P_s = \overline{E}_s c_s$	Sound wave energy flux per unit area
$R = k_B N_A$	Gas constant (in SI: $8.314\,462\ \text{J} \cdot \text{K}^{-1} \cdot \text{mol}^{-1}$)
R_{el}	External electrode radius
R_{Na}, R_{K}, R_L	Sodium, potassium and leakage membrane resistance per unit area
R_M	Resistance times unit length of the myelinated segment
$R_\parallel = r_\parallel / \pi a^2$	The electrolyte resistance in axon per unit length
T	Temperature
U	Potential above the membrane surface
V	Voltage on the membrane
V_{ap}	Action potential

V_R	Resting potential
V_{Na}, V_{K}, V_L	Resting voltages for sodium, potassium, and chloride ions (leakage) in the Hodgkin–Huxley equations
V_{th}	Threshold for the excitation of the action potential
V_d	Drift velocity of transmembrane protein channels
W_{ef}	Binding energy of the negative ion to the membrane surface
W_s	Energy absorbed by unit volume per unit time
Z	Charge number (value of charge in elementary charges)
a	Axon radius
a_s, a_{MW}	ultrasonic and microwave attenuation lengths in water
a_h	Distance between dipole heads in the membrane
b_{skin}	Thickness of the skin
$c_\varepsilon = c/\sqrt{\varepsilon}$	Speed of light in media
c_s	Speed of sound
c_p [J K^{-1}]	Membrane heat capacity of axon membrane
$c_{0,\,p}$ [J K^{-1}]	Melting membrane heat capacity
$c_{p,\,w}$[J kgK^{-1}]	Specific heat capacity of water
c_l, c_t	Longitudinal and transverse sound velocity in the membrane
d_m	Membrane thickness
d_M	Thickness of the myelinated layer
d_R	Diameter of the node of Ranvier
e	Elementary charge (in SI: $1.6021 \cdot 10^{-19}$ C)
f	Frequency of electromagnetic wave
f	Volume fraction of water in membrane
f_s [s^{-1}]	Frequency of sound waves in membrane
$f_{r,\,p}$[s^{-1}]	Resonant frequency of transverse pth acoustic harmonic in the membrane
k_B	Boltzmann's constant (in Si: $1.380649 \cdot 10^{-23}$ J $\cdot$ K^{-1})
$\vec{k}$, $\vec{k_s}$	Wave vectors of the electromagnetic and sound waves
$k_n = \pi n/L_{\text{IS}}$	Wave number of the standing acoustic wave in the initial segment
n	Refractive index
n, m, h	Coefficients used in the Hodgkin and Huxley equations
n_{ch}	Density of the protein channels per unit membrane area
$n_{\text{ch},\,0}$	Equilibrium density of the protein channels per unit membrane area
n_{ion}	Ion density
n_∞	Unperturbed ion density in water
p_{Na}, p_{K}, p_{Cl}	Membrane permeabilities of sodium, potassium, and chloride ions
q	Particle charge
r_p	Effective radius of the ion channel in the coagulation model
$r_\parallel$	Specific electrolyte resistance (in SI: [$\Omega \cdot$ m])
r_h	Radius of the dipole head
r_{ion}	Ion radius
t_M	Time of action potential propagation along the myelinated segment
t_s, $\tilde{t}_s$	Time of stimulated channel redistribution
t_{tr}	Charging time of the capacitor
$\vec{u}$	Displacement vector
v_{ap}	Action potential propagation velocity
ΔE_s	Energy absorbed by unit volume of medium

ΔT_s	Change in water temperature due to ultrasonic absorption
$\Delta V_{\text{th}} = V_{\text{th}} - V_R$	Action potential excitation threshold relative to resting potential
Δt_{ex}	Time required to initiate an action potential
α_n, β_n, α_m, β_m, α_h, β_h	Coefficients used in the Hodgkin and Huxley equations
$\delta_M = 0.5(d_M - d_R)$	Thickness of the myelinated sheath
δ_s	Thickness of the skin layer in the electrolyte for microwave radiation
δV_m	Perturbation of the membrane potential
ε	Relative dielectric permittivity of the media
ε_0	Vacuum permittivity (in SI: $8.854 \cdot 10^{-12}$ [$\text{F} \cdot \text{m}^{-1}$])
ε_m	Relative dielectric permittivity of membrane
$\varepsilon_{\text{skin}}$	Relative dielectric permittivity of skin
λ_s	Wavelength of sound waves in membrane
λ_D	Debye length
μ_L	Lateral mobility of the transmembrane protein channels
ν	Kinematic viscosity in water
ρ_0	Water density
ρ_m	Mean membrane density
ρ_p	Average density of a particle (ion channel) in the membrane
σ	Conductivity in intercellular electrolyte
σ_m	Surface charge of the membrane
τ_M	Maxwell time
φ	Electrical potential
$\omega = 2\pi f$	Cyclic frequency of the electromagnetic wave
$\omega_s = 2\pi f_s$	Cyclic frequency of the sound wave

IOP Publishing

Low-Intensity Control of Nerve Tissue Activity

Mikhail N Shneider and Mikhail Pekker

Chapter 1

Historical review

This section briefly outlines the history of the development of our knowledge of the stimulation, propagation, and observation of excitations in nerve fibers. We dwell only on the critical moments that have qualitatively changed our understanding of the mechanisms underlying the propagation of the action potential. The purpose of this introductory chapter is to emphasize the role of general knowledge in generating ideas for solving scientific problems, since new ideas generally lie at the intersection of two areas of knowledge that may seem unrelated at first glance. One such example is the use of cable equations describing signal propagation in a distributed electrical circuit to characterize the action potential in the squid giant axon (see section 1.4 of this chapter: model of squid axon proposed by Hodgkin and Huxley).

1.1 'Living' electricity

The birth of science begins with the formulation of a physical model of natural phenomena in terms accessible to mathematical description. Classical mechanics can serve as an example: its appearance was associated with Newton's formulation of the three laws of mechanics and the development of the apparatus of integral–differential calculus.[1] Another example is Mendel's genetics, in which Mendel associated color, grain shape, and other features with microparticles in cells and used the apparatus of probability theory to predict the likelihood of a given trait occurring during sexual interbreeding. Microparticles, which Mendel called 'factors,' are not

[1] Before Newton formulated the laws of mechanics, science was dominated by the Aristotelian view of motion: if no effort is applied to a body, then it will stop, since rest is the natural state of any body, and the fall of bodies to earth is explained by their love for Mother Earth: the more massive the body, the stronger the love, and the faster the body falls to the ground.

'contaminated' by subsequent generations but are inherited.[2] Almost 40 years later, the development of Mendel's ideas led to the chromosome theory of inheritance, created independently by Walter Sutton (1877–1916) and Theodor Boveri (1862–1915).

Neurobiology is no exception. Despite its long prehistory, most scholars consider that its development began with a series of works by Alan Lloyd Hodgkin (1914–98) and Andrew Fielding Huxley (1917–2012), who, together with John Carew Eccles, won the 1963 Nobel Prize in Physiology or Medicine. In these works, Hodgkin and Huxley constructed a physical model of action potential propagation along the squid giant axon [1–16], based on nonlinear telegraph equations well known in electrical engineering and empirical parameters taken from experiments. Later, Goldman modified the Hodgkin–Huxley model for myelinated nerve fibers [17].

The originality and revolutionary nature of Hodgkin and Huxley's approach cannot be fully appreciated without a brief historical overview.

In 1780, in the laboratory of the 43-year-old physiologist Luigi Galvani (1737–98) in Bologna, his young wife Lucia Galeazzi Galvani, the daughter of Galvani's teacher, was turning the handle of the electrostatic generator (an electrophorus machine),[3] as shown in figure 1.1(A). Lucia observed how a spark jumped between the balls from time to time. Suddenly, she noticed that during the spark, the leg of the dead frog, which Galvani's assistant had dissected, twitched whenever the assistant's scalpel touched the frog's body. Lucia was interested in science—she was not only a loving wife but also the daughter of a scientist—so she immediately connected these two completely different phenomena, namely the sparking in the electrophorus machine and the twitching of the frog's leg, and drew her husband's attention to them. Thus, we can without doubt consider that Galvani's wife was the coauthor of this great discovery.

As shown below, the operational principle of the ion pumps built into the membranes of neurons and other cells is, in many ways, similar to the operation of an electrostatic generator; therefore, the working principle of the electrophorus machine is shown and explained in figure 1.1(B).

After Galvani published the results of his research [19], a revolution in biology began. Experiments with 'animating dead animals with electricity' became popular among physiologists, physicists, and doctors. The undisputed leaders in the study of 'animal electricity' were Galvani and Alessandro Volta (1745–1827), the inventor of the voltaic column, which was the forerunner of all modern batteries and accumulators. The peak of the popularity of the study of 'animal electricity' can

[2] Gregor Johann Mendel (1822–84) worked as an assistant for Christian Doppler (the Doppler effect is named after him) while studying at the University of Vienna. In 1900, almost 35 years after Mendel reported the results of his experiments to the Brünn Society of Naturalists and published them in the proceedings of that society, they were independently rediscovered by Hugo de Vries (1848–1935), Carl Correns (1864–1933), and Erich von Tschermak-Seysenegg (1871–1962). The exceptional decency of these scientists should be noted, since their articles recognized Mendel's priority in formulating the laws of genetics, although they had not heard anything about Mendel before conducting their experiments.

[3] Most readers are more familiar with the later version of the electrostatic generator, the so-called Wimshurst machine, which appeared in 1880 and is still used in school demonstrations today.

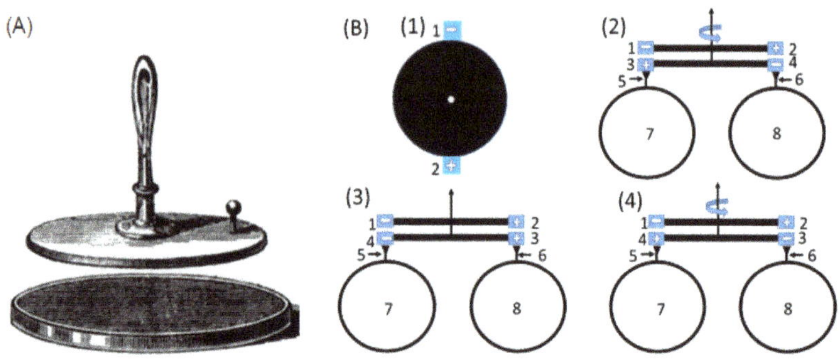

Figure 1.1. (A) Electrophorus machine [18] similar to that used in Galvani's experiments. This image [Electrophorus_device] has been obtained by the author(s) from the Wikimedia website, where it is stated to have been released into the public domain. It is included within this book on that basis. (B) The principle of operation of the electrophorus machine: (1) Top view of the electrophore machine; 1 and 2 are negatively and positively charged metal sections of the upper nonconducting disk, respectively. (2–4) Side views of the electrophore machine. The upper disk is stationary; the lower one, coaxial with the upper one, can rotate around its axis. On the lower rod, there are metal sections 3 and 4, which, through metal brushes five and six, are connected to large metal balls that store a charge. Section 3 has a charge opposite to the charge in section 1, and section 4 has a charge opposite to the charge in section 2. (3) The moment is shown when, after rotating the lower rod by 180 degrees, the positions of the sections with the same charge signs (1, 4 and 2, 3) coincide. The charges in sections 1 and 4 are negative; in sections 2 and 3, they are positive. Accordingly, the negative charge from section 4 passes through metal brush five and flows into ball seven. In turn, we can assume that the positive charge from this ball charges section 4. Similarly, the positive charge from section 3 flows through brush six into ball eight and is itself charged negatively. After turning another 180 degrees, section 3 is opposite section 1, and section 4 is opposite section 2. The process is then repeated. Thus, with each rotation of the lower disk by 180 degrees, a positive charge is transferred from ball seven to ball eight and a negative charge is transferred from ball eight to ball seven. It is clear that to rotate the lower disk 180 degrees, work must be done against the electric field, the effect of which is to separate charges of different signs.

be considered the demonstration of Volta in 1801 in the presence of Napoleon Bonaparte, which consisted of an artificial electric organ imitating the natural electric organ of an eel or a stingray (figure 1.2).

Galvani explained the discovered phenomenon of the mechanical reaction of the frog's legs to an electrical voltage impulse (figure 1.3(A)) by the fact that electricity is concentrated between the inner and outer surfaces of the muscle fibers; that is, the muscle is a kind of battery of capacitors, such as the Leiden jar, shown in figure 1.3 (B), in which animal electricity could be stored.[4] To support the veracity of his hypothesis, Galvani proposed taking into account that 'the muscle fiber, although at first glance very simple, however, consists of various solid and liquid parts, which causes a considerable variety of substances in it' [19]. Filling Leiden jars with electricity (in modern language, charging capacitors), Galvani explained, was

[4] The Leiden jar was the first electrical capacitor. It was invented independently in 1745 by the Dutch scientists Pieter van Musschenbroek and Andreas Cunaeus in Leiden and by the German cleric Ewald Georg von Kleist.

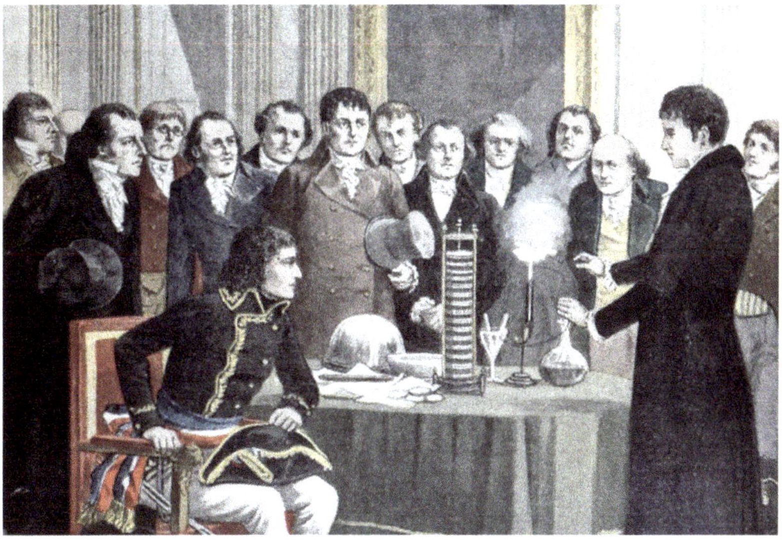

Figure 1.2. Alessandro Volta (right) demonstrates before Napoleon (left) the voltaic column that he invented, the forerunner of all modern batteries. This image [Volta présente son invention à Napoléon] has been obtained by the author(s) from the Wikimedia website, where it is stated to have been released into the public domain. It is included within this book on that basis.

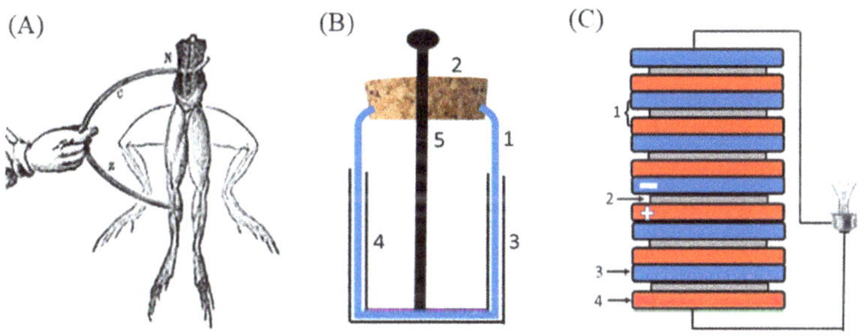

Figure 1.3. (A) When touched by zinc and copper rods, the legs of a dead frog rise. Reprinted with permission from [20]. (B) The first capacitor was the Leiden jar: 1—glass jar (insulator), 2—nonconductive stopper (insulator), 3—outer tin foil (first plate of the capacitor), 4—inner tin foil (second plate of the capacitor), and 5—iron rod touching the inner foil. (C) A voltaic column consists of elementary galvanic elements connected to each other: 1—a galvanic cell or voltaic cell, which is an electrochemical cell in which an electric current is generated from spontaneous oxidation–reduction reactions, 2—electrolytic pad, and 3 and 4—a zinc plate and a copper plate, respectively.

achieved due to the existence of internal mechanisms that cause one type of electric fluid to focus on the outside of the muscle fibers and the other on the inside.[5] Thus,

[5] In 1733, Charles François de Cisternay du Fay (1698–1739) established the existence of two types of 'electric liquid': 'vitreous,' or positive, and 'resinous,' or negative.

Galvani predicted to some extent the existence of ion pumps located on cell membranes, creating a potential difference inside and outside the cell.

Unlike Galvani, who had mainly a medical education, Volta was skilled in mathematics and was well educated in the natural sciences of physics, chemistry, and biology. Volta was the author of many inventions that are still widely used today. Also, the unit of electrical potential difference, the volt, is named after him. As for 'animal electricity,' having read the work of Galvani, 'Commentary on the Effect of Electricity on Muscular Motion,' published in the 1791 issue of the memoirs of the Bologna Institute, Volta was impressed. It seemed to him that Galvani had really found the source of life hidden from us. However, having repeated Galvani's experiments, he came to the conclusion that the frog muscle was most likely only an indicator of electricity: 'an electrometer tens of times more sensitive than even the most sensitive electrometer with gold leaves' [19]. As a result analyzing experimental studies, he showed that the tremor of the frog's muscles observed by Galvani when its leg and body were touched by two different types of copper and zinc wire (figure 1.3(A)) was the same phenomenon as if two plates of different materials had been placed in a jar of saline solution through which an electric current flowed. Volta's discovery led to the loss of interest by the scientific community in the study of 'animal electricity,' which, as it turned out, simply does not exist. The scientific community had rendered a verdict: Galvani's experiments could be explained by the good conductivity of the tissues of organisms, such that even small currents initiated by external sources lead to a physiological effect, an example of which is the trembling of the legs of a dead frog. Soon, experiments on 'revitalizing dead bodies with electricity' were used to demonstrate simple concepts like muscle contractions at the medical departments of universities.

However, in science, there are always people who are not subject to established opinions and dogmas, and it is they who make breakthroughs in areas where everything seems to be already established and clear. One of these scientists was Carlo Matteucci (1811–68), an Italian physicist and neurophysiologist who graduated from the University of Bologna, where Galvani once studied and then taught. He apparently carefully studied Galvani's work and decided that if electricity were indeed concentrated in the muscles, then it would be relatively easy to detect. To determine this, it would be enough to short-circuit the outer membrane of the muscle with the inner membrane through the galvanometer.[6] If the needle did not deviate, no current would flow through the galvanometer, and then Galvani's guess would be shown to be incorrect, meaning that there was no electricity in the muscles. However, if it deviated, that is, there was a potential difference between the inner and outer surfaces of the membranes, then Galvani was right. Matteucci cut the muscle, inserted one galvanometer probe into the cut, and connected the second to the outer surface of the muscle, as shown schematically in figure 1.4. The experiment showed that the galvanometer needle deviated, and the potential on the inner

[6] A galvanometer is a device for measuring small currents and voltages.

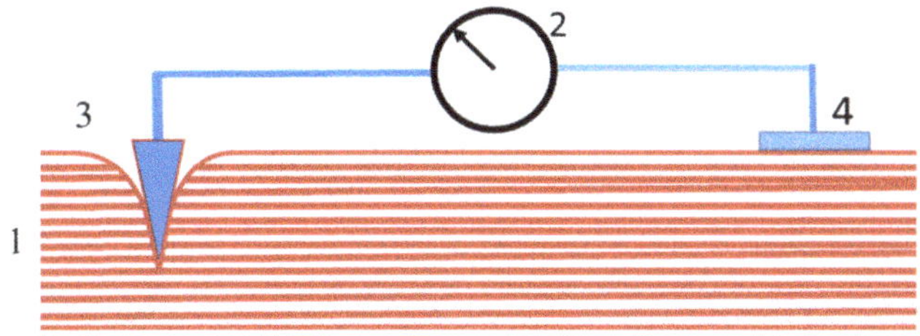

Figure 1.4. Scheme of Matteucci's experiments on currents measured when cutting muscle tissue: 1—muscle, 2—galvanometer, 3—probe located in the area of the muscle incision, and 4—probe located away from the area of the muscle incision. Since the potential in the neuron axon and muscle cell is negative at approximately −90 mV relative to the potential outside them, when the muscle is cut, currents appear to pass through the galvanometer. Naturally, when cutting a muscle, the axons of the neurons are also cut, which also have a negative potential of −90 mV.

surfaces of the muscle fibers turned out to be negative relative to the potential on the outer surface.

Matteucci's experiments clearly showed, as Galvani predicted, that electricity is indeed concentrated in muscle tissue. In addition, the conclusion followed that an internal charge separation mechanism exists in muscles. At the same time, the nature of this mechanism and the principles of its operation remained absolutely unclear, not only to Matteucci.

Matteucci's results immediately attracted the attention of Johannes Müller (1801–58), one of the most prominent physiologists of the time. In 1841, Müller asked his Swiss student Emil du Bois-Reymond (1818–96) to repeat Matteucci's experiments. The brilliant experimenter du Bois-Reymond not only repeated the findings of Matteucci but also showed that during muscle stimulation, the potential difference measured between the external and internal probes decreases. Since the muscles are connected to the brain by nerve fibers, Müller and du Bois-Reymond decided to repeat their experiments with the nerve going from the frog's brain to its leg. As you might guess, the results were the same as for the muscle: the potential in the section was negative, and when the nerve fiber was stimulated, the potential difference recorded by the galvanometer sharply decreased [21].

Du Bois-Reymond interpreted the voltage drop on the galvanometer during nerve stimulation as a signal leading to muscle contraction. This was a huge breakthrough in neurophysiology because, as du Bois-Reymond said, 'I have succeeded in realizing the hundred years' dream of physicists and physiologists, to wit, the identity of the nervous principle with electricity' [21].

However, not all scientists accepted the results obtained by du Bois-Reymond as proof that the propagation of nerve impulses is associated with currents flowing through the nerve fibers, since only a small drop in current was observed in the experiments. Du Bois-Reymond associated the inability to see the shape of the current signal with the inertia of the galvanometer.[7] Also, it was necessary to prove

[7] The duration of the nerve impulse (action potential) is on the order of several milliseconds, which is much shorter than the reaction time of galvanometers existing at that time.

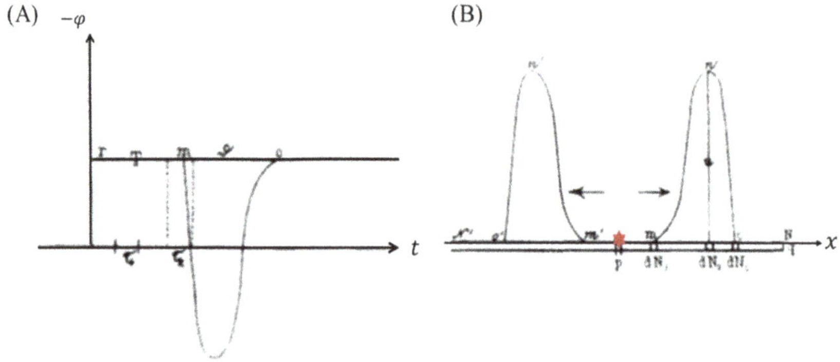

Figure 1.5. Results of Bernstein's experiments [23]. (A) Time dependence of the potential in the area of nerve incision. (B) Potential distribution along the nerve. The presence of two peaks indicates that, when excited, the impulse spreads in both directions from the site of excitation. The location of nerve excitation is shown with a star; arrows indicate the direction of movement of the action potential. Reprinted by permission from Springer Nature Customer Service Center GmbH: [Springer], [European Journal of Physiology] [23], Copyright (1868).

that the speed of propagation of the electrical signal was $\sim$30 m s^{-1}, which would coincide with the speed of propagation of the signal in the nerve fiber causing muscle contraction, measured in 1849 by the outstanding scientist Hermann von Helmholtz (1821–94),[8] a former student of Müller. Du Bois-Reymond began to create a suitable measurement apparatus. After the death of his teacher, Müller, du Bois-Reymond headed his laboratory, although he had to combine scientific research with teaching and administrative work. However, as often happens, something went wrong with the apparatus, and du Bois-Reymond, due to his busy schedule, completely transferred the problem to his student Julius Bernstein (1839–1917).

We will not talk about all the experimental techniques that Bernstein had to resort to in order to measure the shape of the action potential and the speed of its movement along the nerve fiber. This is well documented in [22] and in the original work of du Bois-Reymond [21]. Let us just say that it took Bernstein almost five years of hard experimental work to get convincing results. A historical graph of the nerve impulse (action potential) versus time obtained by Bernstein [23] is shown in figure 1.5.

Thus, through the efforts of Müller, du Bois-Reymond, Helmholtz, and Bernstein, it was shown that:

1. At rest, the potential inside the nervous tissue is negative (rest potential negative).

[8] Hermann Ludwig Ferdinand von Helmholtz was an outstanding German scientist. From 1849 to 1855, he worked as a professor of physiology and general anatomy in Königsberg and later in a similar position in Bonn and Heidelberg. In 1871 he was invited to take the position of professor of physics at the University of Berlin. His breadth of scientific interest was impressive. Among his outstanding discoveries and inventions were the ophthalmoscope and the Helmholtz resonator for decomposing complex sound signals into harmonics. Based on empirical data, he developed the theory of color vision, the theory of sound perception by the ear, pointed out the importance of the unconscious in decision-making, and made great contributions to thermodynamics, electromagnetism, and hydrodynamics.

2. When nerve tissue is stimulated, an electrical impulse (action potential) propagates through it at a speed of about 30 m s^{-1}.
3. An electrical impulse (action potential) leads to the stimulation of muscle tissue contractions.

However, the mechanisms of charge separation in nerve and muscle fibers and what constitutes an action potential remained an absolute mystery. Many scientists believed that since the speed of propagation of an action potential is many orders of magnitude less than the speed of light, the action potential could not be electrical in nature but was rather the result of certain chemical reactions.[9] Only in 1902 did Bernstein hypothesize that both the resting potential and the action potential are associated with the selective permeability of the membranes separating cells from the external environment [24]. In his article [24], he relied on the results of Nernst's research,[10] which we will discuss in the next part of this chapter.

1.2 Nernst potential and Bernstein hypothesis

Let us begin by imagining a vessel that is divided into two parts by a membrane (figure 1.6). An electrolyte made from the same reagent is poured into the vessel, but each part of the vessel receives a different concentration. Let us consider, for example, ordinary table salt NaCl, which, when dissolved in water, dissociates into positive sodium ions and negative chloride ions. As a result, electrolyte solutions are formed in different parts of the vessel with ion densities of $[Na^+]_l$, $[Cl^-]_l$ and $[Na^+]_r$, $[Cl^-]_r$ on the left and right sides of the membrane, respectively.

Let the probability of the passage of sodium ions through the membrane in both directions—from left to right and from right to left—be the same and proportional to p_{Na}. Also, let the same assumption be true for the probability of passage of chloride ions, p_{Cl}. Taking into account the assumptions made about the probabilities

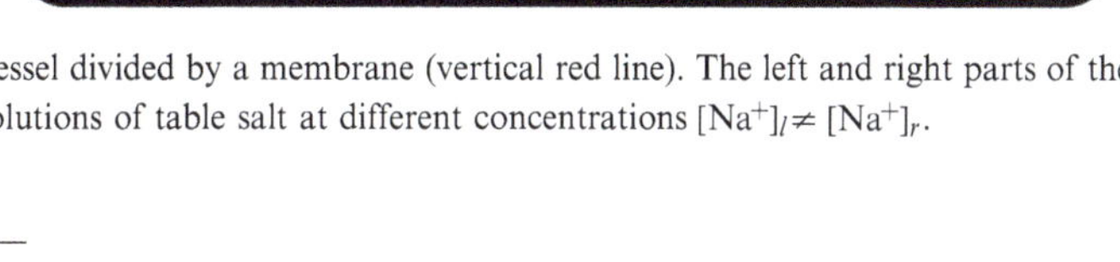

Figure 1.6. A vessel divided by a membrane (vertical red line). The left and right parts of the vessel are filled with aqueous solutions of table salt at different concentrations $[Na^+]_l \neq [Na^+]_r$.

[9] If we assume that nerve fibers are wires through which current flows, then the speed of propagation of the action potential should be close to the speed of light.

[10] Walther Hermann Nernst (1864–1941) was a German physicist and physical chemist. He contributed greatly to the development of thermodynamics, physical chemistry, electrochemistry, and solid-state physics. For his formulation of the third law of thermodynamics, Nernst received the Nobel Prize in Chemistry in 1920.

of passage through the membrane, $p_{\mathrm{Na}}[\mathrm{Na}^+]_l$ sodium ions and $p_{\mathrm{Cl}}[\mathrm{Cl}^-]_l$ chloride ions pass through a unit area of the membrane from left to right per unit time. In this case, the total charge flowing through a unit area per unit time from the left side of the vessel to the right is equal to:

$$Q_l = Ze(p_{\mathrm{Na}}[\mathrm{Na}^+]_l - p_{\mathrm{Cl}}[\mathrm{Cl}^-]_l), \tag{1.1}$$

and from the right side to the left, respectively, is equal to

$$Q_r = Ze(p_{\mathrm{Na}}[\mathrm{Na}^+]_r - p_{\mathrm{Cl}}[\mathrm{Cl}^-]_r). \tag{1.2}$$

In (1.1) and (1.2), $e = 1.602 \cdot 10^{-19}$ C is the elementary charge (the proton charge equal to the absolute value of the electron charge), and Z is the ion charge in units of proton charge. For the considered solution of table salt, in which all ions are singly ionized, $Z = 1$.

If the concentrations of solutions in the left and right parts of the vessel are equal, then there is no charge transfer, since for every ion that passes from left to right, there is an ion that passes from right to left. If the initial concentrations of ions on the left and right are different, then, as a result of charge transfer, a potential difference φ appears on the membrane, limiting the transfer of charge from one part of the vessel to another figure 1.7.

Let us assume, for the sake of certainty, that $[\mathrm{Na}^+]_l > [\mathrm{Na}^+]_r$ and the temperatures T of the electrolyte solutions are equal on both sides of the membrane. In this case, the probability that a sodium ion from the left side of the vessel will end up on the right side is $p_{\mathrm{Na},l} = p_{\mathrm{Na}} e^{\frac{Ze\varphi}{k_B T}}$, where $k_B = 1.38 \cdot 10^{-23}$ J · K^{-1} is Boltzmann's constant, and T is the temperature of the electrolytes on the left and right. As for the transfer of chloride ions from the left side, the probability of them ending up on the right side of the vessel does not depend on the electric field, since the electric field does not prevent the passage of chloride ions from the left side of the vessel to the right, therefore $p_{\mathrm{Cl},l} = p_{\mathrm{Cl}}$. Now let us move on to the ions on the right side of the vessel. Since in that case the electric field does not prevent the passage of sodium ions from the right side of the vessel to the left, $p_{\mathrm{Na},r} = p_{\mathrm{Na}}$, but slows down chloride ions, $p_{\mathrm{Cl},r} = p_{\mathrm{Cl}} e^{\frac{Ze\varphi}{k_B T}}$. Replacing p_{Na} and p_{Cl} with $p_{\mathrm{Na},l}$ and $p_{\mathrm{Cl},l}$ in (1.1), and with

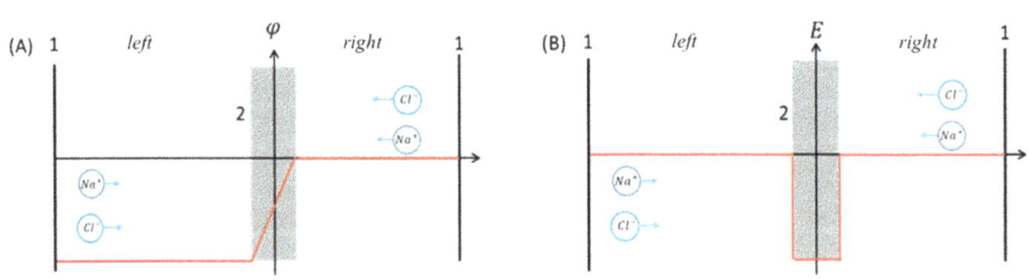

Figure 1.7. (A) and (B) are the potential and electric field distributions, respectively. For example, let us assume that the concentration of NaCl salt in the left part of the vessel is greater than in the right. Segment 1 indicates the walls of the vessel, and rectangle 2 indicates the membrane. A sodium ion located on the left side of the vessel is slowed down by the electric field in the membrane, whereas the chloride ion is accelerated.

$p_{Na,r}$ and $p_{\mathrm{Cl},r}$ in (1.2), we obtain the charge flux from the left part of the vessel to the right:

$$Q_l = Ze\left(p_{\mathrm{Na}} e^{\frac{Ze\varphi}{k_B T}} [\mathrm{Na}^+]_l - p_{\mathrm{Cl}} [\mathrm{Cl}^-]_l\right), \tag{1.3}$$

and, respectively, from right to left,

$$Q_r = Ze\left(p_{\mathrm{Na}} [\mathrm{Na}^+]_r - p_{\mathrm{Cl}} e^{\frac{Ze\varphi}{k_B T}} [\mathrm{Cl}^-]_r\right). \tag{1.4}$$

Equating (1.3) and (1.4), we obtain:

$$p_{\mathrm{Na}} e^{\frac{Ze\varphi}{k_B T}} [\mathrm{Na}^+]_l - p_{\mathrm{Cl}} [\mathrm{Cl}^-]_l = p_{\mathrm{Na}} [\mathrm{Na}^+]_r - p_{\mathrm{Cl}} e^{\frac{Ze\varphi}{k_B T}} [\mathrm{Cl}^-]_r. \tag{1.5}$$

The established potential difference across the membrane, called the Nernst potential [25], follows from (1.5):

$$\varphi = \frac{k_B T}{Ze} \ln\left(\frac{p_{\mathrm{Na}} [\mathrm{Na}^+]_r + p_{\mathrm{Cl}} [\mathrm{Cl}^-]_l}{p_{\mathrm{Na}} [\mathrm{Na}^+]_l + p_{\mathrm{Cl}} [\mathrm{Cl}^-]_r}\right) = \frac{RT}{ZF} \ln\left(\frac{p_{\mathrm{Na}} [\mathrm{Na}^+]_r + p_{\mathrm{Cl}} [\mathrm{Cl}^-]_l}{p_{\mathrm{Na}} [\mathrm{Na}^+]_l + p_{\mathrm{Cl}} [\mathrm{Cl}^-]_r}\right), \tag{1.6}$$

where $F = eN_A \approx 9.64853 \times 10^4$ C·mol^{-1} is Faraday's constant, $N_A \approx 6.022 \times 10^{23}$ mol^{-1} is Avogadro's number, and $R = k_B N_A \approx 8.31446$ J·K^{-1}·mol^{-1} is the gas constant.

The potential energies of the sodium and chloride ions in the left part of the vessel, referred to as $k_B T$ (in the right, they are equal to zero), have the form:

$$\frac{W_{\mathrm{Na}}}{k_B T} = \frac{e\varphi}{k_B T} = \ln\left(\frac{p_{\mathrm{Na}} [\mathrm{Na}^+]_r + p_{\mathrm{Cl}} [\mathrm{Cl}^-]_l}{p_{\mathrm{Na}} [\mathrm{Na}^+]_l + p_{\mathrm{Cl}} [\mathrm{Cl}^-]_r}\right) = \ln\left(\frac{p_{\mathrm{Na}} [\mathrm{NaCl}]_r + p_{\mathrm{Cl}} [\mathrm{NaCl}]_l}{p_{\mathrm{Na}} [\mathrm{NaCl}]_l + p_{\mathrm{Cl}} [\mathrm{NaCl}]_r}\right), \tag{1.7}$$

$$\frac{W_{\mathrm{Cl}}}{k_B T} = -\frac{e\varphi}{k_B T} = \ln\left(\frac{p_{\mathrm{Na}} [\mathrm{Na}^+]_l + p_{\mathrm{Cl}} [\mathrm{Cl}^-]_r}{p_{\mathrm{Na}} [\mathrm{Na}^+]_r + p_{\mathrm{Cl}} [\mathrm{Cl}^-]_l}\right) = \ln\left(\frac{p_{\mathrm{Na}} [\mathrm{NaCl}]_l + p_{\mathrm{Cl}} [\mathrm{NaCl}]_r}{p_{\mathrm{Na}} [\mathrm{NaCl}]_r + p_{\mathrm{Cl}} [\mathrm{NaCl}]_l}\right). \tag{1.8}$$

Let, for example, $p_{\mathrm{Na}} \ll p_{\mathrm{Cl}}$ and $[\mathrm{NaCl}]_l \sim [\mathrm{NaCl}]_r$. In this case, the flow of sodium ions through the membrane is insignificant, and the left and right parts of the vessels exchange only chloride ions, respectively:

$$\frac{W_{\mathrm{Cl}}}{k_B T} \approx \ln\left(\frac{[\mathrm{NaCl}]_r}{[\mathrm{NaCl}]_l}\right). \tag{1.9}$$

It is clear from (1.9) that if the density of chlorine salt on the right is greater than on the left, then $\frac{W_{\mathrm{Cl}}}{k_B T} > 0$, and if less, $\frac{W_{\mathrm{Cl}}}{k_B T} < 0$. In other words, the Nernst potential is always a potential barrier that prevents the flow of ions at a higher density into an area with a lower one. It is easy to see that if we assume that $p_{\mathrm{Na}} \gg p_{\mathrm{Cl}}$ and $[\mathrm{NaCl}]_l \sim [\mathrm{NaCl}]_r$, the result is the same, and the Nernst potential prevents the flow of Na^+ ions from a region where there are more of them to a region where there are fewer of them.

If the electrolyte contains several types of salts (for example, in addition to the NaCl salt, KCl salt is present), then the potential difference across the membrane takes the form:

$$\varphi = \frac{RT}{ZF}\ln\left(\frac{p_{\mathrm{Na}}\,[\mathrm{Na}^+]_r + p_{\mathrm{K}}\,[\mathrm{K}^+]_r + p_{\mathrm{Cl}}\,[\mathrm{Cl}^-]_l}{p_{\mathrm{Na}}\,[\mathrm{Na}^+]_l + p_{\mathrm{K}}\,[\mathrm{K}^+]_l + p_{\mathrm{Cl}}\,[\mathrm{Cl}^-]_r}\right). \tag{1.10}$$

Following [26], let us estimate the probability of a charged particle passing through a membrane separating two electrolytes. The potential energy of a charged particle of radius r_p and charge $q = Ze$ in a liquid with relative dielectric permittivity ε is equal to:

$$W_Z = \frac{(Ze)^2}{4\pi\varepsilon_0\varepsilon r_p}, \tag{1.11}$$

where $\varepsilon_0 = 8.854 \cdot 10^{-12}\ \mathrm{F\,m^{-1}}$ is the dielectric constant of vacuum. From now on, in all cases, we use the 'dielectric constant' of a medium to refer to the relative dielectric constant.

The difference between the energy of a charged particle in the membrane and its energy in water is equal to:

$$\Delta W_Z = \frac{(Ze)^2}{4\pi\varepsilon_0\varepsilon_m r_p} - \frac{(Ze)^2}{4\pi\varepsilon_0\varepsilon_w r_p}, \tag{1.12}$$

where ε_w and ε_m are the dielectric constants of water and the phospholipid membrane, respectively. Therefore, the estimate of the probability of ion transfer from water to the membrane has the following form:

$$p \sim \exp\left(-\frac{\Delta W_Z}{k_B T}\right) = \exp\left(-\frac{(Ze)^2}{4\pi\varepsilon_0 r_p k_B T}\left(\frac{1}{\varepsilon_w} - \frac{1}{\varepsilon_m}\right)\right). \tag{1.13}$$

Using formula (1.13), we can obtain estimates of the probabilities p_{K}, p_{Na}, and p_{Cl} in (1.10). Taking into account the dielectric constants $\varepsilon_w \approx 81$ and $\varepsilon_m \approx 2.5$ and the radii of singly charged potassium, sodium, and chloride ions, which are 0.13, 0.1, and 0.18 nm [27], respectively, we obtain the following probability estimates for p_K, p_{Na}, and p_{Cl}:

$$p_{\mathrm{K}} \sim e^{-\frac{\Delta W_{\mathrm{K}}}{k_B T}} = 10^{-70},\ p_{\mathrm{Na}} \sim e^{-\frac{\Delta W_{\mathrm{Na}}}{k_B T}} = 10^{-91},\ p_{\mathrm{Cl}} \sim e^{-\frac{\Delta W_{\mathrm{Cl}}}{k_B T}} = 10^{-51}. \tag{1.14}$$

Note that since the Nernst potential always works against the flow of ions from an area of higher ionic density to an area of lower density, it can only further complicate the transfer of ions through the membrane. Thus, the diffusive transfers of potassium ions, sodium ions, chloride ions, and other ions through an ideal membrane are impossible; there must be another mechanism for the transfer of ions from one electrolyte to another. We will explore this further in section 1.5 of this chapter.

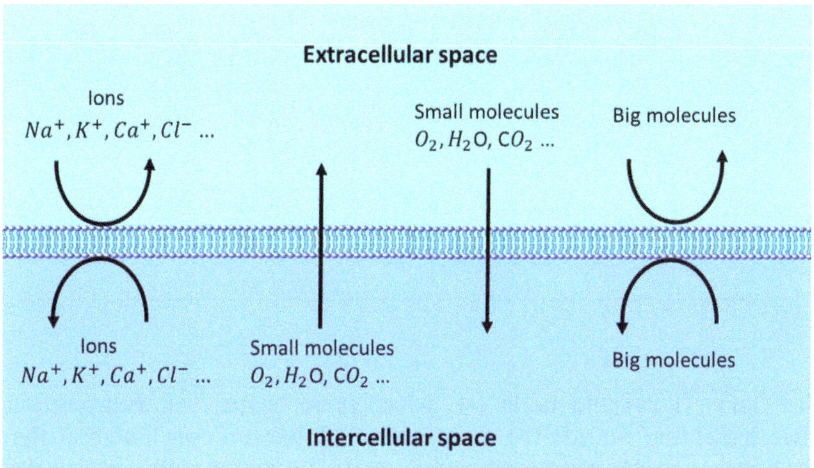

Figure 1.8. Schematic representation of the relative permeability of a phospholipid membrane to various ions and molecules.

Figure 1.8 shows a schematic representation of the relative permeability of an ideal defect-free phospholipid membrane to various ions and molecules.

Based on the simplest theory of ion transport across a membrane discussed above, Bernstein proposed the first theory of the action potential based on the following three facts, experimentally established by that time:

1. The density of potassium ions inside muscle cells and nerve cells is greater than outside.
2. The potential inside muscle and nerve tissue (resting potential) is always negative.
3. When a nerve impulse is initiated, the potential in the area where the impulse passes falls to zero.

Following Nernst's theory, Bernstein proposed that the resting potential discovered by Matteucci in muscles and by du Bois-Reymond in nerve tissues is associated with a potential difference across the cell membrane, which ensures equality of ion fluxes across the membrane. The resting potential is approximately equal to:

$$V_R = \frac{RT}{ZF} \ln\left(\frac{[\mathrm{K}^+]_{\mathrm{out}}}{[\mathrm{K}^+]_{\mathrm{in}}}\right) < 0. \tag{1.15}$$

Since the propagation of the action potential in nerve fibers is initially accompanied by a decrease in $|\Delta\varphi|$ at the point of passage of the nerve impulse and then restored to the previous value in accordance with (1.15), this means that in the area of passage of the action potential, $[\mathrm{K}^+]_{\mathrm{in}}$ drops to the value of $[\mathrm{K}^+]_{\mathrm{out}}$ and then returns to the original value. Bernstein explained that such a local change in the density of potassium ions was due to a change in the conductivity of the membrane separating the internal electrolyte of the cell from the external one. However, if we turn to

Table 1.1. Intracellular and extracellular ion densities [28].

Ion	Intercellular (mmol l^{-1})	Extracellular (mmol l^{-1})
Na^+	50	460
Ka^+	400	10
Ca^{2+}	...	10
Mg^+	10	54
Cl^-	135	560
$(A)^-$	345	...

formulas (1.11)–(1.14) and table 1.1, which presents the ionic composition of the electrolyte inside and outside the squid axon [28], we can conclude that the resting potential is determined by the concentration of Cl^- ions and should be positive, since p_{Cl} is 20 orders of magnitude higher than p_K and 40 orders of magnitude higher than p_{Na}, and the concentrations of K^+, Na^+, and Cl^- ions inside and outside the axon differ by no more than two orders of magnitude. A possible answer to the question of why Bernstein did not consider the Na^+ and Cl^- ions in his theory of the action potential can be found in the coincidence of the resting potential value with formula (1.15).

A direct experiment linking the action potential to the flow of potassium ions across the cell boundary was not possible because the individual axons were too small (1.5–5 microns) for the insertion of electrodes to measure currents and potentials during the passage of the action potential.

Let us sum up the intermediate results. A theory proposed by Bernstein indicated:

1. The source of 'living electricity' is cells.
2. The propagation of the action potential is associated with a change in membrane conductivity with respect to potassium ions.
3. The propagation of the action potential is associated with a change in membrane conductivity with respect to potassium ions.

However, despite its remarkable success, Bernstein's theory left the following questions open:

1. Why is the resting potential determined exclusively by the ratio of K^+ densities inside and outside the axon, while other ions are not involved?
2. Why is the ability of the membrane to transmit K^+ ions sharply increased during the passage of an action potential?
3. According to Bernstein's theory, the restoration of the resting potential after the passage of the action potential should be accompanied by the pumping of potassium ions from the external electrolyte to the internal one. What is the mechanism of this pumping, and what is the source of its energy?

We will answer these questions in the fifth part of this chapter. But first, let us look at the key experiments with axons that allowed Hodgkin and Huxley to construct an empirical mathematical model of the action potential, which is discussed in section 1.4 of this chapter.

1.3 Squid giant axon

In 1909, the English physiologist Leonard Worcester Williams (1875–1912) published his book *The Anatomy of the Common Squid*, which described a squid axon 1.5 mm in diameter [29]. Figure 1.9 shows illustrations taken from Williams's book, which highlight the giant neurons that form the neural network in the squid's body.

It seems that this was an object on which it would have been possible to test Bernstein's ideas. However, as was the case with Mendelian genetics, the scientific world passed this opportunity by. It was only after almost 30 years that John Zachary Young (1907–97) showed [30] that the two giant axons (GA in figure 1.9) are motor neurons, and their stimulation powers the entire complex system of muscles, that is, the squid's 'jet engine': the squid closes the valve in its head and then, with a sharp contraction of the longitudinal muscles, shoots out a powerful stream of water through the nozzle (a narrow hole at the back). This finding triggered renewed interest in the study of the squid's giant axons [30]. One of the first to understand the possibilities of the squid's giant axon for studying nervous activity was a 25-year-old English biophysicist, Hodgkin.[11] After reading Young's paper, he

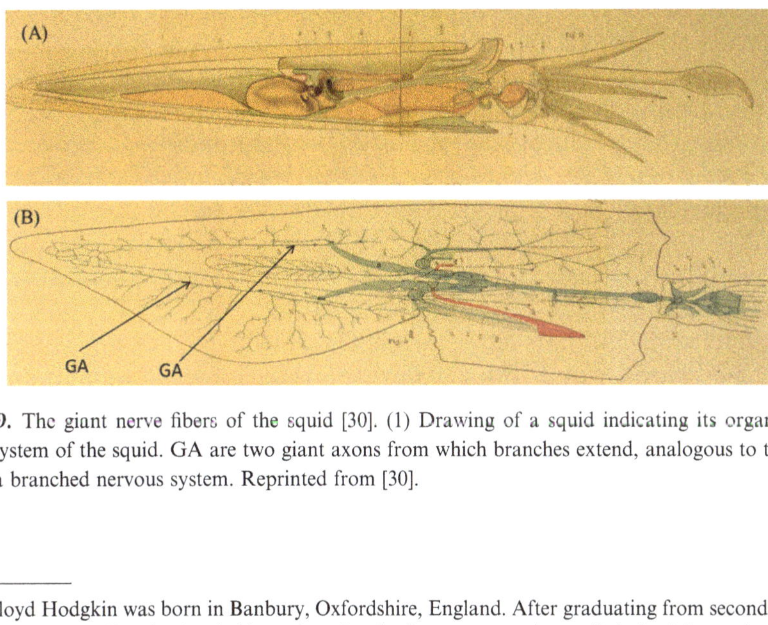

Figure 1.9. The giant nerve fibers of the squid [30]. (1) Drawing of a squid indicating its organs. (2) The nervous system of the squid. GA are two giant axons from which branches extend, analogous to tree trunks, forming a branched nervous system. Reprinted from [30].

[11] Alan Lloyd Hodgkin was born in Banbury, Oxfordshire, England. After graduating from secondary school, he entered Trinity College in Cambridge, where for the first two years he studied physiology, chemistry, and zoology. On the advice of Karl Planty, his future supervisor, instead of a zoology course, he took courses in physics and mathematics. In the physiology laboratory, where he studied frog nerves, Hodgkin became acquainted with cable theory, which allowed him, together with Andrew Fielding Huxley, to develop a new approach to the study of the propagation of action potentials in nerve fibers. He also studied electronics, the knowledge of which allowed him to design equipment with Huxley for experiments. His university friends were John Raven, who later became an outstanding researcher of ancient philosophy, Michael Grant, who became the author of many books on ancient history, Richard L M Synge, who received the Nobel Prize in Chemistry in 1952 for the invention of chromatography, John Humphrey, and Polly and David Hill. In 1935, after graduating from college, Hodgkin began scientific work under the guidance of his university teacher Karl Planty.

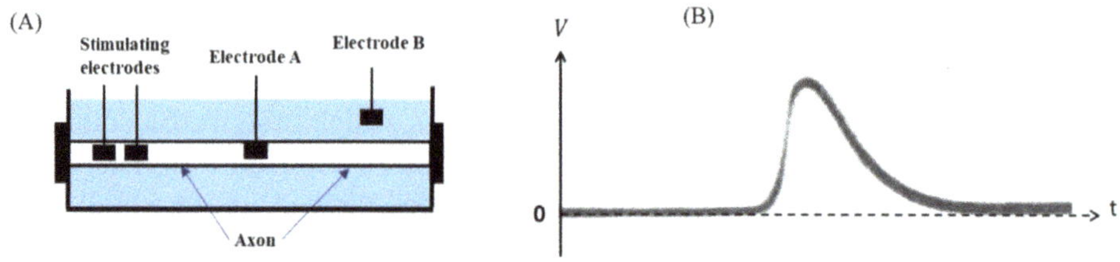

Figure 1.10. Action potential measurements in squid axons. (A) Electrodes on the surface of the membrane. [9] John Wiley & Sons. © 1939 The Physiological Society. (B) The measurement result corresponding to (A).

realized that the large radius of the axon would allow him to measure the action potential on a single nerve cell. Therefore, immediately after returning to Cambridge from the Rockefeller Institute in New York, where he had spent two postdoctoral years and learned to dissect squid axons, Hodgkin began work in 1938 on creating a setup for measuring action potentials in squid axons. Soon, he was able to show that action potentials are excited in the squid axon, as in other nerve fibers, and to measure the speed of their propagation [9]. However, the electrodes in Hodgkin's early experiments touched the surface of the axon and were not small enough or tailored enough to be placed inside the axon. The locations of the electrodes and the results of measuring the action potential are shown in figure 1.10(A, B). In 1939, Hodgkin invited his graduate student Huxley[12] to join him in his research on the electrical properties of the squid axon. The collaboration between the two young scientists immediately bore fruit; they were able to construct a microelectrode that allowed them to 'look inside the axon' by placing the electrodes inside the squid axon (figures 1.11(A) and (B)) and directly measuring the resting potential and action potential in it [12].[13]

The creative collaboration between Hodgkin and Huxley as young scientists was interrupted by World War II. Both Hodgkin and Huxley began working on defense

[12] Andrew Fielding Huxley was born in Hampstead, London. After graduating from secondary school in 1935, he entered Trinity College in Cambridge, dreaming of becoming a physicist. At college, he took the entire set of required courses in physics, chemistry, and mathematics. On the advice of a friend, Huxley chose physiology because he hoped to work in the medical field after college. One of his teachers was Hodgkin, whose research he joined in 1939, after Hodgkin's return from America. After the end of World War II, from 1946 to 1951, Huxley continued with Hodgkin to study the electrical properties of the squid axon and, in parallel, with Robert Stämpfli, to study myelinated nerve fibers. In 1952, Huxley's scientific interests shifted to another important problem, muscle fiber contraction. He invented an interference microscope, which made it possible to understand how muscle contraction occurs.

[13] In their experiments, Hodgkin and Huxley used the giant axon of the longfin inshore squid (*Doryteuthis*, formerly *Loligo*, *pealeii*), which has the largest neurons known.

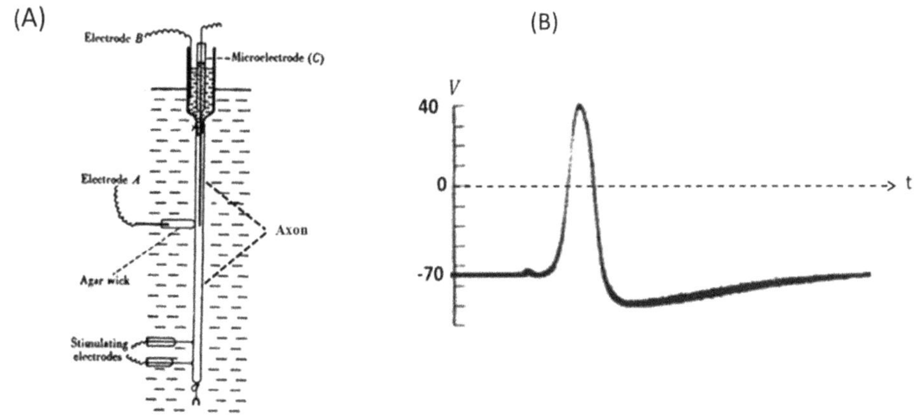

Figure 1.11. (A) The measuring electrodes located inside the axon. Reprinted by permission from Springer Nature Customer Service Center GmbH: [Nature], [13], Copyright (1939). (B) Measurement result corresponding to (A) [12] John Wiley & Sons. © 1945 The Physiological Society.

at the outbreak of war: Hodgkin began developing various systems for airborne radar on fighter planes used for night missions, and Huxley, when the college was closed due to bombing, began doing research for artillery. Another biophysicist who drew attention to the possibility of measuring action potentials without cutting nerve tissue was Kenneth Cole (1900–84).[14] In 1939, he and Howard Curtis (1900–84)[15] measured the action potential in the squid axon [31] using a different approach than that of Hodgkin and Huxley. If we measure the longitudinal and transverse impedances of the axon during the passage of the action potential along the fiber, the equivalent electrical circuit of which is shown in figure 1.12, then knowing the change in potential along the fiber, it is possible to calculate the action potential based on cable theory. Cole and Curtis developed the method shown in figure 1.13, which allowed action potential measurements to be carried out automatically. Below, we will only touch on cable theory when we begin to discuss the mathematical model of the action potential of Hodgkin and Huxley and the experiments they carried out. In 1939, Cole and Curtis, independent of Hodgkin and Huxley, measured the action potential by inserting an additional electrode inside the axon [31]. They published more precise measurements of the resting

[14] Kenneth Stuart Cole was classically trained in physics and engineering. His abilities as an experimenter and theorist were revealed when studying the impedance of biological membranes. In 1947, Cole told Hodgkin about his experiments in controlling the voltage between an internal electrode inserted into a squid axon and an external one. Hodgkin also told Cole about experiments he and Katz had conducted on squid nerves in 1947, establishing that action potentials were generated by sodium ions injected into the axon along a concentration gradient. Thus, Hodgkin confirmed Cole's assumption about the role of sodium ions in exciting the action potential.

[15] Howard James Curtis, following in his father's footsteps, received his PhD from Yale in 1932. In 1935, he began collaborating with Kenneth Cole on research into nerve excitation and conduction. During World War II, he took an active part in the Manhattan Project as a biophysicist dealing with the effects of radiation on living organisms and the development of protection against them.

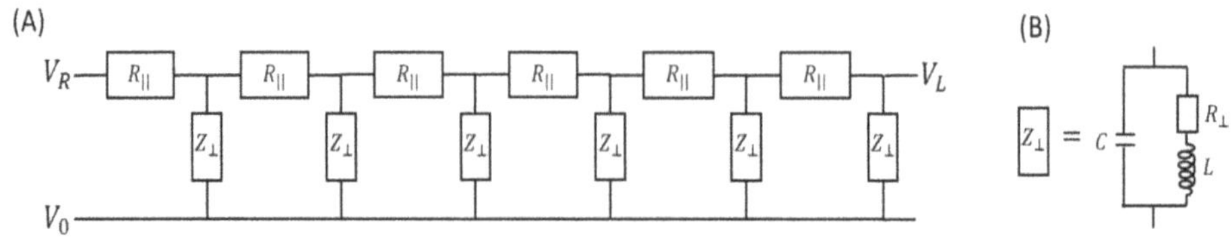

Figure 1.12. (A) section of a cable line simulating a membrane. (B) A separate element corresponding to the perpendicular impedance of the membrane. If $V_R = V_L = 0$, then V_0 corresponds to the resting potential. The propagation of the action potential corresponds to $V_R \neq V_L$. In experiments [31], cable line parameters were measured during the passage of an action potential, and the action potential was reconstructed based on the measurements.

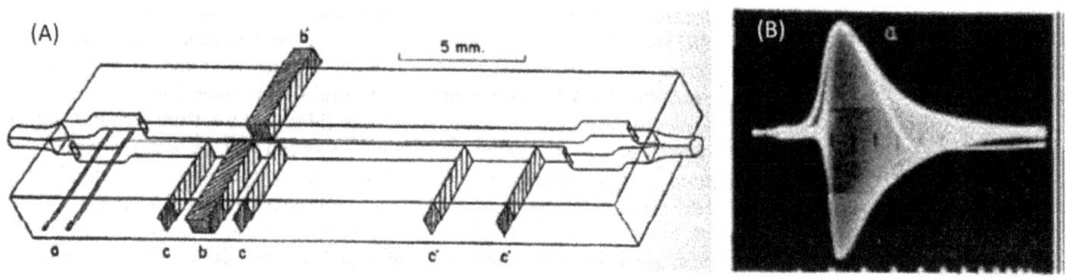

Figure 1.13. (A) Measuring cell for a squid axon. The central trough is for the axon, and the connection for circulating sea water is at each end. The axon is stimulated with electrode a, the transverse impedance is measured with electrodes b and b', and the action potential is measured by various combinations of electrodes b, c, and c'. (B) Photograph from an oscilloscope after signal processing by electronics; the white line shows the action potential. The time intervals at the bottom are 1 ms. Parts (A) and (B) reproduced with permission from [31].

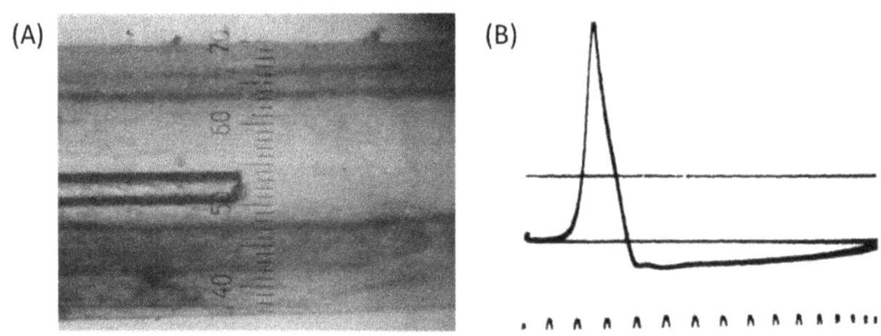

Figure 1.14. (A) Photograph of a chamber with an axon in the trough between an impedance electrode and a metallic capillary electrode in axoplasm at the left [13] John Wiley & Sons. © 1945 The Physiological Society. (B) Membrane action potential of the squid axon. The resting potential in this axon was 58 mV. Thus, the upper horizontal line approximately represents a zero potential difference across the membrane, the lower line represents the resting potential (outside positive), and the action potential, starting from the resting potential, swings to 110 mV (outside negative). The time intervals at the bottom are 0.2 ms [33] John Wiley & Sons. Copyright © 1942 The Wistar Institute of Anatomy and Biology.

potential and the action potential in 1942 [32]. Figure 1.14 shows a photograph of a thin electrode inserted into a squid axon [32] and the measured action potential [33].

In the view of Hodgkin, Huxley, Cole, Curtis, and other biophysicists of that time, the membrane of nerve and other cells was a thin, homogeneous phospholipid shell separating the electrolyte inside the cell from the electrolyte outside. The membrane is weakly permeable to ions; therefore, due to the difference in the ionic compositions of electrolytes inside and outside the cell (see data given in table 1.1), a potential difference corresponding to formula (9) is established across the membrane. When an action potential passes, the permeability of the membrane for ions changes, and ions from the external electrolyte can freely move into the internal one, while ions from the internal electrolyte can move freely to the external one. After the ionic compositions of the external and internal electrolytes equalize, the potential difference across the membrane should become zero. The question of why the action potential, starting from the resting potential, overshoots zero, falls below the resting potential, and is only restored to the resting potential over time has no solution within the framework of these ideas about the membrane.

Now let us ask ourselves: were Hodgkin and Huxley able to study the membrane in detail during the initiation and passage of an action potential and find the reason for its changed properties? The answer is obvious: no. The thickness of the membrane was less than 10 nm, and it was not yet possible to make nanometer electrodes at that time. The use of electron microscopes in biology was problematic; despite their super-resolution, the electron beams of the microscopes destroyed biological objects. A breakthrough was achieved in 1981 when Nobel Prize winners Jacques Dubochet and Alasdair McDowall created cryo-electron microscopy as a means of improving the preservation of specimens. The biological sample is placed in water or a buffer solution, and by being rapidly frozen, reaches the temperature of liquid nitrogen (90 K), at which the stability of samples examined with electron microscopes increases markedly. For more information about the history of the development of the use of electron microscopes in biology, see [34].

This is what Hodgkin and Huxley wrote in their article about the possibility of studying the membrane to understand the origin of the action potential: ‘At present the thickness and composition of the excitable membrane are unknown. Our experiments are therefore unlikely to give any certain information about the nature of the molecular events underlying changes in permeability. The object of this section is to show that certain types of theory are excluded by our experiments and that others are consistent with them’ [1].

Studying the properties of the membrane required a different approach, which was formulated by Cole. He proposed considering the propagation of an action potential similar to the propagation of an electrical signal in a cable line, an element of which is shown in figure 1.12. His studies with Curtis showed that during the passage of an action potential, the longitudinal ohmic resistance changes by approximately 10%, while the transverse resistance drops by 200 times [33], which explains the reason for the drop in the absolute value of the potential across the membrane. This approach has proven to be very fruitful for constructing a mathematical model of action potential propagation.

It should be noted that a dispute initially arose between Hodgkin and Huxley on one hand and Cole and Curtis on the other about the role of sodium ions in the development of the action potential. Hodgkin and Huxley argued that sodium ions do not play a significant role in the development of the action potential because the potential difference across the membrane corresponds to the logarithm of the ratio of the potassium ion densities outside and inside the cell, which is why the resting potential is negative. However, if the resting potential were determined by sodium ions, then, since there are more sodium ions in the external electrolyte than in the internal electrolyte, the potential would be positive. Cole responded to this argument with the counter-argument that when the potential difference across the radial resistance changes (see figure 1.12), the permeability of sodium ions p_{Na} can increase sharply, making it greater than p_{K}, which then leads to a flow of sodium ions from the external electrolyte without a flow of potassium ions from the cell outward. Accordingly, the potential difference should be determined by the modified formula (1.10):

$$\varphi(t) = \frac{RT}{ZF}\ln\left(\frac{p_{\mathrm{Na}}(t)([\mathrm{Na}^{+}]_{\mathrm{out}} - \Delta[\mathrm{Na}^{+}]_{\mathrm{out}}) + p_{\mathrm{K}}[\mathrm{K}^{+}]_{\mathrm{out}} + p_{\mathrm{Cl}}[\mathrm{Cl}^{-}]_{\mathrm{in}}}{p_{\mathrm{Na}}(t)([\mathrm{Na}^{+}]_{\mathrm{in}} + \Delta[\mathrm{Na}^{+}]_{\mathrm{out}}) + p_{\mathrm{K}}[\mathrm{K}^{+}]_{\mathrm{in}} + p_{\mathrm{Cl}}[\mathrm{Cl}^{-}]_{\mathrm{out}}}\right). \quad (1.16)$$

In (1.16), $\Delta[\mathrm{Na}^{+}]_{\mathrm{out}}$ is the amount of sodium ions flowing from the external electrolyte to the internal one. Since the volume of electrolyte outside the cell is much larger than the volume of electrolyte inside, the change in the density of ions outside the cell can be neglected. The initial amount of Na^{+} in the cell can also be neglected. In this case, (1.16) takes the form:

$$\varphi(t) = \frac{RT}{ZF}\ln\left(\frac{p_{\mathrm{Na}}(t)[\mathrm{Na}^{+}]_{\mathrm{out}} + p_{\mathrm{K}}[\mathrm{K}^{+}]_{\mathrm{out}} + p_{\mathrm{Cl}}[\mathrm{Cl}^{-}]_{\mathrm{in}}}{p_{\mathrm{Na}}(t)\Delta[\mathrm{Na}^{+}]_{\mathrm{out}} + p_{\mathrm{K}}[\mathrm{K}^{+}]_{\mathrm{in}} + p_{\mathrm{Cl}}[\mathrm{Cl}^{-}]_{\mathrm{out}}}\right). \quad (1.17)$$

Since $\Delta[\mathrm{Na}^{+}]_{\mathrm{out}} \leqslant [\mathrm{Na}^{+}]_{\mathrm{out}}$, it is quite possible that at some point in time the denominator in (1.17) may become less than the numerator, leading to a change in the sign of φ. When the flow of sodium ions from the outside to the inside stops upon reaching $\Delta[\mathrm{Na}^{+}]_{\mathrm{out}} \approx [\mathrm{Na}^{+}]_{\mathrm{out}}$, then due to the fact that $[\mathrm{K}^{+}]_{\mathrm{in}} \gg [\mathrm{K}^{+}]_{\mathrm{out}}$, the potential φ again becomes negative. Cole qualitatively explained why the action potential goes from negative to positive and then to negative again. However, this did not explain why the action potential returns to the initial value (equal to the resting potential) over time.

It should be noted that the entire small group of scientists involved in research on the excitation and propagation of action potentials in nerve cells not only considered their colleagues as competitors but also maintained trusting and friendly relationships with each other and shared their results with each other, even before writing and publishing articles. In 1947, Cole, in his letter to Hodgkin, spoke about a device that allows, through feedback, control of the potential difference inside the squid axon. And Hodgkin, during a visit to America before his article was submitted to a journal [15], informed Cole about his experiments, which he carried out together with George Marmont with an electrode inserted inside the squid axon. In turn, the conversation with Cole and Marmont encouraged Hodgkin, Huxley, and Bernard Katz (1911–2003) (joint winner of the 1970 Nobel Prize in Physiology or Medicine) to create a similar device for their research, the results of which were published in 1949 [6].

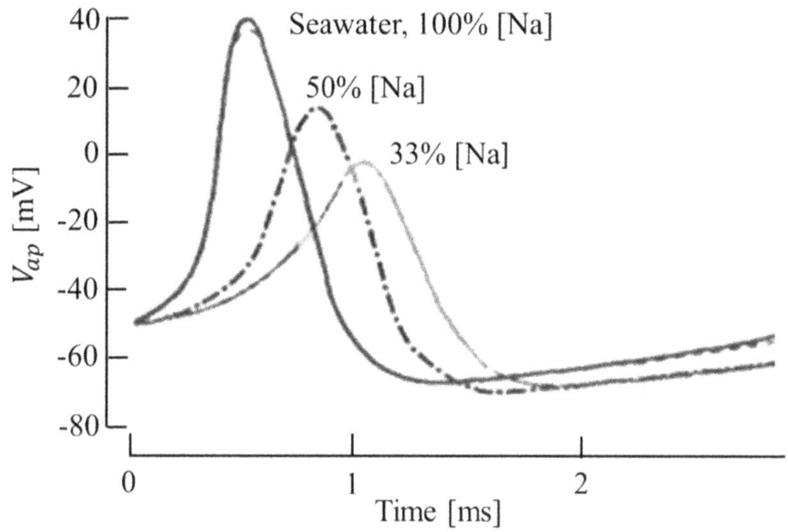

Figure 1.15. Action of sodium-deficient solutions on the resting and action potentials [15] John Wiley & Sons. © 1949 The Physiological Society.

Figure 1.15 shows the results of measuring the action potential as a function of the density of sodium ions in the surrounding electrolyte.

Before we proceed to consider the results of Hodgkin and Huxley's work, we draw the reader's attention to the importance of a comprehensive education in science. If we turn to the scientific biographies of all participants who were involved in determining the nature of nervous activity, we find that all of them, starting with Volta, first received a good education in physics, engineering, and electronics, and only after that did they turn to biology. The question is whether a scientist always acquires enough knowledge during their university studies to reach the correct conclusions about the phenomena that they will encounter in their scientific and professional activities. The answer is: not always.

Professional biologists of the late 19th century and the first half of the 20th century did not have the knowledge necessary to formulate ideas in the fields of nervous activity and genetics. One of the rare examples of a scientist who received only a classical education in biology but managed to write his name in the history of biology of the 20th century is James Watson. Having no idea about organic chemistry or crystallography and not knowing physics (Watson received a PhD in ornithology), thanks to his intuition, Watson realized that the science that would allow one to prove that it is the DNA molecule that is the carrier of genetic information would be crystallography, so he undertook incredible efforts to join a group engaged in crystallographic research in biology. His enthusiasm was transmitted to Francis Crick (1916–2004), a physicist by training who worked in protein crystallography. The collaboration between Watson and Crick turned out to be very fruitful. They managed to decipher the structure of DNA and thereby answer the main questions of genetics: what genes are, how hereditary information is transmitted from generation to generation, and how hereditary information is transformed into the basis of life—proteins. For the results of these studies, Watson and Crick were awarded the Nobel Prize in Physiology or Medicine in 1962.

A small book by one of the founders of quantum mechanics, Erwin Schrödinger (1887–1961), *What Is Life? The Physical Aspect of the Living Cell*, played a huge role in popularizing interest in biology among physicists.[16] In this book, Schrödinger clearly formulated the concept of a code as a sequential recording of information on the production of proteins and formulated a condition for the molecule on which it should be written. Another physicist who made an exceptional contribution to unraveling the genetic code was George Gamow (1904–68).[17] He predicted that the basic element of the genetic code should consist of three letters. Gamow noticed that all proteins in living organisms consist of 20 types of amino acids, from which he concluded that there are only 20 words in the protein dictionary, so three of the four nucleotides included in the DNA molecule are enough to encode them.

Now, when almost 100 years have passed since the famous work of Hodgkin and Huxley [1], which summarizes the results of 13 years of hard experimental work, it seems that there is nothing special in it; everything is in plain sight. The student opens the textbook, quickly flips through the pages describing the experiments, and lets their gaze fall on the equations describing the propagation of the action potential in the axons of nerve cells. If the student is inquisitive, they will naturally pay attention to the complexity of the equations and ask themselves how such equations could be obtained on the basis of experimental data and return to the history of the problem.

1.4 Model of squid axon proposed by Hodgkin and Huxley

An electrical circuit proposed by Hodgkin and Huxley, which simulates the propagation of the action potential, is shown in figure 1.16. It takes into account only the currents of sodium and potassium ions. Currents of other types of ions passing through the membrane (see table 1.1) are not reflected in this model electrical circuit, since Hodgkin and Huxley, in their experiments, did not observe the penetration of other ions through the membrane of the squid axon during the passage of the action potential. As for the leakage current I_L, Hodgkin and Huxley did not know its nature and associated it with small flows of chloride ions or other ions. They introduced leakage current into their model because, without it, the potential difference across the membrane could not be guaranteed to return to the resting potential after an action potential had passed. In fact, the leakage current is associated with ion pumps that transport excess sodium ions inside the axon outward, re-establishing the lack of potassium ions inside and pumping them out

[16] Erwin Rudolf Josef Alexander Schrödinger was one of the fathers of quantum mechanics and the winner of the 1933 Nobel Prize in Physics. In 1944, he published a small book, *What Is Life? The Physical Aspect of the Living Cell*, which forever inscribed his name in the history of biology and biophysics.

[17] George Gamow, a Soviet and American polymath, theoretical physicist, and cosmologist. He discovered alpha decay via quantum tunneling, proposed the Big Bang theory (expanding universe), and formulated the concept of the genetic code.

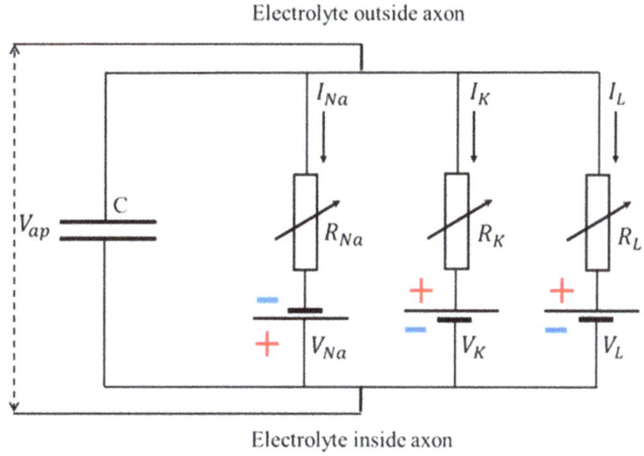

Figure 1.16. The electrical circuit proposed by Hodgkin and Huxley imitates the electrical properties of the squid axon membrane [1]. V_{ap} is the potential difference between internal and external electrolytes.

from the external environment. In the next section, we will describe ion channels and ion pumps built into the membranes of nerve cells. Note that ion channels and pumps are also present in other cells.

The fundamental difference between the electrical circuits shown in figures 1.16 and 1.12 is the presence of voltage sources in the Hodgkin–Huxley model. It is easy to see that when $V_{ap} < V_{Na}$, the direction of the current associated with sodium ions reverses. The same applies to the case when $V_{ap} < V_K$ and $V_{ap} < V_L$.

The differential equation corresponding to the electrical circuit is shown in figure 1.16:

$$C_m \frac{dV_{ap}}{dt} + g_{Na}(t, V_{ap})(V_{ap} - V_{Na}) + g_K(t, V_{ap})(V_{ap} - V_K) + g_L(V_{ap} - V_L) = 0, \quad (1.18)$$

$$g_{Na} = 1/R_{Na}, \; g_K = 1/R_K, \; g_L = 1/R_L. \quad (1.19)$$

The unknown quantities in equation (1.18) are g_{Na}, g_K, and g_L, while the membrane capacitance C_m is known.

The key to the success of Hodgkin and Huxley was the creation of a device that made it possible to record the potential inside the squid axon and measure the time dependences of g_{Na}, g_K, and g_L at a fixed value of the membrane potential V_{ap}.

Figure 1.17 shows a schematic diagram of Hodgkin and Huxley's measurements. Since electrodes 1 and 2 are connected to each other through a conductive liquid, their potential is constant and equal to the potential of the electrolyte inside the axon. Electrode 3 is grounded, so the potential of the external electrolyte is always zero. The voltage source 7 and amplifier 8 make it possible to maintain a constant potential difference between the internal electrolyte and the external one. Since electrode 2 passes through the entire axon, there is no longitudinal potential gradient during measurements; therefore, the currents from the external to the internal

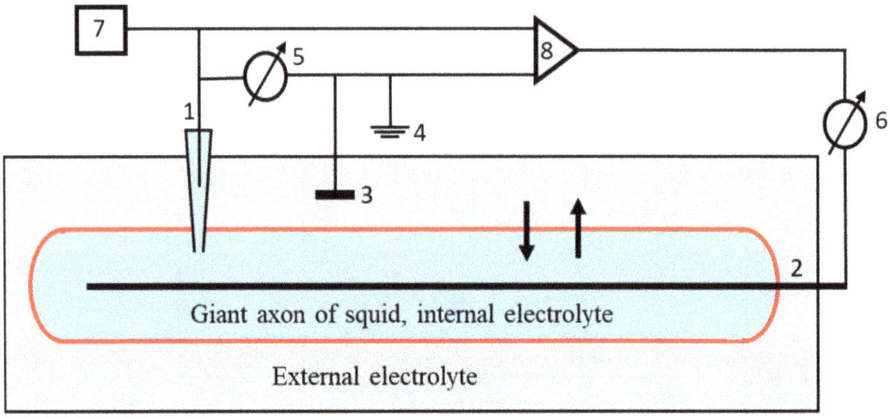

Figure 1.17. Schematic diagram of measurements made in Hodgkin and Huxley's experiments [1–9]: 1. electrode for measuring the potential inside the squid axon, 2. electrode inserted inside the axon, 3. electrode located in the external electrolyte, 4. ground, 5. voltmeter, 6. ammeter, 7. constant voltage source, and 8. current amplifier. The arrows indicate the direction of currents either from the external to the internal electrolyte or from the internal to the external electrolyte.

electrolyte, as well as from the internal to the external electrolyte, are the same along the entire length of the axon.

Obviously, in order to find the parameters of the electrical circuit shown in figure 1.16, namely the dependence of the functions g_{Na}, g_K, and g_L in equation (1.18) on time and the potential difference across the membrane, it was desirable to consecutively turn off two of the three circuits, so that the current flowed through only one circuit.

To find g_K, Hodgkin and Huxley used an external electrolyte as an electrolytic liquid in which Na^+ ions were replaced by choline$^+$ ions (the membrane is impermeable to choline$^+$ ions). Choline is a cation with the chemical formula $[(CH_3)_3NCH_2CH_2OH]^+$.

At a fixed value of $V_{ap} = V_0$, the ammeter (6) in figure 1.17 measured the current:

$$I_K = g_K(t,\ V_0)(V_0 - V_K). \tag{1.20}$$

In (1.20), we excluded the current associated with g_L, since it is small and does not play a role at the stage of excitation of the action potential. Knowing the dependence of I_K on time, it is easy to find $g_K(t,\ V_0)$ and V_K.

To find the dependence of g_{Na} on time and V_{Na} for seawater (taken as an external electrolyte), Hodgkin and Huxley acted quite logically: they subtracted the currents I_K from the current values I measured by the ammeter (6):

$$I = I_{Na} + I_K = g_{Na}(t,\ V)(V_0 - V_{Na}) + I_K. \tag{1.21}$$

Figure 1.18 shows the results of measuring membrane conductivity with respect to sodium and potassium ions.

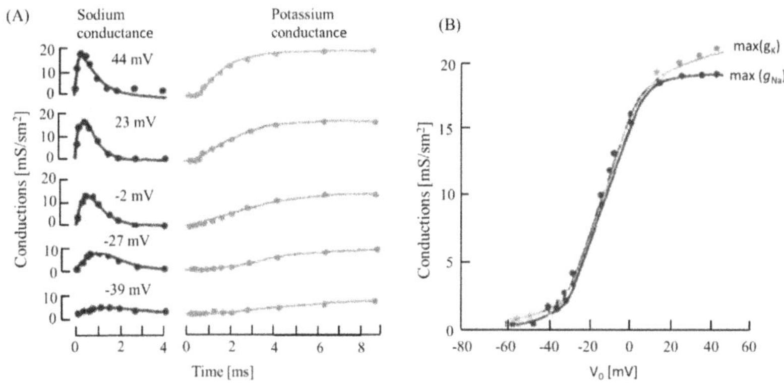

Figure 1.18. Time dependences of membrane conductivity during various stimulating jumps in the potential difference on the membrane. (A) Time dependences of membrane conductivity with respect to sodium and potassium ions. (B) Dependences of the maximum membrane conductance values with respect to sodium and potassium ions on the potential inside the squid axon (the potential outside the axon is zero) for different values of V_0. Parts (A) and (B) reproduced from [1] John Wiley & Sons. © 1952 The Physiological Society..

It is striking that, as shown in figure 1.18(A), with a jump in potential, the conductivity of the membrane for potassium ions smoothly reaches a stationary state, while the conductivity for sodium ions quickly increases and then quickly drops to zero. How can there be such a 'dislike' for sodium ions in the membrane, since they are no different from potassium ions except for their size? It seems as if there is a guard in the membrane who, recognizing that sodium ions are rushing through the gate, quickly closes the gate in front of them. Neither Hodgkin, Huxley, Cole, nor their colleagues had any idea why such selectivity occurs in the membrane. We would like to point out that, according to the measurement results shown in figure 1.18(B), the maximum conductivity values of the membrane with respect to potassium and sodium ions are almost the same; however, the time taken to reach the maximum conductivity for sodium ions is shorter than for potassium ions, and, with increasing amplitude of the voltage surge, this difference decreases. Thus, at $V_0 = -27$ mV, the maximum conductivity value for sodium ions is achieved after 1 ms and for potassium ions after 8 ms, while at $V_0 = 23$ mV, the maximum conductivity of sodium ions is again achieved after 1 ms but for potassium ions after 4 ms. In other words, if the voltage surge is less than 23 mV and lasts less than 1 ms, then the main contribution to the current passing through the membrane is determined by sodium ions. However, if, for example, the voltage surge is +44 mV and lasts for 5 ms, then the total current passing through the membrane is determined by potassium.

After processing the measurements, Hodgkin and Huxley found that:

$$V_{Na} = -115\,\text{mV}, \quad V_K = 120\,\text{mV}, \quad V_L = -10\,\text{mV}, \tag{1.22}$$

$$g_L = 3\,\Omega^{-1}\text{m}^{-2}, \tag{1.23}$$

$$C_m = 10^{-2}\text{F m}^{-2}. \tag{1.24}$$

As for the conductivities $g_{Na}(t, V_{ap})$ and $g_K(t, V_{ap})$, they presented them in this form:

$$g_K = G_K n^4, \quad g_{Na} = G_{Na} m^3 h, \tag{1.25}$$

where $G_K = 36\ \Omega^{-1}\ m^{-2}$, $G_{Na} = 1200\ \Omega^{-1}\ m^{-2}$, and $G_L = g_L = 3\ \Omega^{-1}\ m^{-2}$ and the functions n, m, and h are described by the following empirical equations:

$$\frac{dn}{dt} = \alpha_n(1 - n) - \beta_n n, \tag{1.26}$$

$$\frac{dm}{dt} = \alpha_m(1 - n) - \beta_m m, \tag{1.27}$$

$$\frac{dh}{dt} = \alpha_h(1 - n) - \beta_h h, \tag{1.28}$$

$$\alpha_n = (V_{ap} + 10)/\left(\exp\left(\frac{V_{ap} + 10}{10}\right) - 1\right), \quad \beta_n = 0.125\exp\left(\frac{V_{ap}}{80}\right), \tag{1.29}$$

$$\alpha_m = 0.1(V + 25)/\left(\exp\left(\frac{V_{ap} + 25}{10}\right) - 1\right), \quad \beta_m = 4\exp\left(\frac{V_{ap}}{18}\right), \tag{1.30}$$

$$\alpha_h = 0.07\exp\left(\frac{V_{ap}}{20}\right), \quad \beta_h = 1/\left(\exp\left(\frac{V_{ap} + 30}{10}\right) + 1\right). \tag{1.31}$$

Accordingly, equation (1.18) takes the following form:

$$C_m\frac{dV_{ap}}{dt} + G_K n^4(V_{ap} - V_K) + G_{Na} m^3 h(V_{ap} - V_{Na}) + G_L(V_{ap} - V_L) = 0. \tag{1.32}$$

Let us write down the asymptotic stationary values of n, m, and h in (1.26)–(1.28), which are achieved for $t \to \infty$ and a fixed value of $V_{ap} = V_0$:

$$m_\infty(V_0) = \frac{\alpha_m(V_0)}{\alpha_m(V_0) + \beta_m(V_0)}, \tag{1.33}$$

$$n_\infty(V_0) = \frac{\alpha_n(V_0)}{\alpha_n(V_0) + \beta_n(V_0)}, \tag{1.34}$$

$$h_\infty(V_0) = \frac{h_n(V_0)}{h_n(V_0) + h(V_0)}. \tag{1.35}$$

Figure 1.19 shows the dependences of the stationary values m_∞, n_∞, and h_∞ on V_0, and figure 1.20 shows the dependence of the action potential on time.

We will give an interpretation of equation (1.32) in the next subsection of this chapter. Now let us move on to deriving the equation for the propagation of the

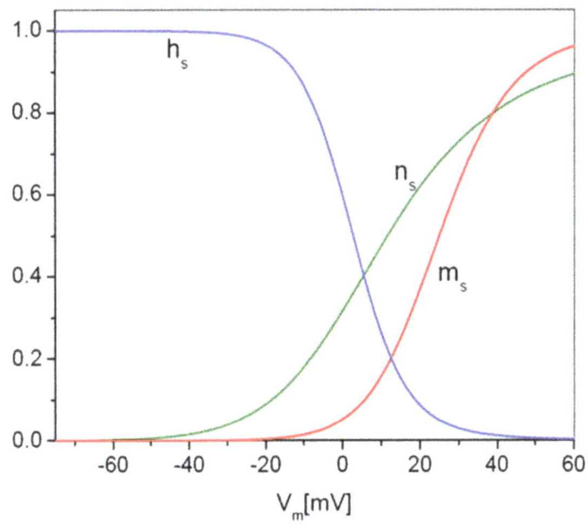

Figure 1.19. Dependences of the stationary values m_∞, n_∞, and h_∞ on V_0.

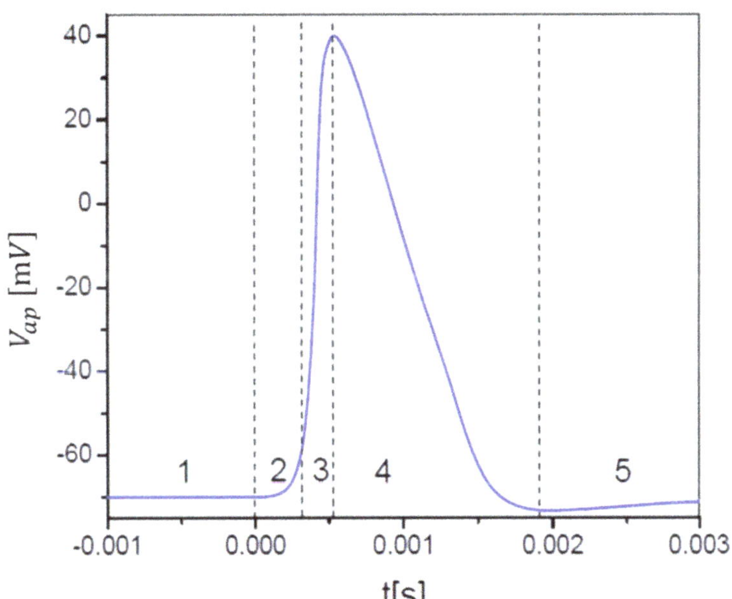

Figure 1.20. Action potential in the squid axon. Time dependence with characteristic time intervals: 1. resting potential; 2. the voltage across the membrane (due to charging currents) rises by 10–30 mV; 3. sodium ions enter the neuron and the potential difference on the membrane increases to +40 mV; 4. potassium ions exit the axon, and the potential difference falls below the resting potential level; and 5. potassium and sodium ions stop passing through the membrane. The stage of restoration begins to restore the nonequilibrium ion density.

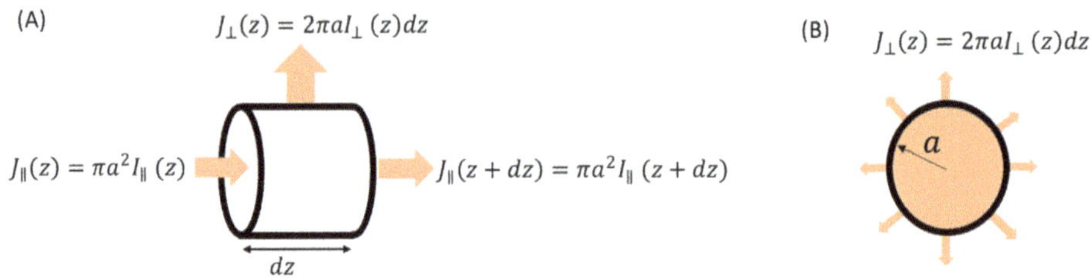

Figure 1.21. System of currents in an axon element. The thick black lines show the membrane, and a is the radius of the axon. In (A), $J_{\|}(z)$ is the current flowing into the cylinder (axon), while $J_{\|}(z + \mathrm{d}z)$ is the current flowing out of the cylinder (axon) through the end. Accordingly, $I_{\|}(z) = J_{\|}(z)/\pi a^2$ is the current flowing into the cylinder (axon) per unit area, and $I_{\|}(z + \mathrm{d}z) = J_{\|}(z + \mathrm{d}z)/\pi a^2$ is the current flowing from the end of the cylinder (axon) per unit area. In (A) and (B), $J_{\perp}(z)$ is the current flowing through the boundary of the cylinder (membrane), and $I_{\perp}(z) = J_{\perp}(z)/2\pi a dz$ is the current flowing through the boundary of the cylinder (membrane) per unit area.

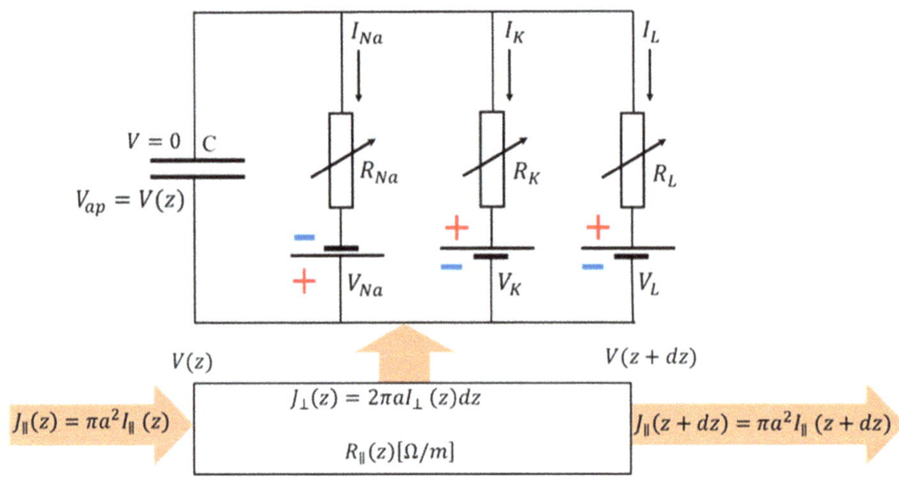

Figure 1.22. Currents in the schematic electrical circuit of an axon element proposed by Hodgkin and Huxley [1].

action potential along the squid axon. The longitudinal and transverse components of currents during the passage of an action potential in a squid axon are shown in figures 1.21 and 1.22.

In accordance with the law of current conservation:

$$J_{\|}(z + \mathrm{d}z) - J_{\|}(z) = J_{\perp}(z). \tag{1.36}$$

Substituting $J_{\|} = \pi a^2 I_{\|}$ and $J_{\perp} = 2\pi a I_{\perp}\mathrm{d}z$ into (1.36), we obtain:

$$\pi a^2 (I_{\|}(z + \mathrm{d}z) - I_{\|}(z)) = 2\pi a I_{\perp}(z)\mathrm{d}z \tag{1.37}$$

or

$$\pi a^2 \frac{\mathrm{d}I_{\|}(z)}{\mathrm{d}z} = 2\pi a I_{\perp}(z). \tag{1.38}$$

Since the longitudinal resistance of the membrane is orders of magnitude higher than the resistance of the electrolyte in the axon, the potential difference is determined exclusively by the currents flowing inside the axon.[18] The voltage drop in an electrical circuit is equal to its current multiplied by its resistance. Therefore, in accordance with figure 1.22:

$$\mathrm{d}V(z) = V(z + \mathrm{d}z) - V(z) = J_{\|}R_{\|}\mathrm{d}z \tag{1.39}$$

or

$$\frac{\mathrm{d}V(z)}{\mathrm{d}z} = J_{\|}R_{\|} = \pi a^2 R_{\|} I_{\|}(z), \tag{1.40}$$

where $R_{\|}$ [$\Omega\ \mathrm{m}^{-1}$] is the electrolyte resistance per unit length.

Differentiating the left and right sides of equation (1.40) with respect to dz and considering (1.36), we get:

$$\frac{\mathrm{d}^2V(z)}{\mathrm{d}z^2} = R_{\|}\pi a^2 \frac{\mathrm{d}I_{\|}(z)}{\mathrm{d}z} = 2\pi a R_{\|} I_{\perp}(z) \tag{1.41}$$

or

$$\frac{1}{2\pi a R_{\|}} \frac{\mathrm{d}^2V(z)}{\mathrm{d}z^2} = I_{\perp}(z). \tag{1.42}$$

Expressing $R_{\|}$ in terms of the specific resistance $r_{\|}\left[\Omega \cdot \mathrm{m}\right]$ and letting $R_{\|} = r_{\|}/\pi a^2$, we obtain:

$$\frac{a}{2r_{\|}} \frac{\mathrm{d}^2V(z)}{\mathrm{d}z^2} = I_{\perp}(z). \tag{1.43}$$

In accordance with the electrical diagram shown in figure 1.22, the current $I_{\perp}(z)$ is the sum of the displacement current passing through the capacitance C_{m} and the currents passing through the active resistances R_{Na}, R_{K}, and R_L:

$$I_{\perp}(z) = I_C(z) + I_{\mathrm{Na}}(z) + I_{\mathrm{K}}(z) + I_L(z). \tag{1.44}$$

Taking into account (1.32), (1.33), and (1.44), we obtain:

$$\frac{a}{2r_{\|}} \frac{\partial^2 V_{\mathrm{ap}}(z, t)}{\partial z^2} = C_{\mathrm{m}} \frac{\partial V_{\mathrm{ap}}}{\partial t} + G_{\mathrm{K}} n^4 (V_{\mathrm{ap}} - V_{\mathrm{K}}) + G_{\mathrm{Na}} m^3 h (V_{\mathrm{ap}} - V_{\mathrm{Na}}) + G_L (V_{\mathrm{ap}} - V_L). \tag{1.45}$$

Figure 1.23 shows the solution to equation (1.45) at a fixed time moment.

The dependence of the action potential excitation threshold on the duration of excitation, obtained using the Hodgkin and Huxley model, is shown in figure 1.24. It can be seen that if the excess of the excitation potential over the resting potential is

[18] In fact, the potential difference is determined by the currents in the internal electrolyte and the external one. The problem of the distribution of currents in an external electrolyte will be considered in chapter 2, in which we will discuss ephaptic coupling.

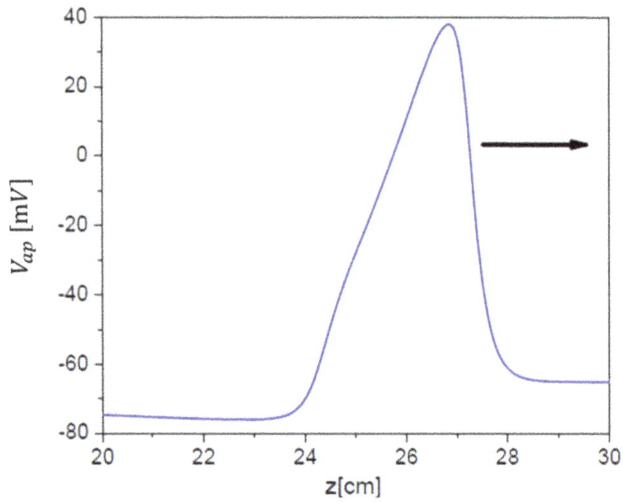

Figure 1.23. The instantaneous longitudinal structure of the action potential in the squid axon. The arrow designates the direction of propagation.

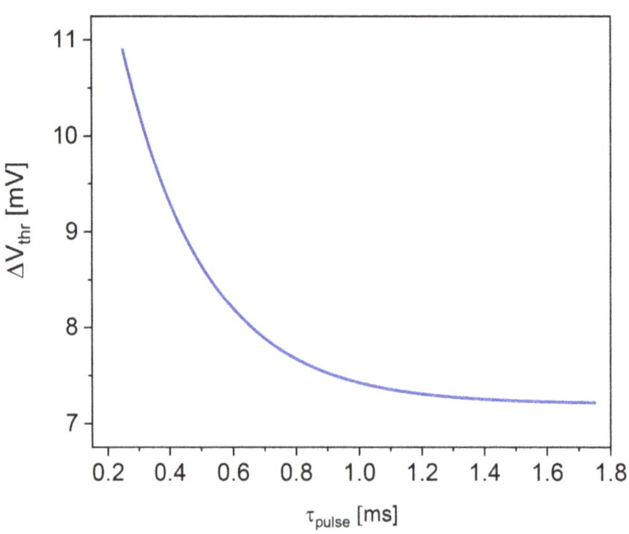

Figure 1.24. Dependence of the excitation threshold of the action potential on the excitation duration.

less than 7 mV, then the action potential is not excited, regardless of the duration of the excitation.

To estimate the propagation velocity of the action potential, in accordance with [1], we neglect the current of potassium ions I_K and the leakage current I_L in equation (1.45), and we consider the current density of sodium ions to be constant and equal to $G_{Na} V_{ap}$. In this case, equation (1.45) looks like:

Table 1.2. Selected diameters, conduction velocities, and functions of nerves [35].

Type of fiber	Radius (μm)	Velocity ($m\,s^{-1}$)	Function
A (α)	6–10	70–120	Somatic motor, proprioception
A (β)	2.5–6	30–70	Touch, pressure
A (γ)	1.5–3	15–30	Motor to muscle spindle
A (δ)	1–2.5	12–30	Pain and temperature
B	<1.5	3–15	Preganglionic autonomic
C dorsal root	0.2–1.6	0.5–2	Pain and temperature
C sympathetic	0.15–1.6	0.7–2.3	Postganglionic sympathetic

$$\frac{a}{2r_{\|}G_{\text{Na}}}\frac{\partial^2 V_{\text{ap}}(z,\,t)}{\partial z^2}=\frac{C_m}{G_{\text{Na}}}\frac{\partial V_{\text{ap}}}{\partial t}+V_{\text{ap}}. \tag{1.46}$$

From here, based on dimensional considerations, an estimate of the speed of propagation of the action potential follows:

$$v_{\text{ap}}\approx\sqrt{\frac{a}{2r_{\|}G_{\text{Na}}}}\frac{G_{\text{Na}}}{C_m}=\frac{1}{C_m}\sqrt{\frac{aG_{\text{Na}}}{2r_{\|}}}. \tag{1.47}$$

Substituting $C_m=10^{-2}\text{F m}^{-2}$, $G_{\text{Na}}=1200\,\Omega^{-1}\,\text{m}^{-2}$, and $a=0.238\cdot10^{-3}$m into (1.47) and letting $r_{\|}=0.35\,\Omega\cdot\text{m}$, we get $v_{\text{ap}}\approx 63\text{ m s}^{-1}$. If, instead of G_{Na}, we choose G_{K}, we then get the velocity of propagation of the action potential, $v_{\text{ap}}\approx 35\text{ m s}^{-1}$. The value of the action potential propagation speed calculated on the basis of equation (1.45) is 18.8 m s^{-1}, which differs slightly from the measured experimental value of 21.2 m s^{-1} [1].

The radii of the neural axons of vertebrates (including humans) vary from 0.1 to 10 μm. Therefore, in accordance with the estimation (1.47), the propagation velocity of the action potential in axons should be in the range of 0.1–1 m s^{-1}. In fact, the propagation velocity of the action potential in living organisms reaches values of ~100 m s^{-1}. This value is determined by the radius of the axon and the functional purpose of the corresponding nerve cells, for which the conditional classification given in table 1.2 is adopted. Such high propagation velocities of the action potential in thin axons, listed in table 1.2, are associated with the presence of myelinated sections along the axon. We will consider myelinated axons in section 1.6 and, in more detail, in chapter 2, section 2.1.

Before we move on to the next part of this introductory chapter, we note that the power supplies introduced by Hodgkin and Huxley into the electrical circuit shown in figure 1.16 essentially simulate the operation of ion channels that open at a certain potential difference between the electrolytes inside and outside the cell. In modern language, we would say that Hodgkin and Huxley built a phenomenological model of an excitable membrane.[19]

It should be said that the construction of phenomenological theories, that is, theories devised without detailed knowledge of the mechanism behind a given phenomenon, has always played a significant role in the development of science. An example is the phenomenological theory of superconductivity proposed in 1950 by Ginzburg and Landau [36]. Later, in 1957, Bardeen, Cooper, and Schrieffer developed a detailed microscopic theory of superconductivity [37].

1.5 Ion channels and pumps

Measurements carried out in various types of cells showed that the absolute value of the resting potential varied from 10 to 100 mV. Figure 1.25 shows a summary of the

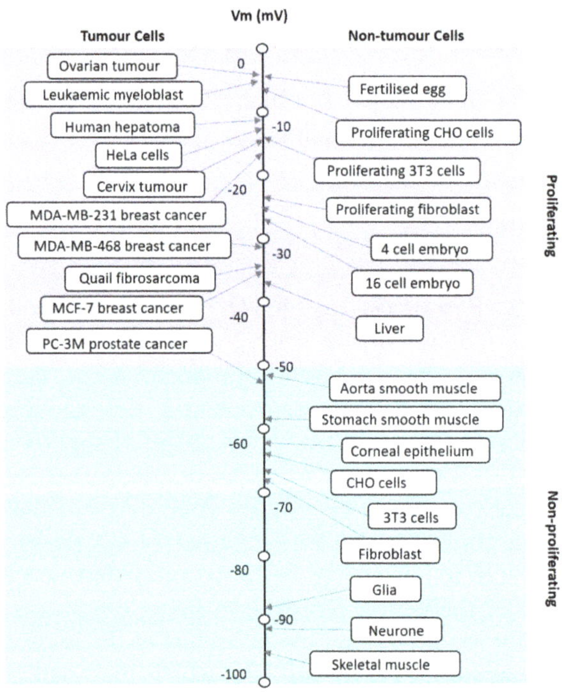

Figure 1.25. Different functions and the cell types associated with these functions that are regulated by the resting membrane potential. Reproduced from [38]. CC BY 4.0.

[19] Phenomenological theory comes from the word 'phenomenon.' Such theory is built on the basis of the phenomenon itself and therefore, unlike microscopic theory, it does not provide an exact cause. An example of a phenomenological theory is the caloric theory, in which heat was considered a kind of liquid flowing from a warm body to a cold one. Within the framework of Maxwell's kinetic theory, heat is one of the manifestations of atomic motion. Another example of a phenomenological theory is Aristotle's theory of gravity. In it, the falling of bodies to the ground demonstrates their love for Mother Earth. Within the framework of Newton's laws, the fall of bodies to the ground is one of the manifestations of the universal law of attraction.

resting potential values [38]. It is problematic to explain such a large spread in the values of resting potentials and, accordingly, the ionic compositions inside cells solely by differences in the permeability of the phospholipid membrane. In the continuous 'phospholipid fence' separating the cell from the outside world, there must be 'gates' that either open or close according to certain signals. But what they are, where they are, and what controls them remained completely unclear for a long time.

An indication of the existence of ion channels was provided by experiments with tetrodotoxin contained in puffer fish and tetraethylammonium. In their experiments, Kao and Fuhrman showed that tetrodotoxin blocks the passage of sodium ions through the membrane without affecting its permeability with respect to potassium ions [39], while Ichiji Tasaki (1910–2009) had previously shown that tetraethylammonium blocks the passage of potassium ions through the membrane without affecting its permeability with respect to sodium ions [40]. The physics of the effect of tetraethylammonium and tetrodotoxin on the permeability of a membrane with respect to sodium and potassium ions is quite simple; the molecules of tetrodotoxin and tetraethylammonium, due to their size and structure, get stuck in the corresponding channels and thereby interfere with the function of nerves.

The binding of the radiolabeled sodium channel blocker tetrodotoxin made it possible to measure the density of sodium channels. It turned out that there were about 500 sodium channels per square micrometer of squid axon surface. The real breakthrough in the study of ion channels is associated with two German scientists, physicist Erwin Neher and physician Bert Sakmann [41]. They managed to create a special pipette (the patch clamp), which was suctioned to the membrane in such a way that there was only one channel inside it, and they specially created equipment that made it possible to measure currents passing through one channel. The paper published by Neher and Sakmann in 1976 [41] was received with great enthusiasm by the biological science community, as it provided the first direct evidence for the existence of ion channels. In 1991, Neher and Sakmann received the Nobel Prize in Physiology for their discoveries concerning the function of single ion channels in cells.

Figure 1.26 shows a circuit for measuring currents flowing through a single channel proposed and implemented by Neher and Sakmann. Measurements by Neher and Sakmann showed that the channels operate in either an 'open' or a 'closed' mode. Moreover, the time interval between the open and closed modes is random. The amplitude of the current passing through the channel depends on the potential difference between the electrolytes on opposite sides of the membrane and the potassium concentration.

The results of measuring the current through the potassium channel at the same concentration of potassium ions in the pipette and outside it, equal to 150 mmol l^{-1}, are shown in figure 1.27.

Figure 1.28 shows the results of measuring the potassium current passing through the channel when the concentration of potassium ions in the pipette is close to the concentration of ions in the cytoplasm of the cell, which is $[N_k^+]_{in} = 90$ mmol l^{-1},

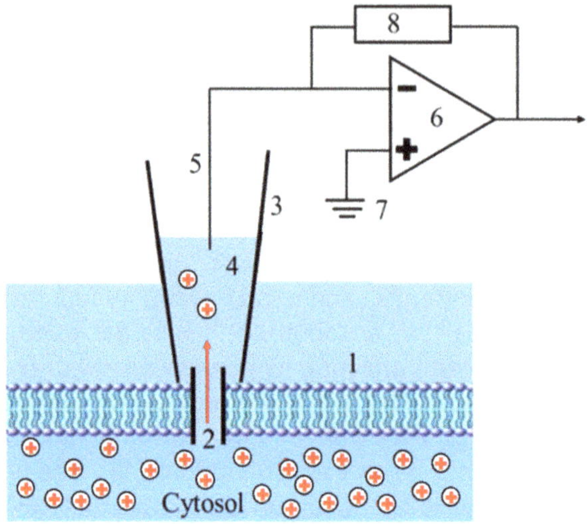

Figure 1.26. Schematic diagram of a circuit for measuring currents in a single channel: 1—membrane, 2—ion channel, 3—patch pipette, 4—pipette solution, 5—electrode, 6—operating amplifier, 7—earth, 8—feedback resistor, pluses—ions.

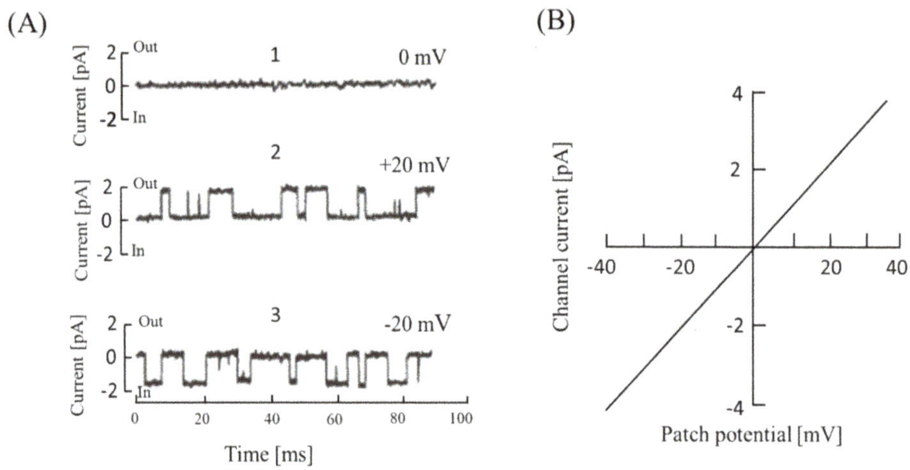

Figure 1.27. The results of measuring the current passing through the potassium channel when the concentration of potassium ions in the pipette is the same as that outside it: $[N_k^+]_{in} = [N_k^+]_{out} = 150\ \mathrm{mmol\ l^{-1}}$. (A) Dependence of currents on time through a single channel: 1. at zero potential on the pipette; 2. at +20 mV on the pipette; and 3. at −20 mV on the pipette. (B) Dependence of the average current through the channel on the voltage on the pipette. Parts (A) and (B) reproduced with permission from [42].

and outside the pipette the concentration of potassium ions in the extracellular fluid, which is $[N_k^+]_{out} = 3\mathrm{mmol\ l^{-1}}$.

Figure 1.29 shows the results of measuring sodium currents through single channels [43]. To inactivate sodium channels, the potential inside the cell was

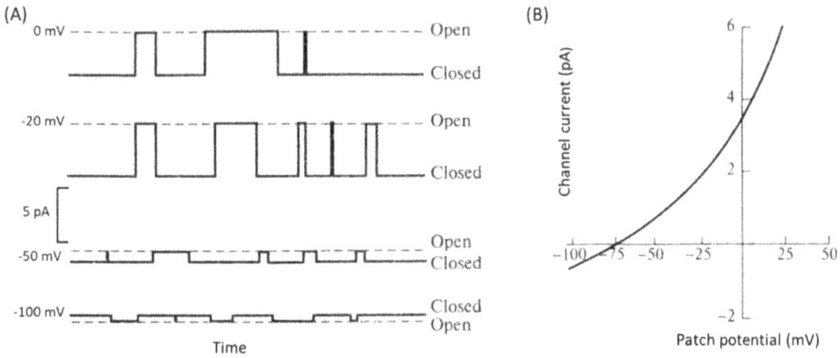

Figure 1.28. Time dependence of currents flowing through one channel. The density of potassium ions in the pipette is $[N_k^+]_{in} = 90\text{mmol l}^{-1}$, and it is $[N_k^+]_{out} = 3\text{mmol l}^{-1}$ outside it. (A) Time dependence of currents passing through a single channel at different voltages on the pipette: at zero potential on the pipette, the current flows from an area with a higher concentration of sodium ions to an area with a lower concentration; at a potential of -20 mV on the pipette, the current amplitude increases; at a potential of -50 mV on the pipette, the current amplitude decreases; and at a potential of -100 mV on the pipette, the current changes direction. (B) Dependence of the average current passing through the channel on the applied voltage on the pipette. At a voltage of -75 mV, the current passing through the channel is zero. Parts (A) and (B) reproduced with permission from [42].

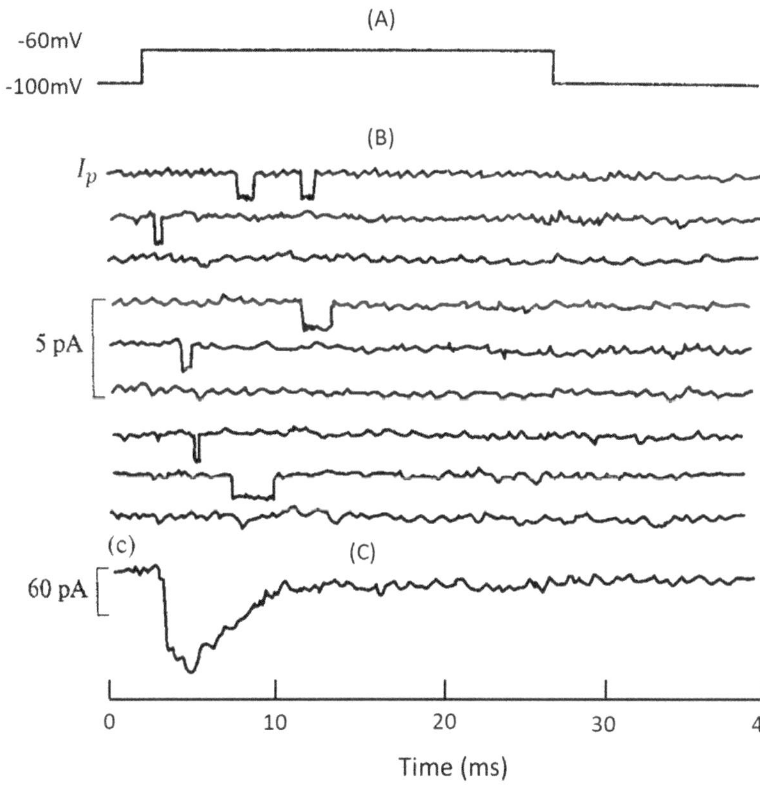

Figure 1.29. Time dependence of currents passing through sodium channels. (A) Voltage on the internal electrolyte. (B) Current versus time in several sodium channels. (C) Summed current for 300 sodium channels. Parts (A)–(C) reprinted by permission from Springer Nature Customer Service Center GmbH: [Nature], [43], Copyright (1980).

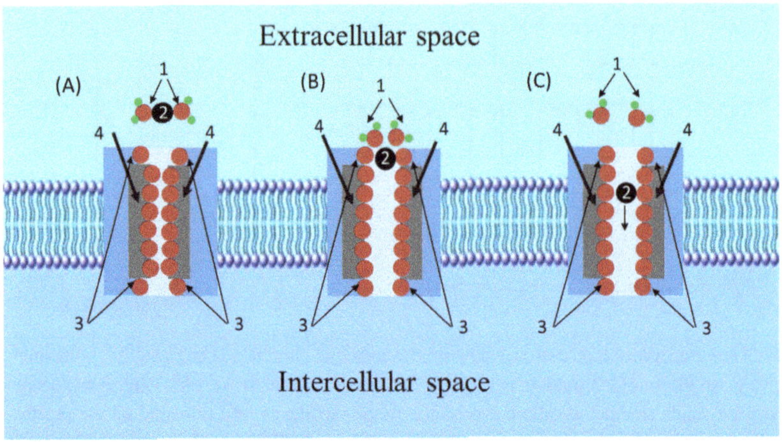

Figure 1.30. Scheme of operation of a potassium channel built into the axon membrane. (A) Channel is closed; hydrated potassium ions cannot pass through the channel. (B) Channel is open; dehydration of potassium ions at the entrance to the channel. (C) Transfer of potassium ions along the channel: 1—water molecules, 2—potassium ions, 3—oxygen atoms on the inner surface of the channel, and 4—gating mechanism. In (A), the gating mechanism is closed, preventing ions from entering the channel. In (B) and (C), the gating mechanism is open, and potassium ions can pass through the channel. The energy of dehydration of the potassium ion is close to zero.

decreased to −100 mV, after which it increased abruptly to 40 mV and remained for 20 ms. During this time, some of the channels opened and remained in the open state for an average of 0.7 ms, after which they closed and remained in the closed state for 20 ms. The average current passing through the open channel was 1.6 pA. Figure 1.29(C) shows the sum of the currents passing through 300 sodium channels. It should be noted that sodium channels, unlike potassium channels, actually opened once in a 20 ms period.

The next breakthrough in the study of ion channels came from the research of Roderick MacKinnon. In 1998, MacKinnon obtained the three-dimensional molecular structure of the potassium channel and unraveled the reason for its selectivity [44, 45]. By growing crystals of the potassium channel protein and exposing them to *x*-rays, he was able not only to see the structure of each channel molecule but also to trace the movement of a potassium ion along the channel. He determined that channel selectivity is ensured by two factors: the pore diameter of 0.3 nm is close to the potassium ion diameter of 0.27 nm and the spacing of the oxygen atoms present on the channel walls. This allows the potassium ion to squeeze into the channel and throw off the water shell almost without energy expenditure, as shown schematically in figure 1.30. As for the sodium ion, its diameter is 0.19 nm, so it is not able to create sufficiently tight contact with the four oxygen atoms inside the channel and therefore remains hydrated. However, in the hydrated state, the sodium ion is too large to pass through the narrow channel.

In his work, MacKinnon experimentally showed that potassium ion channels contain molecular structures capable of local displacements (conformations) inside

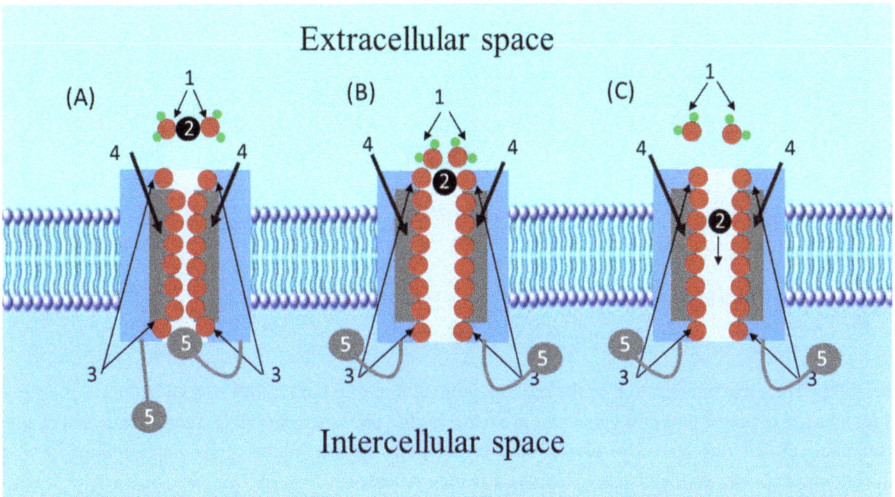

Figure 1.31. Scheme of operation of the sodium channel with the 'balls on strings' inactivation mechanism. (A) The channel is open, and the hydrated sodium ions cannot pass through the channel due to inactivation of the channel. (B) The channel is open, and the ion dehydrates upon entering the channel. (C) Ion transport along the channel: 1. water molecules, 2. sodium ion, 3. oxygen molecules built into the internal surface of the channel, 4. gating mechanism, and 5. inactivation of the channel is carried out by 'balls on strings.'

the channel in response to the action of an electric field. These structures, called 'gate mechanisms,' either close (inactivate) the channel, as shown in figure 1.30(A), or open (activate) it, as shown in figure 1.30(B,C). The probability of activation of the gate mechanism (opening of the channel) depends on the magnitude of the electric field. When a depolarizing field appears, the probability of opening a channel increases as the coefficient n in equation (1.32) increases. The opening of ion channels is accompanied by a sharp increase in electric current through the membrane. The permeability of the channels ranges from 10^6 to 10^8 ions per second, which is significantly higher than the transport of ions through ion pumps, which we will discuss below.

Sodium channels differ from potassium channels in that they have an inactivation mechanism that operates independently of the gating mechanism (figure 1.31). In Hodgkin and Huxley's equations, the inactivation mechanism is reflected by the coefficient h. In figure 1.19, it can be seen that at an internal electrolyte potential of $V_0 = V_R < -80$ mV, the inactivation mechanism is disabled. The balls in figure 1.30 do not close the input channel, $h \approx 1$, but when the potential is close to zero, they block it completely, $h \approx 0$. Since the coefficient h depends on time (equation (1.28)), a rapid change in the action potential triggers a flow of sodium ions from the external electrolyte to the internal one, even at $V_{\text{ap}} > 30$ mV.

In [46], it is shown that if the strings are 'cut', then sodium channels work like potassium channels. The dependence of the activation of the sodium channel on the potential difference between the internal and external electrolytes when the collar

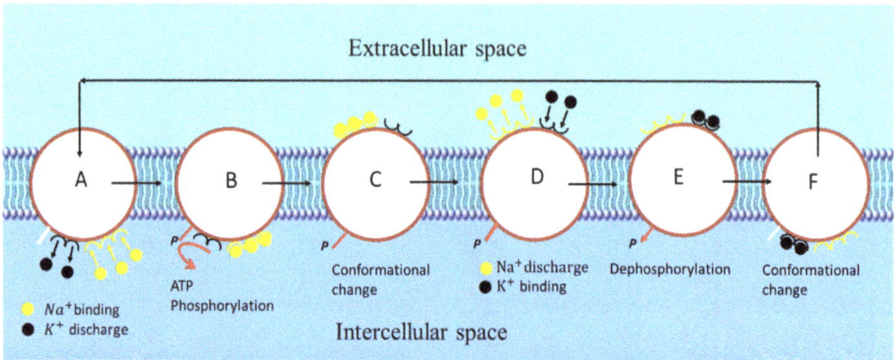

Figure 1.32. The cycle of operation of the sodium–potassium pump built into the squid axon membrane. A—sodium ions are captured and potassium ions are released. B—phosphorylation. C—conformational change of the channel. D—sodium ions are released and potassium ions are captured. E—dephosphorylation. F—conformational change of the channel. The cycle is then repeated.

mechanism is open corresponds to the curve m_∞ in figure 1.19, while inactivation corresponds to the curve h_∞.

Figure 1.32 shows the cycle of operation of the sodium–potassium pump in transporting sodium ions from the inside of the cell to the outside and potassium ions from the outside to the inside, as built into the membrane of the squid axon. In step (A), the sodium–potassium pump takes up sodium ions and releases potassium ions. At stage (B), phosphorylation occurs, and then at stage (C), a conformational change of the channel happens, that is, the channel rotates 180 degrees. Next, in step (D), sodium ions are released and potassium ions are captured. At stage (E), dephosphorylation occurs, and then at stage (F), a conformational change of the channel occurs. The cycle is then repeated.

Note that the sodium–potassium pump shown in figure 1.32 has a certain similarity to the operation of the electrophore machine shown in figure 1.1. If the electrophore machine transfers a positive charge from the right reservoir to the left and a negative charge from the left to the right, then the sodium–potassium pump transfers sodium ions from the axon electrolyte to the external electrolyte and potassium ions from the external electrolyte to the inside of the axon. Since the sodium–potassium pump works against the density gradients of sodium and potassium ions, it, like an electrophore machine, requires energy.

Now let us return to the Hodgkin and Huxley model and describe the excitation of the action potential through the dynamics of processes in ion channels. At the first stage of action potential excitation, the sodium channel is turned on and excess sodium from the external environment is pumped into the squid axon; the action potential grows and changes from negative to positive (the potential outside the axon is assumed to be zero). When the action potential reaches a certain positive value, the sodium channels close and the potassium channels turn on, causing excess potassium ions to flow out of the axon. The drop in potential intensifies, and, at some point in time, the potassium channels also close. At this moment, there is an excess of sodium ions inside the squid axon and an excess of potassium ions outside. It is then that the sodium–potassium pump turns on, which pumps sodium ions out of the axon and pumps in potassium ions. In this way, the equilibrium density of sodium and potassium ions in the axon, corresponding to its unexcited state, is restored.

Here, we will stop and will not describe the features of various channels regulating the ionic composition in cells, since they fit either into the category of passive channels, which do not require energy expenditure, or active ones, which require energy expenditure. A fairly detailed modern description of ion channels and their processes can be found in many reviews and books, for example, in the monograph [42].

After the discovery of transmembrane protein channels, it was found that many types of ion channels are not tied to their locations but can move in the protein channel under the influence of the thermal effect of membrane phospholipids, performing the so-called lateral diffusion movement. The range of values of the lateral diffusion coefficient of transmembrane ion channels lies in the range $D_L \sim 10^{-12} - 10^{-14}\ \mathrm{m^2\,s^{-1}}$ [47–50]. Lateral diffusion prevents the appearance of local inhomogeneities in the density of ion channels; therefore, without external influence, the distribution of ion channels susceptible to lateral diffusion is almost uniform.

Before we move on to consider the possibility of restructuring the distribution of transmembrane ion channels in the membrane, we must note that in the equation of Hodgkin and Huxley (1.45), the variables G_K, G_{Na}, and G_L can be interpreted as values characterizing the densities of potassium and sodium channels and sodium–potassium pumps pumping the corresponding ions through the axon membrane, which have the values n, m, h, V_K, V_{Na}, and V_L as their parameters. As for the values of C and $r_{\|}$, they characterize the membrane capacitance and the conductivity of the electrolyte inside the axon, respectively.

The threshold for excitation of the action potential depends on the ratio of the densities of Na^+ channels and the pumps that pump sodium ions out. Indeed, the greater the density of the sodium channels (at a fixed density of sodium–potassium pumps), the more negative the potential value on the internal electrolyte (if it is assumed that the external electrolyte has zero potential) at which the action potential starts. This is due to the fact that the voltage dependence of the membrane permeability toward different ions on the membrane does not change abruptly but has a smooth character, as can be seen, for example, in figure 1.19, which shows the dependence of the parameters m_∞, h_∞, and n_∞ on the potential difference between the internal and external electrolytes of the squid axon. Figure 1.33 shows the dependence of the threshold $\Delta V_{th} = V_{th} - V_R$ (where V_{th} is the potential at which the action potential is excited) on G_{Na} values. It can be seen that with increasing G_{Na}, the threshold falls, and, at $G_{Na} \approx 1550\ [\Omega^{-1}\,\mathrm{m^{-2}}]$, the threshold is close to zero, and the action potential is excited at the resting potential. The calculations were carried out based on the Hodgkin and Huxley model by varying the values of G_{Na}, leaving other parameters unchanged, and assuming that the duration of the exciting pulse is 1 ms.

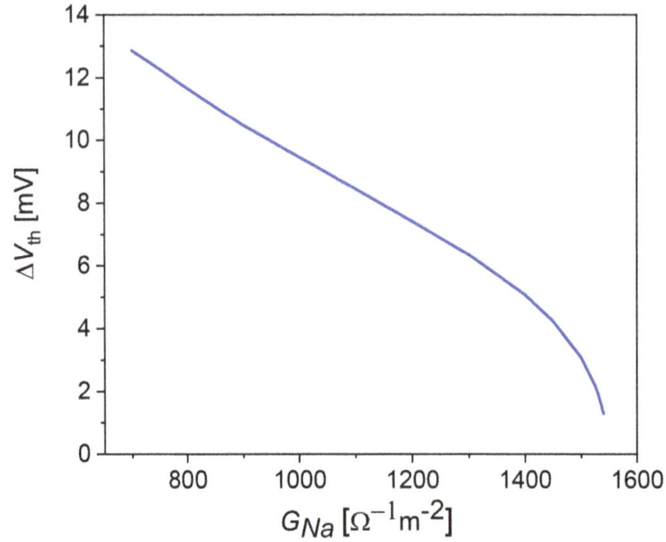

Figure 1.33. Dependence of the action potential excitation threshold $\Delta V_{\text{th}} = V_T - V_{\text{rest}}$ on the G_{Na} values calculated using the Hodgkin and Huxley axon model. The duration of the exciting pulse is assumed to be 1 ms.

The calculated dependences of the threshold voltage V_T on the ratio $\tilde{g}_{\text{Na}}/\tilde{g}_L$ $\tilde{g}_{\text{Na}} = \max(g_{\text{Na}})$ and $\tilde{g}_L = G_L$ for various types of nerve cells are shown in figure 1.34, which is taken from [51].

A well-known fact in acoustics is that suspended particles in the field of a standing acoustic wave are collected in the antinodes or in the nodes (see, for example, [57]). The direction of the suspended particles' displacement is determined by their density relative to the density of the medium. Since ion channels diffuse freely in the lateral directions of the membrane, the excitation of longitudinal vibrations in it should lead to the appearance of inhomogeneities in the densities of transmembrane ion channels along the membrane of the axon. Changing the ion channel density alters the transport of ions between the external and internal electrolytes, which leads to a change in the resting potential and the excitation threshold of the action potential, in accordance with the expected changes in the excitation thresholds shown in figure 1.34. The mechanism of redistribution of transmembrane proteins, including voltage-gated ion channels and ionic pumps, was proposed in [58, 59]. To put it briefly, the mechanism is associated with the acoustic pressure on the transmembrane proteins caused by a longitudinal ultrasonic (traveling or standing) wave excited in the axon's membrane. The redistribution of transmembrane proteins leads to the appearance of regions with a high density of transmembrane proteins and regions with transmembrane protein depletion. Such redistribution of voltage-gated Na^+ ion channels can stimulate or block the propagation of action potentials along the axon. A possible source of forced oscillations of the membrane is the interaction of an external microwave electromagnetic field with the charged surfaces of the axon membrane. In chapter 4, we consider this mechanism in detail and outline the conditions necessary for its implementation.

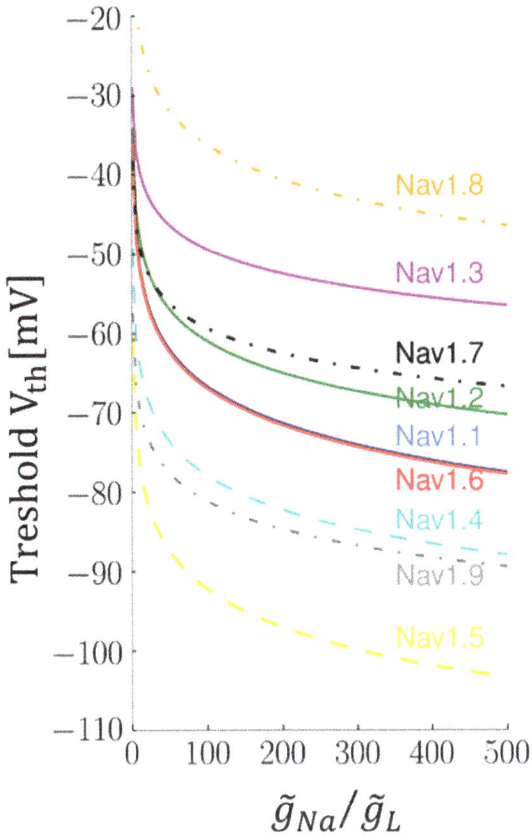

Figure 1.34. Influence of Na activation characteristics on the spike threshold. The threshold is a function of the ratio $\tilde{g}_{Na}/\tilde{g}_L$ ($\tilde{g}_{Na}$ = max (g_{Na}) and $\tilde{g}_L = G_L$) for the nine types of voltage-gated sodium channels [52] with characteristics reported in [53]. For each channel type, the threshold obtained across the data set is plotted. Nav1.{1–3,6} are expressed in the central nervous system, Nav1.{4,5} are expressed in cardiac and muscle cells, and Nav1.{7–9} are expressed in the peripheral nervous system. Nav1.6 is expressed at the action potential initiation site [54–56]. Here, V_T is the voltage on the membrane at which the action potential starts. Obviously, the higher the density of the sodium channels (for a fixed density of the sodium–potassium pumps), the more negative the potential value at the internal electrolyte (if the external electrolyte is assumed to have zero potential) that initiates an action potential. Reproduced from [51]. CC BY 4.0.

1.6 Myelinated nerve fibers, ephaptic coupling

A typical structure of a neuron with a myelinated axon is shown in figure 1.35. The axon is a long, slender projection of a neuron along which the nerve impulses travel from the body of the nerve cell (soma) to the innervated organs and other nerve cells. Dendrites are short and highly branched extensions of a neuron that serve as the main sites for the excitatory and inhibitory synapses affecting the neuron (different neurons have a different ratio of axon lengths to dendrite lengths); they transmit excitation to the neuron's body. A neuron can have several dendrites and usually

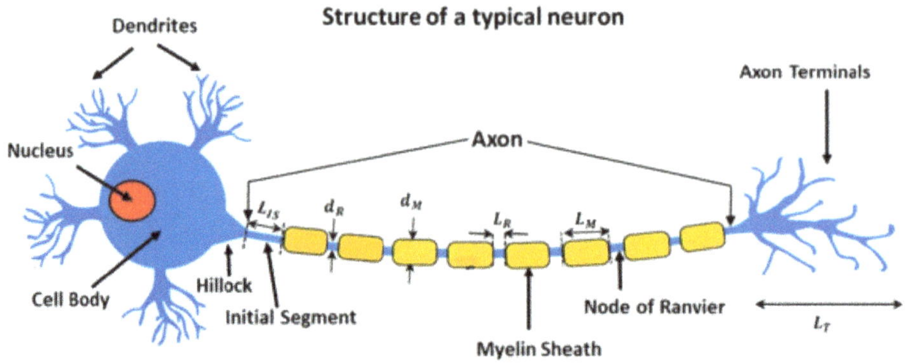

Figure 1.35. A neuron, showing the characteristic elements of a myelinated axon. The most excitable part of a neuron is the section after the axon hillock (where the axon exits the cell body), which is called the axon initial segment. Typically, the length of the initial segment L_{IS} is in the range of 20–70 μm (but it can reach 75 μm and even 200 μm), the length of the node of Ranvier L_R is 1–2.5 μm, the length of the myelin sheath L_M is $\sim$ 1–5 mm, and the length of the axon terminal L_T is $\sim$ 10–200 μm [60]. The diameter of the node of Ranvier d_R varies widely from 1–2 to 20 μm, and the thickness of the myelinated layer, formed by the Schwann cell, is $\delta_M = 0.5(d_M - d_R) \sim$ 3–5 μm. Excitation of the action potential in the myelinated axon occurs in the initial segment.

only one axon. One neuron can have connections with many (up to 20 000) other neurons.

The myelin coating of isolated sections of the axon is formed by the so-called Schwann cells, which are wrapped in several layers around the axon and reliably separate the internal electrolyte of the axon from the external one. Therefore, the exchange of ions between the axon and the external environment occurs only in places lacking 'isolation,' that is, in the nodes of Ranvier and the initial segment. The system of currents passing through ion channels in the nodes of Ranvier is shown in figure 1.36. Ions spreading over the outer surface of the myelinated fiber lead to surface charge but do not lead to the generation of an action potential, since, in the myelinated sections, there are no ion channels connecting the external electrolyte to the internal one. In this case, the action potential is transferred in the so-called saltatory conduction way, by 'jumps' from one node of Ranvier to another. Thus, axon myelination allows high action potential propagation velocities (up to 150 m s^{-1}) to be achieved at very small axon diameters. The saltatory mechanism of action potential propagation in myelinated nerve fibers was discovered and studied by Ichiji Tasaki [40, 61, 62].

Experimentally, saltatory transfer was first demonstrated in 1941 by Tasaki [62] and later by Huxley and Stämpfli [63]. Figure 1.37 shows a schematic of Tasaki's experiments [62]. A myelinated axon was placed in three baths of saline solution, the middle, narrower one being separated from the others by an air gap. The baths were connected by an external electric circuit. Therefore, the current was not blocked by the air gap as it flowed through the resistor R. The voltage drop across the resistor allowed the magnitude and direction of the currents to be measured.

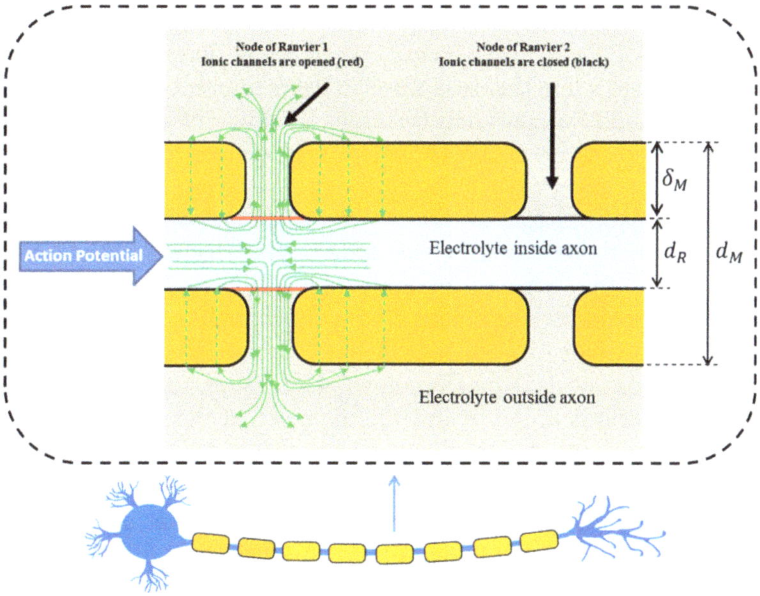

Figure 1.36. Schematic of the longitudinal structure of the myelinated axon. The action potential propagates from left to right. In the active phase of node of Ranvier 1, the ion channels are open, and currents induced inside and outside the axon (shown by green arrows) charge the membrane of the adjacent myelinated section. When the potential difference at the right end of the myelinated segment (node of Ranvier 2) reaches the threshold for initiation of the action potential (for example, at ~20 mV above the resting potential), sodium ion channels in node 2 open and the action potential starts in node 2. In general, as a result of the finite conductivity of the Schwann cells, a small conduction current (leakage current) flows through the myelin sheath in addition to the displacement current.

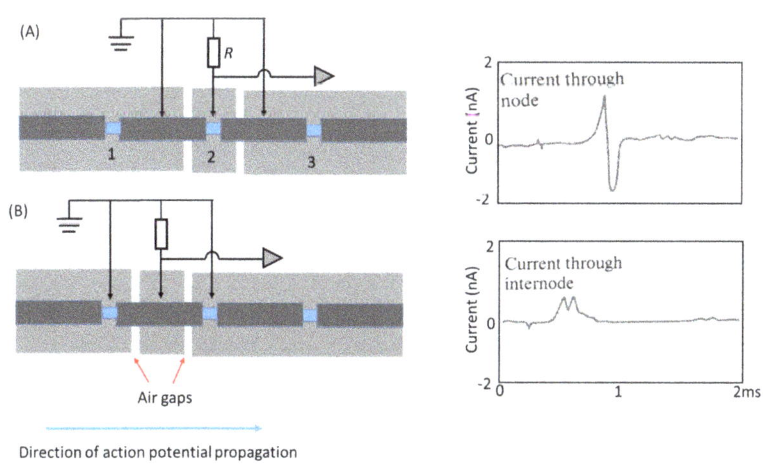

Figure 1.37. Current flow through a myelinated axon. (A) With Ranvier's node in the central bath. (B) With a myelinated axon segment in the central bath. Currents recorded through the resistor R are shown on the right. Adapted from [62].

The case where the node of Ranvier was in the central bath is shown in figure 1.37(A). Upon the passage of the action potential, the current across the resistance R first increases (ions Na^+ flow into the axon through the membrane of the node of Ranvier) and then decreases and becomes negative (ions K^+ flow out of the axon through the membrane of the node of Ranvier). The opposite case of current measurement, where the central bath contained a myelinated axon segment, is shown in figure 1.37(B).

Let us estimate the propagation velocity of the action potential in the myelinated fiber, assuming that the potential at the node of Ranvier is a step function with a duration t_R. To do this, we use equation (1.45), in which the capacitance and resistance of the membrane are replaced with the capacitance and resistance of the myelin region. Following [64, 65], we assume, without loss of generality, that we consider certain axons of the frog (Xenopus) nerve tissue, for which the diameter of the myelinated section is $d_M = 15\ \mu\text{m}$, the diameter of the Ranvier interception is $d_R = 9\ \mu\text{m}$, the length of the myelinated segment is $L_M = 92 d_M \approx 1.4$ mm, the specific resistance of the internal electrolyte is $r_{\|} = 1.1\ \Omega \cdot \text{m}$, and the specific resistance of the fiber is $\rho_M = 5.68 \cdot 10^5\ \Omega \cdot \text{m}$. In this case, the equation for the propagation of the action potential along the myelinated fiber is [64–66]:

$$\frac{1}{R_{\|}} \frac{\partial^2 V_M}{\partial z^2} = C_M \frac{\partial V_M}{\partial t} + g_M V_M, \tag{1.48}$$

where

$$R_{\|} = \frac{4 r_{\|}}{\pi d_R^2} = \frac{r_{\|}}{\pi a^2} = 1.7 \cdot 10^{10} [\Omega \cdot \text{m}^{-1}], \tag{1.49}$$

$$C_M = \frac{2\pi \varepsilon_M \varepsilon_0}{\ln\,(d_M/d_R)} = 1.6 \cdot 10^{-9} [\text{F} \cdot \text{m}^{-1}], \tag{1.50}$$

$$g_M = \frac{1}{\rho_M \ln\,(d_M/d_R)} = 0.34 \cdot 10^{-5} [\Omega^{-1} \cdot \text{m}^{-1}]. \tag{1.51}$$

Let us rewrite equation (1.48) as:

$$\frac{1}{g_M R_{\|}} \frac{\partial^2 V_M}{\partial z^2} = \frac{C_M}{g_M} \frac{\partial V_M}{\partial t} + V_M. \tag{1.52}$$

Similar to estimate (1.47) for a non-myelinated fiber, (1.52) yields an estimate of the speed of propagation of the action potential in the myelinated axon:

$$v_{ap} \approx \sqrt{\frac{1}{R_{\|} g_M} \frac{g_M}{C_M}} = \frac{1}{C_M} \sqrt{\frac{g_M}{R_{\|}}}. \tag{1.53}$$

For the parameter values given by (1.49)–(1.51), we obtain $v_{\text{ap}} \approx 9.7\ \text{s}^{-1}$. The exact calculation based on the model described in [64] gives a velocity equal to $11.9\ \text{m s}^{-1}$.

If we consider the myelin sheath to be a perfect insulator ($g_M = 0$), then the velocity of action potential propagation from the excited node to the neighboring node of Ranvier is determined by the length of the myelin segment. Indeed, according to the diffusion equation (1.48) (the $g_M V_M$ term is omitted), at time t the action potential propagates over a distance $z \sim \sqrt{\frac{t}{R_{\|} C_M}}$. Accordingly, the propagation velocity of the action potential $v_{\text{ap}} \sim \frac{\mathrm{d}z}{\mathrm{d}t} \sim \frac{1}{2}\sqrt{\frac{1}{R_{\|} C_M t}}$. Given an estimate of the propagation time of the action potential along the myelin segment to the next node of Ranvier, $t_M \approx R_{\|} C_M L_M^2$, we obtain

$$v_{\text{ap}} \approx \frac{1}{2 L_M C_M R_{\|}}. \tag{1.54}$$

Upon substituting the value $L_m = 1.4$ mm and the values of C_M, $R_{\|}$ from (1.49) and (1.50) into (1.54), we obtain $v_{\text{ap}} \approx 14.9 \text{ m s}^{-1}$. Note that if we take $L_M = 2$ mm, as in the calculations given in [64], then $v_{\text{ap}} \approx 10.4 \text{ m s}^{-1}$.

The system of currents generated by the action potential in the intercellular medium can charge not only the myelin sheaths closest to the excited interception of Ranvier (figure 1.36) but also the axon membranes of neighboring neurons. If the neighboring neuron is sufficiently close to the excited one, then when the potential difference across the membrane of the nodes of Ranvier in the neighboring neuron exceeds the threshold, an action potential is also initiated in it (figure 1.38). This process of transferring excitation from an active neuron to neighboring ones is called ephaptic coupling. In the next chapter, we take a closer look at this important process.

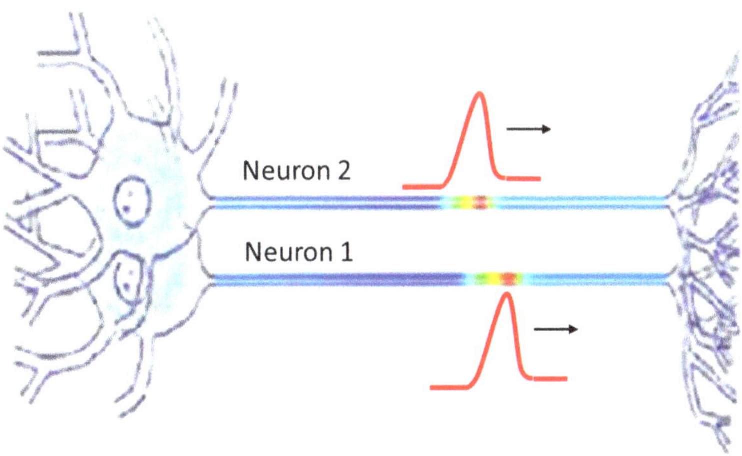

Figure 1.38. Ephaptic coupling. An action potential propagating in the axon of the lower neuron initiates an action potential in the upper neuron. Since there is a delay in the excitation of the action potential in the initiated neuron, its signal lags behind the initiating one. The arrows indicate the direction of action potential propagation.

1.7 Synapses

The previous parts of this chapter have been devoted to critical moments in the history of the development of our knowledge of the stimulation and propagation of action potentials in nerve fibers. In particular, we noted the role of physicists and engineers in formulating the fundamental ideas on the basis of which the modern biophysics of nervous tissues is still developing. In this section, we discuss the discovery of contacts between neurons and other cells. The main roles in this discovery were played by three classical physiologists: the Italian Camillo Golgi (1843–1926), the Spaniard Santiago Ramón y Cajal (1852–1934), and the German Otto Loewi (1873–1961). For their outstanding research results, they all became Nobel laureates, Golgi and Cajal in 1906 and Loewi in 1936.

In 1873, the Italian physiologist Golgi revealed that if a section of nervous tissue is immersed in a weak solution of silver nitrate, the neurons turn black. He described this discovery in his article [67]. The drawing from this article is shown in figure 1.39 (A). Later, in 1875, he published an article 'On the Fine Structure of the Olfactory Bulb,' in which he detailed his method of visualizing nervous tissue [68]; the drawing from this article is shown in figure 1.39(B). However, as was usually the case, his articles went unnoticed by physiologists of that time. It was only after he published his book, *On the Fine Anatomy of the Central Organs of the Nervous System* in 1886 [69], that the method of visualizing the fine structure of nervous tissue was recognized by the entire physiological community. Illustrations from this famous book by Golgi are shown in figure 1.40.

We do not know what prompted Golgi to use silver nitrate in his research, but we can assume that the incentive was the development of photography. In fact, silver iodide is used in photography, not silver nitrate. Apparently, Golgi tried many silver salts until he found what he was looking for. The scientist who contributed most to the dissemination of Golgi's imaging technique was Cajal. However, in the sections of nervous tissue they obtained, they saw different things: Golgi saw the nervous tissue as a single system of channels connected to each other (figure 1.41(A)),

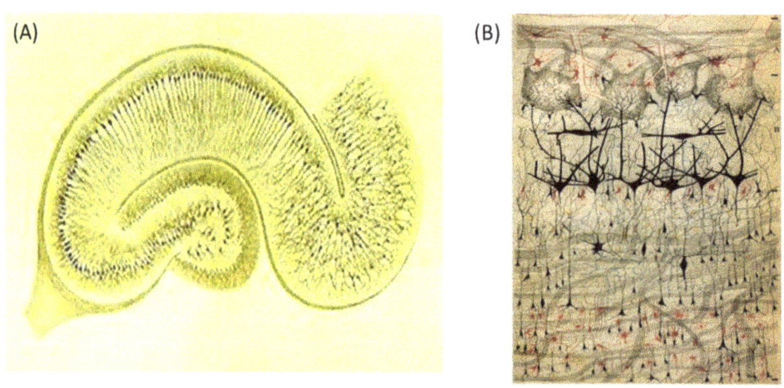

Figure 1.39. (A) The structure of the gray matter of the brain. Reproduced with permission from [68]. (B) Visualization of the nervous system of the dog's olfactory bulb. Reproduced from [69].

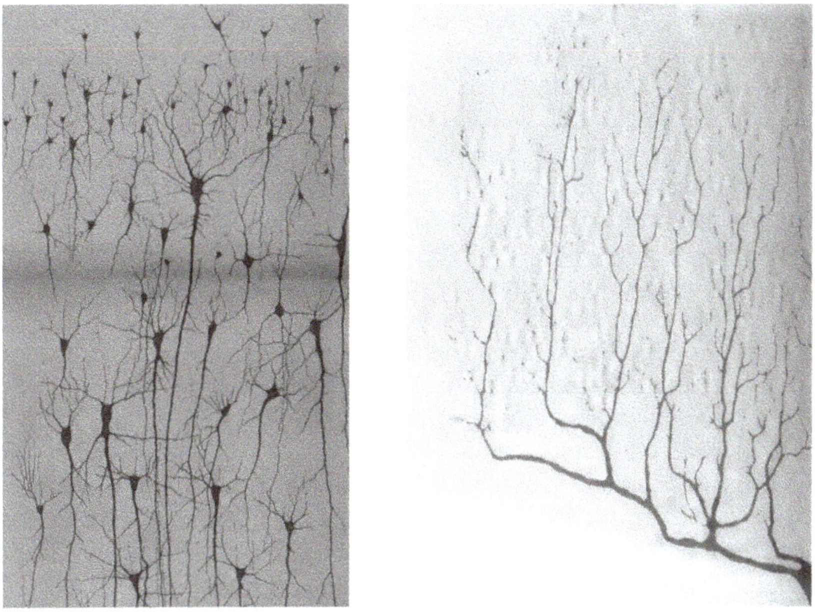

Figure 1.40. Drawings of various elements of nervous tissue. Reprinted from [69].

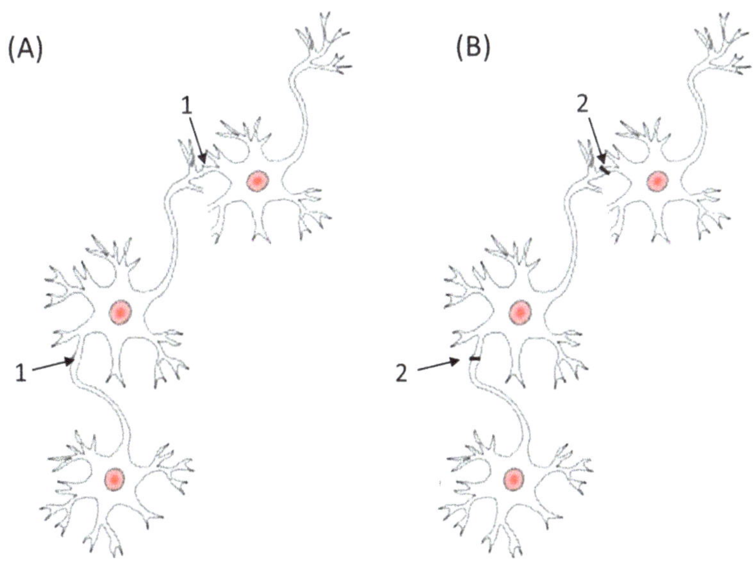

Figure 1.41. (A) Nerve cells and target cells are connected to each other by protoplasmic gates, so that substances from one cell can easily flow into others. 1—junction of two cells. (B) Nerve cells and target cells are independent units separated from each other by membranes. 2—synapses, the places where cells touch each other.

whereas Cajal saw a system of independent cells touching each other (figure 1.41(B)). Or, in other words, Golgi believed that nerve cells and target cells have a common cytoplasm, and Cajal believed that between the cells of the nervous system, there are thin gaps, that is, synapses,[20] separating cells from each other [71]. The dispute between the two scientists reached such intensity that, even in his Nobel speech, Golgi harshly criticized the views of Cajal, with whom he shared the Nobel Prize in Physiology or Medicine in 1906.

Eventually, neurophysiology established the view that nervous tissue consists of individual cells, or neurons,[21] that are in contact with each other and with target cells through electrical contacts, namely synapses. With such electrical contacts, impulses can propagate both from neuron A to neuron B, and in the opposite direction, from neuron B to neuron A.

It should be noted that not all physiologists unconditionally adhered to the theory of electrical contacts. There was another view: the connection between neurons and muscles occurs due to the secretion at the ends of nerve endings of special molecules that cause muscle contraction. Nevertheless, this view had a significant flaw. The fact is that the time between the initiation of a nerve impulse and muscle contraction is ~0.1–0.2 s. This time seemed too short for a certain chemical agent to be released from the nerve ending and cause muscle contraction. However, the idea of a chemical agent was supported by the facts that signal transmission through the ciliary ganglion can be blocked by nicotine [72] and that secreted adrenaline produces the same effect on target cells as the stimulation of sympathetic nerves associated with them [73].

The question of whether excitation is transmitted from neurons to muscles through electrical contact (electrical synapse) or chemical contact (chemical synapse) was resolved in 1921 by the work of Loewi [74], which supported chemical contact. Loewi was sure that the connection between neurons and muscle cells was carried out by some kind of chemical agent, but he was unsure how to test this. Then, one day, Loewi had a dream in which he saw an experimental diagram that allowed him to test the hypothesis about the existence of a chemical synapse (contact). The idea was so clear and simple that he decided to wait until the morning to experiment and simply sketched it on a piece of paper. Naturally, in the morning, he did not remember anything except that he had a brilliant idea. He was not upset, because he knew that he had drawn the experimental diagram the previous night. Imagine his disappointment when he looked at the paper with the sketch and did not understand anything in it. The next night he had the same dream again. This time, Loewi decided not to postpone the experiment until the morning. He immediately went to the laboratory and conducted the experiment, the idea of which is shown in figure 1.42. He took two beating frog hearts, leaving one of them with the nervus

[20] The term 'synapse' was introduced into biology in 1897 by English neurophysiologist Charles Sherrington in a textbook on physiology [70]. The word was derived from the Greek 'synapsis' (σύναψις), meaning 'conjunction.'

[21] The term 'neuron' was introduced into physiology by the ardent anti-Golgi anatomist Heinrich Wilhelm Gottfried von Waldeyer-Hartz in 1891.

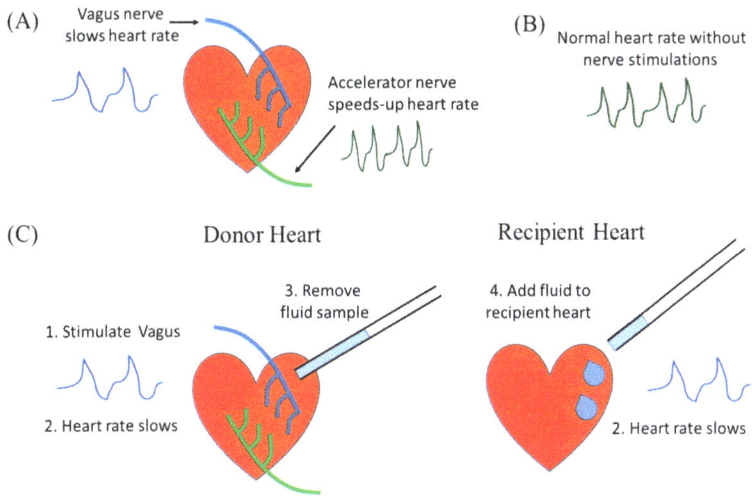

Figure 1.42. Idea of Loewi's experiment [74]. (A) Stimulation of the vagus nerve slows the heart rate. Stimulation of the accelerator nerve accelerates the heart rate. (B) Normal heart rate without nerve stimulation. (C) Schematic of Loewi's experiment.

vagus (vagus nerve), and placed them in separate containers filled with salt water. Then, he electrically stimulated the nerve and found that the heart rate slowed down. After this, he took a little of the solution from the container where the heart with the nerve was located and poured it into the container with the heart without the nerve, and its rhythm also slowed down. Thus, he proved that when nerve fibers are stimulated, a certain chemical substance is released that affects muscle cells. In 1936, Loewi was awarded the Nobel Prize for his discovery.[22]

After Loewi's convincing proof that signal transmission between neurons and muscles occurs chemically, interest in electrical synapses disappeared. This often happens when a discovery in one area of science undeservedly cuts off consideration of all other possible mechanisms. We saw this in Galvani and Volta's debate about animal electricity. When Volta showed that the frog's body conducts electricity, Galvani's idea of the existence of animal electricity (electricity stored in the bodies of animals and fish) was rejected as completely incorrect.

Since a description of electrical and chemical synapses can be found in almost any modern book devoted to the physiology of nervous tissue (see, for example, books [73, 74]), we only briefly touch on them.

An electrical synapse, or, as it is also called, a gap junction, is shown in figure 1.43. The distance between neurons at a gap junction is about 2–4 nm [75]. This small distance is due to the presence of special connexin proteins that compose a connexon, which are channels that penetrate both membranes. According to

[22] It should be noted that the Nobel Prize literally saved Loewi's life. In 1938, Austria 'voluntarily' joined Germany, and Loewi, as a Jew, was immediately sent to prison with his two sons. In order to leave the country, he had to transfer his Nobel Prize to the 'right' bank.

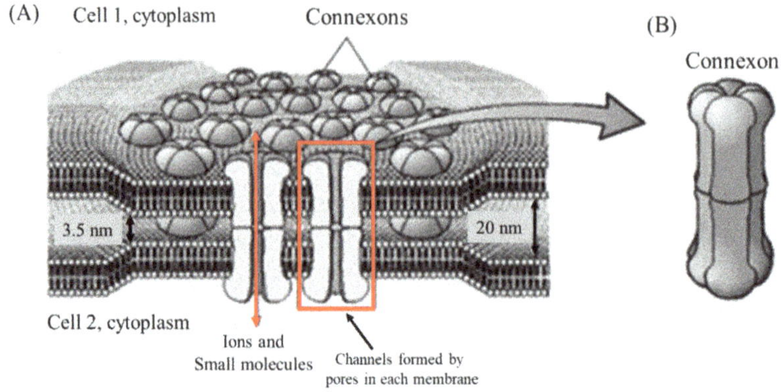

Figure 1.43. (A) The structure of an electrical synapse. (B) Separate connexon. It is believed that during the passage of an action potential, the channel in the connexon widens, allowing ions from one cell to freely pass into the other. This mechanism allows electrical contact between neurons.

established opinion, charge flows from one neuron to another through these channels, which ensures almost instantaneous transmission of an action potential from an excited neuron to an unexcited one. The opening of the contact depends on the potential difference across the connexon. Therefore, electrical synapses can be found in those parts of the nervous system where a quick response is required. It is important to note that an electrical synapse can transmit excitation from neuron A to neuron B, and in the opposite direction, from neuron B to neuron A [75]. Electrical synapses can be found in the neocortex, hippocampus, thalamic reticular nucleus, locus coeruleus, inferior olivary nucleus, mesencephalic nucleus, trigeminal nerve region, olfactory bulbs, retina, and spinal cord of vertebrates. However, it should be noted that in the total number of connections in vertebrates, electrical synapses account for about 1% of all synaptic contacts.

We want to point out that at a gap junction, the neurons are so close to each other that the excitation of an action potential can be caused not only by internal currents but also by external currents, as is the case when an action potential propagates in a myelinated axon. In this case, in our opinion, the connexons act as a kind of rivet that holds the gap in the electrical synapse in a fixed position. We look at this model of the electrical synapse in more detail in chapter 2, section 2.4.

The chemical synapse, schematically depicted in figure 1.44, is found to be much more common, and its structure and functions are fundamentally different from those of the electrical synapse. It consists of a nerve ending with a presynaptic membrane, a postsynaptic membrane of the target cell, and a synaptic cleft between them. The size of the synaptic cleft is about 20–40 nm [76]. The postsynaptic membrane has receptors on its surface that are sensitive to transmitters that are released into the synaptic cleft from the surface of the presynaptic membrane. In the synaptic extension, there are relatively small spherical vesicles containing the transmitter. Their size is about 40–50 nm. The presynaptic membrane is not a smooth surface; it consists of depressions about 10 nm in size, which are ordered into

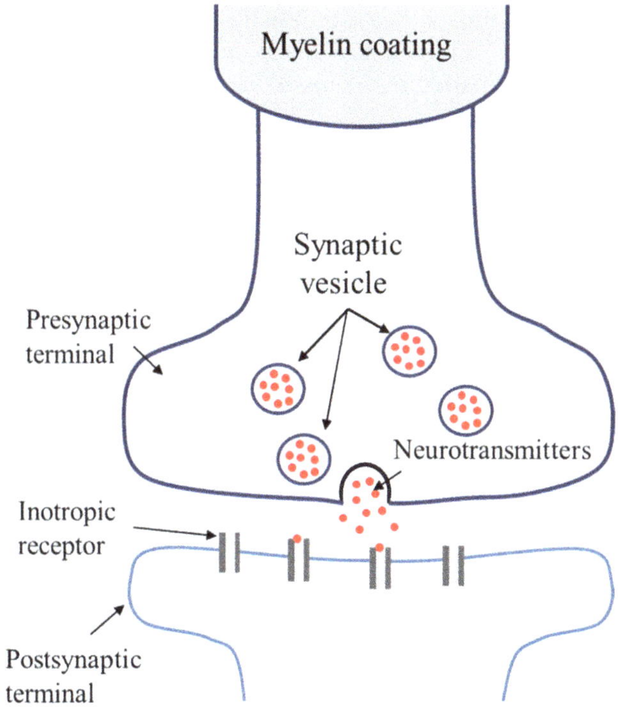

Figure 1.44. Schematic structure of a chemical synapse.

hexagonal clusters. These clusters are attachment sites for vesicles that release the transmitter into the synaptic cleft. An electrical impulse arriving at the nerve ending opens the ion channels for Ca^{2+} ions, which activate the release of the transmitter into the synaptic cleft. Transmitter molecules bind to receptors (acetylcholine ligand-activated channels) on the postsynaptic membrane, which leads to the opening of the transmembrane ion channel. Incoming ions either depolarize the cell, stimulating the excitation of an action potential in it, or, conversely, polarize it, thereby inhibiting the excitation of an action potential. In the first case, the synapse is stimulating, and in the second, it is inhibitory. At a chemical synapse, the action potential does not reach the presynaptic membrane but only stimulates the opening of Ca^{2+} channels. Otherwise, it could cause the direct excitation of an action potential in the postsynaptic membrane. Note that if the fixed size of the gap junction in electrical synapses is maintained by connexons, then in a chemical synapse, the required fixed size of the gap junction is maintained by special proteins that differ from connexons.

1.8 Optogenetics and thermogenetics

Our brain is essentially a black box consisting of almost 90 billion elements (neurons), each of which is connected by synaptic connections to a large number of other neurons (up to about 10 000) [77, 78]. We cannot take our brain apart and, like an ancient watch, after examining and establishing functional connections between its elements, put it back together. We do not have a magic magnifying glass to see which of the nearly 90 billion neurons, each connected to thousands of others, participate in the transformation of the input signal (stimulus) into the output signal (body reaction).

The idea of 'point-wise' control of neurons was first formulated in 1979 by Francis Crick (who was a co-winner of the Nobel Prize for the discovery of the structure of DNA). He suggested that since different types of neurons respond differently to light, it would be possible to selectively affect nervous tissue by using a certain wavelength. Twenty years later, in 1999, he proposed introducing light-sensitive proteins into the neurons of the brain in order to selectively influence them using light fibers. Apparently, Crick assumed that neurons in the retina have special rhodopsin receptors that are photosensitive to light of a certain wavelength.

In practice, there are two ways to deliver the rhodopsin gene into brain cells, implemented, for example, in laboratory mice. The first method is through the introduction of the gene encoding rhodopsin into the mouse body at the stage of embryonic development, which results in all the cells of the body containing it. However, this gene does not work in all cells but only where it is deposited, so genetic engineers attach a special sequence of nucleotides to the rhodopsin gene, which promotes its expression in neurons. However, this method is ineffective, since it takes several months for the embryo to grow into a mouse upon which experiments can be carried out. The second way of delivering the gene into cells works much faster. It uses viruses that carry the rhodopsin gene. If such a virus is introduced into a given part of the brain, it penetrates the neuron and synthesizes rhodopsin. Obviously, viruses that are incapable of reproducing are used for such experiments. It should be noted that the introduction of mammalian rhodopsins into signaling neurons did not yield good and stable results: 'artificial neurons' were activated slowly and unstably under the influence of light.

Single-celled algae also have light-sensitive receptors. It turned out that their light-sensitive proteins not only react to light but are themselves ion channels. In other words, light of a certain wavelength manifests itself as a mediator, similar to acetylcholine molecules that open ion channels in the postsynaptic membranes of chemical synapses. The first channel rhodopsin was discovered in 1971 by Dieter Oesterhelt (1940–2022) and Walther Stoeckenius (1921–2013) [79], but it did not attract the attention of biologists and genetic engineers. In 2002, rhodopsin from the unicellular green alga *Chlamydomonas reinhardtii* was discovered, which became the first channel rhodopsin introduced into neurons using genetic engineering [80]. In 2005, a group led by Hiromu Yawo from Tohoku University in Japan [81] and Edward S. Boyden's group from Stanford University [82] were able to introduce rhodopsin into the mouse brain and act upon it through a light fiber. Subsequently, in the process of studying the rhodopsins of microbes and unicellular algae, light-sensitive proteins were discovered that became capable of conducting sodium ions under the influence of light. Other light-sensitive proteins, when exposed to light, acquired the ability to conduct sodium ions or certain negative ions. Some of them reacted to blue light, while others reacted to red. Therefore, there are rhodopsins that suppress the excitation of the action potential, and there are stimulating ones.

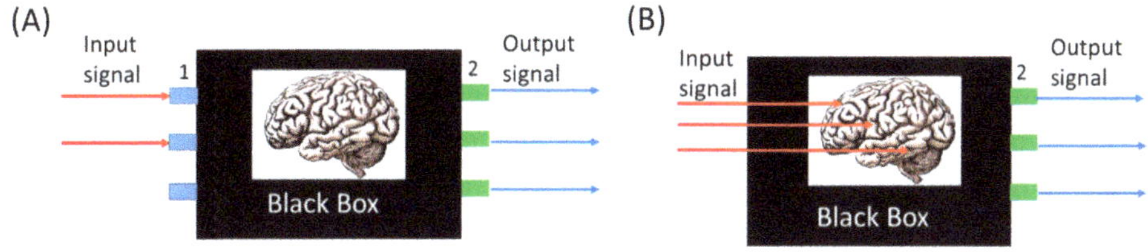

Figure 1.45. The brain is like a black box. (A) Stimulation occurs through sensory organ receptors: 1. fixed signal input locations and 2. fixed signal output locations. (B) The use of optogenetic methods allows scientists to 'turn on' or 'turn off' any neuron or group of neurons in the brain.

Currently, in biology, rhodopsins are divided into two categories: channel and non-channel. The introduction of rhodopsins into brain neurons has revolutionized brain research. Scientists have obtained a tool that allows them to study the neural networks of the brain, and just as a programmer testing a complex program or an electronics engineer testing an electronic system does, they can now 'turn on' or 'turn off' any neuron or group of neurons in the brain (figure 1.45).

We will not discuss here the prospects of optogenetics in brain research and its practical application for therapeutic purposes, since this area is beyond the scope of our book, and, moreover, it is developing too rapidly to indicate its individual achievements. Let us give just one example of research done at the Massachusetts Institute of Technology in the laboratory led by Nobel Prize winner Susumu Tonegawa [83].

Let a mouse be in room A, where it feels quite comfortable and does not feel afraid. The mouse is then taken to room B, where it is given mild electric shocks. After several visits to room B, the mouse experiences fear every time it is brought into the room, even if it is not exposed to an electric shock. Fear causes the mouse to freeze in place and not move. After the mouse is returned to room A, it begins to move around normally without experiencing fear. Neuroscientists have only been able to make light-sensitive neurons that fire when the mouse is in room A, but they do not fire when it is in room B. Now, let us say, while the mouse is again in room B, where it has been subjected to electric shocks, the neurons associated with room A are activated by light. After this, when it is returned to room A, where the mouse has never received an electric shock, it experiences fear. In other words, the experimenter can introduce a false memory into the mouse's consciousness—an event that actually did not happen. This simple example shows how powerful a tool researchers and doctors have received to influence and control the nervous system, the impact of which can help to cure diseases such as spinal cord injury, multiple sclerosis, epilepsy, Alzheimer's disease, Parkinson's disease, and many others [84], that is, many diseases that are considered incurable.

For those who want to become better acquainted with optogenetics and the prospects for its development, as well as the relevant original literature, review articles [85, 86] will be very useful.

In conclusion to this section, we note that, along with ion channels that respond to light, ion channels have been discovered that, depending on temperature, can activate or suppress action potentials in nerve cells. This has led to the development of so-called thermogenetics [86, 87], which is based on local temperature control of certain protein molecules encoded in the genome, called receptors [88, 89]. For the discovery of these receptors, physiologist David Julius and molecular biologist Ardem Patapoutian received the 2021 Nobel Prize in Physiology or Medicine. In practice, local heating, resulting in the stimulation of nervous tissue, can be caused by the absorption of infrared laser radiation, the effect of an alternating magnetic field on cells on the surface of which there are magnetic nanoparticles, or the use of focused ultrasound.

As previously noted in section 1.5, the stimulation of neural tissue activity is not necessarily associated with the absorption of photons or heat. It may also be associated with a lowering of the excitation threshold due to the rearrangement of laterally mobile transmembrane ion channels in weak acoustic fields caused by an external ultrasound source or by weak microwave radiation that irradiates nervous tissue.

1.9 Green fluorescent protein (GFP) diagnostics

Optogenetics makes it possible to control (initiate and suppress) the propagation of an action potential at the level of an individual neuron, but it cannot trace the propagation of the signal in the brain from the point of initiation to the body's response. Nor does optogenetics allow non-perturbative visualization of the processes of excitation and propagation of action potentials in an ensemble of neurons in nervous tissue. As for the Golgi method, discussed in section 1.7, it allows one to see only the connections of an individual neuron with others, but nothing more. Until recently, there were only two methods for actively studying the brain: using electrodes to activate neurons and using chemicals that can selectively inhibit the functioning of certain types of neurons. Each of these methods of influencing the brain has a significant drawback: the implanted electrode, no matter how miniature it is, excites all the nerve cells surrounding it, and the most modern inhibitor affects the cells much longer than the natural stimulus. Therefore, until recently, we did not have the opportunity, like a programmer, to turn on or off individual areas of the brain one by one, while simultaneously avoiding disruption of its structure. The use of GFP has opened up new possibilities for visualizing the dynamics of processes in nervous tissue.

In 1991, the young biologist Douglas Prasher managed to decipher the structure of the gene encoding GFP [90, 91], which he and his colleagues extracted from jellyfish. This protein, unlike other light-sensitive proteins, had a unique ability: it could fluoresce without the participation of a chromophore. Prasher immediately recognized the importance of GFP as a biomarker. If you attach GFP to a protein or gene of interest, the fluorescent signal from GFP instantly and accurately shows where the molecule it tags is located. Moreover, if the GFP gene is introduced into a cell using a virus, it additionally and independently produces GFP, which fluoresces in the presence of Ca^{2+} ions. As noted in section 1.7, the release of acetylcholine at synapses is associated with the influx of Ca^{2+} ions into the synapse; therefore, GFP may be a marker of synapse activation.

Unfortunately, Prasher's two-year grant from the American Cancer Society expired in 1992, and he did not complete the research he had begun. After the end of the project, Prasher sent the DNA of the GFP he had cloned to other laboratories, in particular to the laboratories of Martin Chalfie and Roger Y Tsien, which used the results obtained by Prasher in their studies. Subsequently, Prasher did not find support at the Woods Hole Oceanographic Institution, where he was working at the time, to continue his work on cloning the GFP gene and had to leave the institute. He tried to get a job at other scientific institutions but was unsuccessful. He eventually gave up his job search in science and began working as a shuttle driver to support his family. In 2008, the Nobel Prize in Chemistry was awarded to Osamu Shimomura, Martin Chalfie, and Roger Y Tsien for 'the discovery and development of the green fluorescent protein, GFP.' All three of the 2008 Nobel Chemistry laureates thanked Prasher in their speeches and noted his key role in their successes. Unfortunately, Prasher did not receive the Nobel Prize he deserved, since no more than three people can receive it in this category.

The working principle of the GFP protein is shown schematically in figure 1.46.

To date, there have been many examples of the successful use of GFP to visualize processes in nervous tissue directly in living beings, synchronously with their life activities. We will not delve into the consideration of this extensive and important topic but limit ourselves to mentioning a few excellent works. For example, [92] described the use of GFP for visualizing the nervous system of a living drosophila, and [93, 94] presented the real-time observation of processes in the brain of a zebrafish larva.

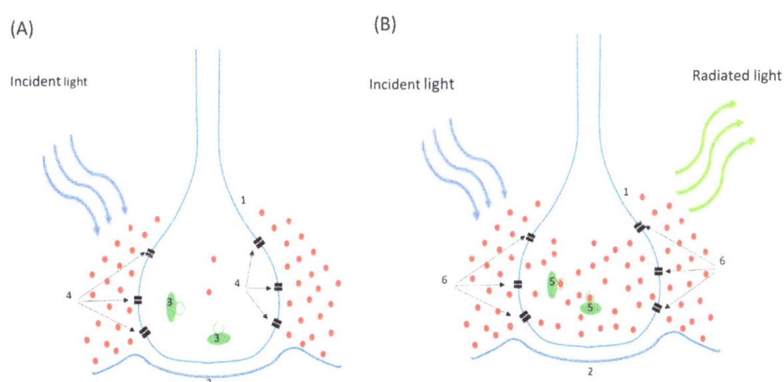

Figure 1.46. The working principle of GFP at the synapse. (A) Action potential is not activated. Ion channels are closed. Ca^{2+} ions are located mainly outside the synapse. GFP exhibits no fluorescence. (B) The action potential opens the calcium channels, and Ca^{2+} ions enter the synapse. Ca^{2+} ions are then captured by GFP, and incident light stimulates the fluorescence of the GFP molecules that have captured the calcium ions. Incident light and emitted GFP fluorescence are shown as wavy blue and green lines, respectively. 1—axon or terminal with a synapse at the edge, 2—postsynaptic membrane, 3—GFP, and 4—calcium channels of the synaptic membrane are closed. Calcium ions are mainly on the outside. 5—GFP-captured ions of Ca^{2+}, and 6—Ca^{2+} channels are open, and a significant number of calcium ions are present within the synapse.

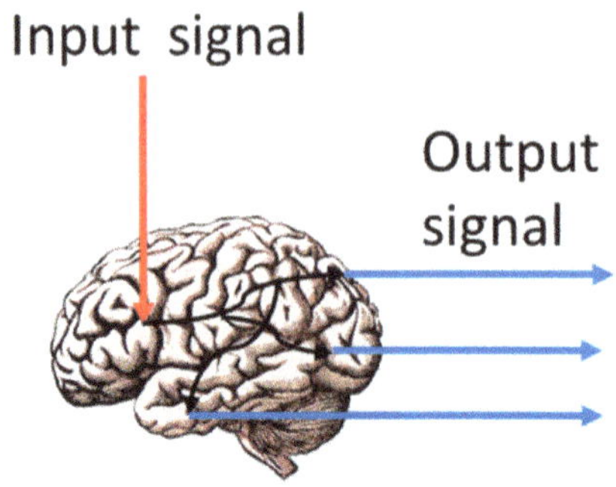

Figure 1.47. Optogenetics combined with GFP-gene-based imaging allows researchers to 'turn on' or 'turn off' any neuron in the brain and trace the entire chain of propagation of action potentials through the new tissue.

Optogenetics combined with GFP-gene-based imaging provides unprecedented opportunities in the study of the brain and nervous system. While remaining an extremely complex object for research, the brain and nervous system are no longer a complete black box for scientists, as shown schematically in figure 1.47.

Without going into detail, we want to note an example of the effective use of the combined method of optogenetics and GFP: local excitation of the brain with radiation transmitted through an optical fiber implanted into the brain of a living mouse to control its reactions and behavior [95, 96].

At the conclusion of this introductory chapter, we note once again that revolutionary ideas in science always lie far from its beaten path, which is why it is so important for a young scientist to have an open mind so that revolutionary ideas can come into their field of vision.

References

[1] Hodgkin A L and Huxley A F 1952 A quantitative description of membrane current and its application to conduction and excitation in nerve *J. Physiol.* **117** 500

[2] Hodgkin A L 1951 The ionic basis of electrical activity in nerve and muscle *Biol. Rev.* **26** 339

[3] Hodgkin A L and Huxley A F 1952 Currents carried by sodium and potassium ions through the membrane of the giant axon of Loligo *J. Physiol.* **116** 449

[4] Hodgkin A L and Huxley A F 1952 The components of membrane conductance in the giant axon of Loligo *J. Physiol.* **116** 473

[5] Hodgkin A L and Huxley A F 1952 The dual effect of membrane potential on sodium conductance in the giant axon of Loligo *J. Physiol.* **116** 497

[6] Hodgkin A L, Huxley A F and Katz B 1949 Ionic currents underlying activity in the giant axon of the squid *Arch. Sci. Physiol.* **3** 129

[7] Hodgkin A L, Huxley A F and Katz B 1952 Measurement of current-voltage relations in the membrane of the giant axon of Loligo *J. Physiol.* **116** 424

[8] Hodgkin A L and Katz B 1949 The effect of temperature on the electrical activity of the giant axon of the squid *J. Physiol.* **109** 240

[9] Hodgkin A L 1939 The relation between conduction velocity and the electrical resistance outside a nerve fiber *J. Physiol.* **94** 560

[10] Hodgkin A L 1947 The membrane resistance of a non-medullated nerve fibre *J. Physiol.* **106** 305

[11] Hodgkin A L 1948 The local electric changes associated with repetitive action in a non-medullated axon *J. Physiol.* **107** 165

[12] Hodgkin A L and Huxley A F 1939 Action potentials recorded from inside a nerve fibre *Nature* **144** 710

[13] Hodgkin A L and Huxley A F 1945 Resting and action potentials in single nerve fibres *J. Physiol.* **104** 176

[14] Hodgkin A L and Huxley A F 1947 Potassium leakage from an active nerve fibre *J. Physiol.* **106** 341

[15] Hodgkin A L and Katz B 1949 The effect of sodium ions on the electrical activity of the giant axon of the squid *J. Physiol.* **108** 37

[16] Baker P F, Hodgkin A L and Show T I 1962 The effects of changes in internal ionic concentration on the electrical properties of perfuse giant axons *J. Physiol.* **164** 355

[17] Goldman L and Albus J S 1968 Computation of impulse conduction in myelinated fibers *J. Biophys.* **8** 596

[18] https://en.wikipedia.org/wiki/Electrophorus

[19] Galvani L 1953 *Commentary on the Effects of Electricity on Muscular Motion* ed M G Foley (Norwalk, CT: Burndy Library) (translated)

[20] David A W 1878 *The Science of Common Things: A Familiar Explanation of the First Principles of Physical Science* (New York: Ivison, Phinney, Blakeman & Co)

[21] du Bois-Reymond E 1849 *Untersuchen ueber thierische Elektricitaet* (Berlin: G. Rennet)

[22] Schuetze S M 1983 The discovery of the action potential *Trends. Neurosci.* **6** 164

[23] Bernstein J 1868 Ueber den zeitlichen Verlauf der negativen Schwankung des Nervenstroms *Pflügers Arch* **1** 173

[24] Bernstein J 1902 Untersuchungen zur Thermodynamik der bioelektrischen Ströme *Pflügers Arch* **92** 521

[25] Wahl D 2005 A short history of electrochemistry *Galvanotechtnik* **96** 1820

[26] Antonov V F, Chernysh A M, Pasechnik V I, Voznesensky S A and Kozlova E A 2000 *Biofizika. Uchebnik dlya vuzov (Biophysics High School Textbook)* (Moscow: Vlados Publising) (in Russian)

[27] https://chem.libretexts.org/Bookshelves/General_Chemistry/Map%3A_Chemistry_-_The_Central_Science_(Brown_et al.)/07%3A_Periodic_Properties_of_the_Elements/7.03%3A_Sizes_of_Atoms_and_Ions

[28] Aidly D J 1998 *The Physiology of Excitable Cells* 4th edn (Cambridge: Cambridge University Press)

[29] Williams L W 1910 The anatomy of the common squid, Loligo Pealii *Lesueur Nat.* **83** 366

[30] Young J Z 1938 The functioning of the giant nerve fibres of the squid *J. Exp. Biol.* **15** 170

[31] Cole K S and Curtis H J 1939 Electric impedance of the squid giant axon during activity *J. Gen. Physiol.* **22** 649

[32] Curtis H J and Cole K S 1940 Membrane potential of the squid giant axon during current flow *J. Cell. Comp. Physiol.* **15** 147

[33] Curtis H J and Cole K S 1942 Membrane resting and action potentials from the squid giant axon *J. Cell. Compar. Physiol.* **19** 135

[34] Masters B R 2009 History of the Electron Microscope in Cell Biology *Encyclopedia of Life Sciences* (New York: Wiley)

[35] http://biologydiscussion.com/human-physiology/nerve-fiber-classificationand-properties-biology/62074
[36] Ginzburg V L and Landau L D 1965 On the theory of superconductivity *Zh. Eksp. Teor. Fiz.* **20** 1064 English translation
Landau L D (ed) *Collected Papers* (Oxford: Pergamon) 546
[37] Bardeen J, Cooper L N and Schrieffer J R Microscopic theory of superconductivit *Phys. Rev.* **106** 162
[38] Kadir L A, Stacey M and Barrett-Jolle R 2018 Emerging roles of the membrane potential: action beyond the action potential *Front. Physiol.* **9** 1661
[39] Kao C Y and Fuhrman F A 1967 Differentiation of the actions of tetrodotoxin and saxitoxin *Toxicon* **5** 25
[40] Tasaki I 1959 Demonstration of two stable states of the nerve membrane in potassium-rich media *J. Physiol.* **148** 306
[41] Neher E and Sakmann B 1976 Single-channel currents recorded from membrane of denervated frog muscle fibres *Nature* **260** 799
[42] Nicholls J G, Martin A R, Fuchs P A, Brown D A, Diamond M E and Weisblat D A 2012 *From Neuron to Brain* 5th edn (Sunderland, MA: Sinauer Associate, Inc. Publishers)
[43] Sigworth F G and Neher E 1980 Single Na^+ channel currents observed in cultured rat muscle cells *Nature* **287** 447
[44] MacKinnon R, Cohen S L, Kuo A, Lee A and Chait B T 1998 Structural conservation in prokaryotic and eukaryotic potassium channels *Science* **280** 1069
[45] Doyle D A, Morais C J, Pfuetzner R A, Kuo A, Gulbis J M, Cohen S L, Chait B T and MacKinnon R 1998 The structure of the potassium channel: molecular basis of K+ conduction and selectivity *Science* **280** 69
[46] Catterall W A 1980 Neurotoxins that act on voltage-sensitive sodium channels in excitable membranes *Ann. Rev. Pharmacol. Toxicol.* **20** 15
[47] Gambin Y, Lopez-Esparza R, Reffay M, Sierecki E, Gov N S, Genest M, Hodges R S and Urbach W 2006 Lateral mobility of proteins in liquid membranes revisited *Proc. Natl Acad. Sci. USA* **103** 2098
[48] Jacobson A I and Inman R 1987 Lateral diffusion of proteins in membranes *Ann. Rev. Physiol.* **49** 163
[49] Almeida P F F and Vaz W L C 1995 Lateral diffusion in membranes *Handbook of Biological Physics* **Vol. 1** ed R Lipowsky and E Sackmann (Amsterdam: Elsevier Science B. V) Elsevier Science B.V.
[50] Ramadurai S, Holt A, Krasnikov V, van den Bogaart G, Killian J A and Poolman B 2009 Lateral diffusion of membrane proteins *J. Am. Chem. Soc.* **131** 12650
[51] Platkiewicz J and Brette R 2010 A threshold equation for action potential initiation *PLoS Comput. Biol.* **6** e1000850
[52] Catterall W A, Goldin A L and Waxman S G 2005 International Union of Pharmacology. XLVII. Nomenclature and structure-function relationships of voltage-gated sodium channels *Pharmacol. Rev.* **57** 397
[53] Angelino E and Brenner M P 2007 Excitability constraints on voltage-gated sodium channels *PLoS Comput. Biol.* **3** 1751
[54] Ogawa Y and Rasband M N 2008 The functional organization and assembly of the axon initial segment *Curr. Opin. Neurobiol.* **18** 307

[55] Hu W, Tian C, Li T, Yang M, Hou H and Shu Y 2009 Distinct contributions of Na(v)1.6 and Na(v)1.2 in action potential initiation and backpropagation *Nat. Neurosci.* **12** 996

[56] Kress G J and Mennerick S 2009 Action potential initiation and propagation: upstream influences on neurotransmission *Neuroscience* **158** 211

[57] Mednikov E 1965 *Acoustic Coagulation and Precipitation of Aerosols* (New York: Springer) https://link.springer.com/book/9781489949318

[58] Shneider M N and Pekker M 2013 Non-thermal mechanism of weak microwave fields influence on nerve fiber *J. Appl. Phys.* **114** 104701

[59] Shneider M N and Pekker M 2014 Initiation and blocking of the action potential in an axon in weak ultrasonic or microwave fields *Phys. Rev.* E **89** 052713

[60] Debanne D, Campanac E, Bialowas A, Carlier E and Alcaraz G 2011 Axon physiology *Physiol. Rev.* **91** 555

[61] Tasaki I 1939 The electro-saltatory transmission of the nerve impulse and the effect of narcosis upon the nerve fiber *Am. J. Physiol.* **127** 211

[62] Tasaki I 1959 Conduction of nerve impulse *Handbook of Physiology* **Vol 1** (Bethesda, MD: American Physiological Society) 75

[63] Huxley A F and Stämpfli R 1949 Evidence for saltatory conduction in peripheral myelinated nerve fibres *J. Physiol.* **108** 315

[64] Goldman L and Albus J S 1968 Computation of impulse conduction in myelinated fibers; theoretical basis of the velocity-diameter relation *Biophys. J.* **8** 596

[65] Fitzhugh R 1962 Computation of impulse initiation and saltatory conduction in a myelinated nerve fiber *Biophys. J.* **2** 11

[66] Shneider M N and Pekker M 2019 Stimulated activity in the neural tissue *J. Appl. Phys.* **125** 211101

[67] Golgi C 1873 Sulla struttura della sostanza grigia del cervello *Gazz. Med. Ital.—Lombardia* **33** 244

[68] Golgi C 1875 Sulla fina struttura dei bulbi olfactorii *Rivista* Sperimentale di Freniatria e Medicina Legale **1** 405

[69] Golgi C 1886 *Sulla fina anatomia degli organi centrali del sistema nervosa* (Libraio: Napoli, Milano, Pisa)

[70] Foster M 1877 *A Text Book of Physiology* (London: Macmillan))

[71] Cajal S R 1906 The structure and connexions of neurons *Nobel Lecture*, December 12, 1906 (https://nobelprize.org/prizes/medicine/1906/cajal/lecture/)

[72] Langley J N and Anderson H K 1892 On the mechanism of the movements of the iris *J. Physiol.* **13** 460

[73] Elliott T R 1904 The action of adrenalin *J. Physiol.* **31** xx–xxi

[74] Loewi O 1921 Überhumorale Übertragbarkeit der Herznervenwirkung. II. Mittei-lung *Pflügers Arch. Ges. Physiol.* **193** 239

[75] Kandel E R, Schwartz J H and Jessell T M 2000 *Principles of Neural Science* 4th edn (New York: McGraw-Hill)

[76] Dale P, Augustine G J, Fitzpatrick D, Hal W C, LaMantia A-S, McNamara J O and White L E 2008 *Neuroscience* 4th edn (Sunderland, MA: Sinauer Associates)

[77] Herculano-Houzel S 2009 The human brain in numbers: a linearly scaled-up primate brain *Frontiers Human Neurosc.* **3** 31

[78] Eryomin A L 2022 Biophysics of evolution of intellectual systems *Biophysics* **67** 320

[79] Oesterhelt D and Stoeckenius W 1971 Rhodopsin-like protein from the purple membrane of halobacterium halobium *Nat. New Biol.* **233** 149

[80] Franklin S, Ngo B, Efuet E and Mayfield S P 2002 Development of a GFP reporter gene for *Chlamydomonas reinhardtii* chloroplast *Plant J.* **30** 733

[81] Araki R, Sakagami H, Yanagawa Y, Hikima T, Ishizuka T and Yawo H 2005 Transgenic mouse lines expressing synaptopHluorin in hippocampus and cerebellar cortex *Genesis* **42** 53

[82] Boyden E S, Zhang F, Bamberg E, Nagel G and Deisseroth K 2005 Millisecond-timescale, genetically targeted optical control of neural activity *Nat. Neurosci.* **8** 1263

[83] Liu X, Ramirez S, Pang P T, Puryear C B, Govindarajan A, Deisseroth K and Tonegawa S 2012 Optogenetic stimulation of a hippocampal engram activates fear memory recall *Nature* **484** 381

[84] Ordaz J D, Wu1 W and Xu X-M 2017 Optogenetics and its application in neural degeneration and regeneration *Neural Regen. Res.* **12** 1197

[85] Emiliani V *et al* 2022 Optogenetics for light control of biological systems *Nat. Rev. Methods Primers* **2** Article number: 55

[86] Bernstein J G, Garrity P A and Boyden E S 2012 Optogenetics and thermogenetics: technologies for controlling the activity of targeted cells within intact neural circuits *Curr. Opin. Neurobiol.* **22** 61

[87] Kitamoto T 2001 Conditional modification of behavior in Drosophila by targeted expression of a temperature-sensitive shibire allele in defined neurons *J. Neurobiol.* **47** 81

[88] Viswanath V, Story G M, Peier A M, Petrus M J, Lee V M, Hwang S W, Patapoutian A and Jegla T 2003 Opposite thermosensor in fruitfly and mouse *Nature* **423** 822

[89] McKemy D D, Neuhausser W M and Julius D 2002 Identification of a cold receptor reveals a general role for TRP channels in thermosensation *Nature* **416** 52

[90] Prasher D C, Eckenrode V K, Ward W W, Prendergast F G and Cormier M J 1992 Primary structure of the *Aequorea victoria* green-fluorescent protein *Gene* **111** 229

[91] Prasher D C 1995 Using GFP to see the light *Trends. Genet.* **11** 320

[92] Sun B, Xu P and Salvaterra P M 1999 Dynamic visualization of nervous system in live Drosophila *Proc. Natl. Acad. Sci. USA* **96** 10438

[93] Naumann E A, Kampff A R, Prober D A, Schier A F and Engert F 2010 Monitoring neural activity with bioluminescence during natural behavior *Nat. Neurosci.* **13** 513

[94] Muto A, Ohkura M, Abe G, Nakai J and Kawakami K 2013 Real-time visualization of neuronal activity during perception *Curr. Biol.* **23** 307

[95] Sparta D R, Stamatakis A M, Phillips J L, Hovelsø N, van Zessen R and Stuber G D 2012 Construction of implantable optical fibers for long-term optogenetic manipulation of neural circuits *Nat. Protoc.* **7** 12

[96] Doronina-Amitonova L V, Fedotov I V, Ivashkina O I, Zots M A, Fedotov A B, Anokhin K V and Zheltikov A M 2013 Implantable fiber-optic interface for parallel multisite long-term optical dynamic brain interrogation in freely moving mice *Sci. Rep.* **3** 3265

IOP Publishing

Low-Intensity Control of Nerve Tissue Activity

Mikhail N Shneider and Mikhail Pekker

Chapter 2

Ephaptic coupling and related phenomena

This chapter discusses processes in neurons and nervous tissue, including the saltatory transmission of excitation in myelinated axons and non-synaptic propagation of excitation from one activated neuron to the nearest neurons, which is known as ephaptic coupling. The model is similar to the saltatory conduction of action potentials between nodes of Ranvier in myelinated axons. Additionally, this chapter considers a model of electrical synapses based on the assumption that the transmission of excitation in them may be, to some extent, a manifestation of ephaptic coupling.

2.1 Estimates of myelin segment length and action potential propagation velocity

Before we move on to consider ephaptic coupling, let us clarify the role of myelin-covered sites in propagating action potentials along axons. To do this, we can write equation (1.48) in the form:

$$\frac{\partial V_M}{\partial t} = \frac{1}{C_M R_\parallel} \frac{\partial^2 V_M}{\partial z^2} - \frac{1}{C_M R_M} V_M, \tag{2.1}$$

where C_M [$\mathrm{F \cdot m^{-1}}$] and $R_M = 1/g_M$ [$\Omega \cdot \mathrm{m}$] are the capacitance per unit length and the conductivity per unit length of the myelinated segment, respectively; $R_\parallel[\Omega \cdot \mathrm{m}^{-1}]$ is the specific resistance per unit length of the fiber. Let us rewrite equation (2.1) in the form of the Goldman–Albus equation [1], which is widely used to model the saltatory propagation of the action potential in myelinated axons. To do so, we let V denote the excess of the potential on the axon membrane over the resting potential, $V = V_M - V_R$, leading to:

doi:10.1088/978-0-7503-6034-0ch2

$$\frac{\partial V}{\partial t} = \alpha \frac{\partial^2 V}{\partial z^2} - \beta V. \tag{2.2}$$

As an example, assume that the constants in the coefficients α and β correspond to the axons of frog (Xenopus) nerve tissue (1.49)–(1.51):

$$\alpha = \frac{1}{C_M R_\parallel} = 0.156 \cdot 10^9 \frac{\pi d_R^2}{r_\parallel} \frac{\ln\left(\frac{d_M}{d_R}\right)}{\ln(1.43)} = 0.052 \quad \mathrm{m^2 s^{-1}}, \tag{2.3}$$

$$\beta = \frac{1}{C_M R_M} = 0.\ 21 \cdot 10^4 \mathrm{s}^{-1}. \tag{2.4}$$

When the numerical values of the coefficients for (2.3) and (2.4) were obtained, all parameters of the myelinated fiber were the same as in chapter 1, section 1.6. In a certain sense, we can say that the coefficients α and β in (2.2) characterize the longitudinal and transverse conductances of the myelinated axon, respectively.

An example of the saltatory propagation of an action potential calculated using the Goldman–Albus equation (2.2) with parameters (2.3) and (2.4) [1, 2] is shown in figure 2.1(A). The action potential pulses $V_{j,\,\mathrm{ap}}(t) = \lim\limits_{z \to jL_M} V_M(z,\,t)$ at the jth node of Ranvier shown in figure 2.1(B) were assumed to be described by the Frankenhaeuser–Huxley theory [3] (figure 2.1).

Figure 2.2 shows a schematic of the currents in the myelin segment of the axon generated by the action potential at the node of Ranvier. Figures 2.2(A) and (B) correspond to the nonconducting case (no charge leakage through myelin layers, $\beta = 0$) and the conducting case (nonzero charge leakage through myelin layers, $\beta > 0$), respectively. Obviously, the charging efficiency (rate) of the conductive myelin segment of the axon must be lower than that of the nonconductive segment, which does not allow for leakage currents.

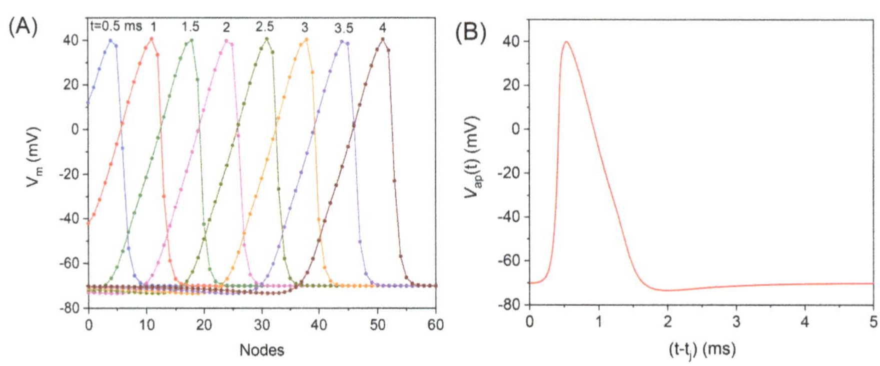

Figure 2.1. (A) Saltatory action potential propagation in normal myelinated fibers [2]. (B) Action potential $V_{j,\,\mathrm{ap}}$ at the jth node of Ranvier, where t_j is the arrival time of the action potential at the jth node, as computed by the Frankenhaeuser–Huxley model [3].

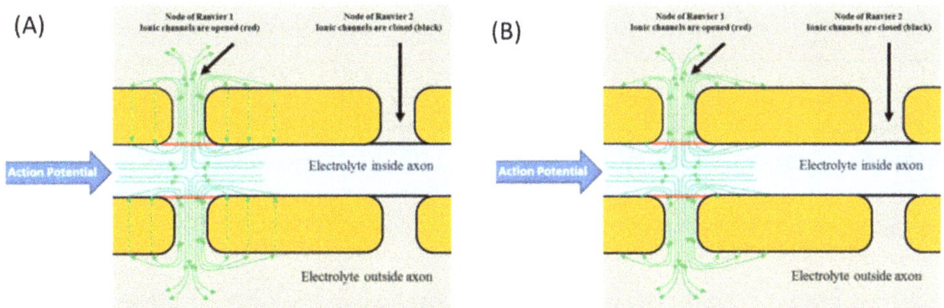

Figure 2.2. Schematic of the charging of a myelin-coated axon through the current generated in the node of Ranvier. (A) A weakly conducting myelin sheath that permits charge leakage, i.e. $\beta > 0$. (B) An ideal insulator myelin coating with no charge leakage, i.e. $\beta = 0$.

The propagation velocity of the action potential depends on the thickness of the myelin sheath and the length of the myelin segment. If we neglect the transverse currents and set $\beta = 0$ in equation (2.2), then, as shown in chapter 1, section 6, we obtain estimate (1.54) for the action potential propagation velocity along the myelin segment. From this estimate, taking into account (2.3), we obtain the dependence of the action potential velocity on the geometric parameters of the myelin segment:

$$v_{\mathrm{ap}} \approx \frac{\alpha}{2L_M} \propto \frac{d_R^2}{2L_M} \ln\left(\frac{d_M}{d_R}\right). \tag{2.5}$$

We use the technique proposed in [4] to estimate the $\frac{d_M}{d_R}$ ratio. For the sake of clarity, assume that the action potential propagates from left to right. Let the potential at the left edge of the myelin section be constant and equal to $\widetilde{V}$. Then, in the stationary case, equation (2.2) has the following form:

$$\alpha \frac{\partial^2 V}{\partial z^2} - \beta V = 0. \tag{2.6}$$

Equation (2.6) has the following solution:

$$V = \widetilde{V} \exp\left(-\sqrt{\beta/\alpha}\, z\right). \tag{2.7}$$

Substituting $z = L_M$ into (2.7), we find the potential at the end of the myelin section:

$$V_{L_M} = \widetilde{V} \exp\left(-\sqrt{\beta/\alpha}\, L_M\right) = \widetilde{V} \exp\left(-k \frac{d_M}{d_R \sqrt{\ln\left(d_M/d_R\right)}} \frac{L_M}{d_M}\right), \tag{2.8}$$

where k is a constant that is independent of the values of d_M and d_R. Next, we determine the ratio d_M/d_R that minimizes the value of the function

$$y = \frac{d_M}{d_R \sqrt{\ln\left(d_M/d_R\right)}}. \tag{2.9}$$

Equating the derivative of function y (2.9) by d_M/d_R to zero, we find that the minimum value of y is reached at:

$$d_M = \exp(0.5)d_R \approx 1.65d_R. \tag{2.10}$$

Substituting the value of d_M from (2.10) into (2.9) and (2.5), we find that the maximum achievable potential at the end of the myelinated segment during the pulse is equal to

$$V_{L_M} = \widetilde{V}\exp\left(-2.33k\frac{L_M}{d_M}\right). \tag{2.11}$$

Figure 2.3 shows the results of the measurements of lengths and diameters of the myelin segments in myelin fibers of adult cats and 16-day-old kittens [5, 6]. These experiments showed that the diameters of myelin segments are proportional to their lengths, $d_M \propto L_M$, and the velocity of action potential propagation in them is proportional to the diameters of the myelinated fibers, $v_{\text{ap}} \propto d_M$. From the analysis of the data given in [7, 8], it follows that in 75% of the measurements, the d_M/d_R ratio is in the range of 1.35–2.13. These data are in agreement with the results of other authors presented in [9–12]. Moreover, in all these works, the mean value of d_M/d_R is approximately equal to 1.65 with an accuracy of 5%, which is in agreement with the

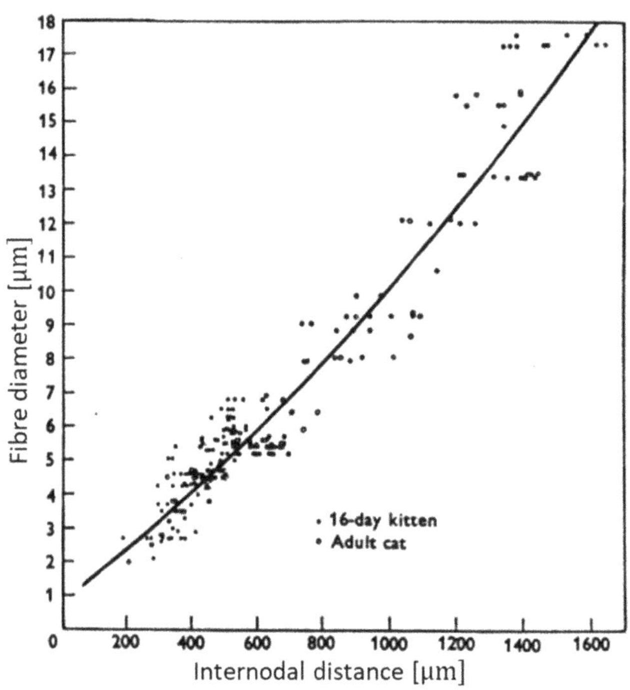

Figure 2.3. Results of the measurements of the dependence of nerve fiber diameter on the length of the myelinated segment for an adult cat and a 16-day-old kitten [5, 6]. Theoretical curve obtained by making observations of $\frac{d_M}{d_R}$ [7, 8] in $\frac{L_M}{d_M} \propto \frac{d_R}{d_M}\sqrt{\ln(d_M/d_R)}$ [4] John Wiley & Sons. © 1951 The Physiological Society.

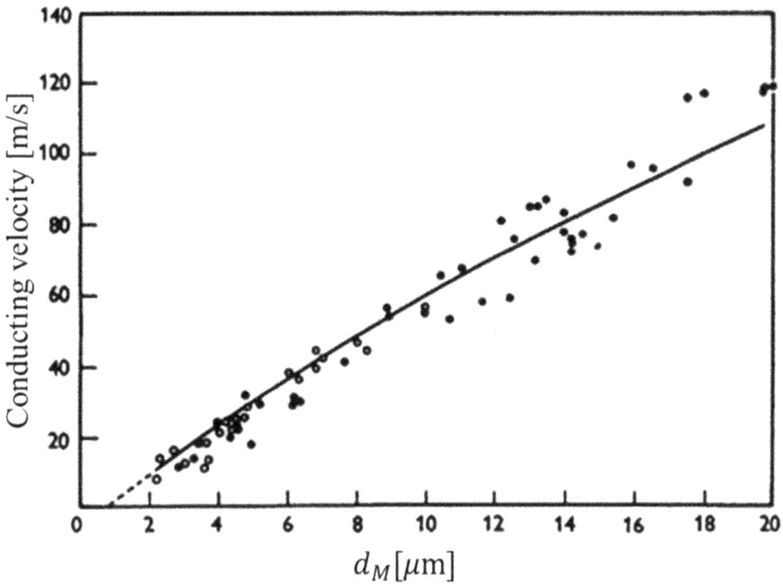

Figure 2.4. Results of measurements performed in [5, 6] on the dependence of action potential propagation velocity on nerve fiber diameter for an adult cat and a 16-day-old kitten [4] John Wiley & Sons. © 1951 The Physiological Society.

above estimate (2.10). It follows that since $L_M \propto d_M \approx 1.65 d_R$, the maximum potential at the right-hand end of the myelinated segment is a constant value determined by formula (2.11), and the rate of action potential propagation is (2.5):

$$v_{\text{ap}} \propto \frac{d_R^2}{2L_M} \ln\left(\frac{d_M}{d_R}\right) \propto d_M \ln\left(\frac{d_M}{d_R}\right). \tag{2.12}$$

Figure 2.4 shows the dependence of the action potential propagation velocity in the myelinated nerve fibers of adult cats and 16-day-old kittens on the axon diameter d_M obtained in [5, 6]. These measurements are in agreement with the above estimate (2.12). Note that Tasaki, in his experiments with myelinated frog fibers [13], later confirmed these observations [5, 6].

We now turn to the mathematical formulation of the problem of action potential propagation along the myelin segment. Let us assume that the node of Ranvier in which the action potential is initiated lies at $z = 0$. Taking into account that $L_M \gg L_R$, the propagation of the potential diffusion wave along the myelinated section can be considered to lie on a semi-axis of $0 \leqslant z \leqslant \infty$ with the following initial and boundary conditions [14, 15]:

$$V(z, t = 0) = 0 \tag{2.13}$$

and

$$V(z = 0, t) = V_0(t) = V_{\text{ap}}(t) - V_{\text{rest}}. \tag{2.14}$$

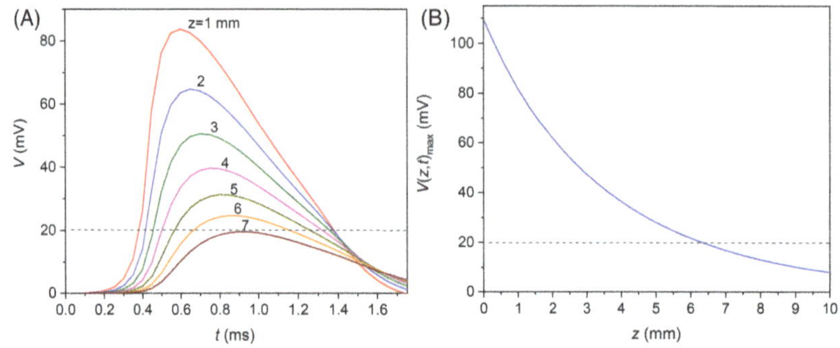

Figure 2.5. (A) Dependence of voltage on time for different values of z; curve n corresponds to $z = n$ mm. (B) Dependence of the maximum voltage on the distance from the active node of Ranvier. The dashed line indicates the potential assumed to be the threshold for excitation of the action potential at the next node of Ranvier.

Here, $V_{ap}(t)$ is the action potential in the node of Ranvier at $z = 0$, and V_R is the resting potential. The action potential $V_{ap}(t)$ at the node of Ranvier, calculated using the Frankenhaeuser–Huxley theory [3], is shown in figure 2.1(B).

The solution of equation (2.2) with the boundary and initial conditions (2.13) and (2.14) has the following form [14, 16, 17]:

$$V(t, z) = \frac{2}{\sqrt{\pi}} \int_{\frac{z}{2\sqrt{at}}}^{\infty} V_{ap}\left(t - \frac{z^2}{4\alpha\mu^2}\right) \exp\left(-\frac{\beta z^2}{4\alpha\mu^2} - \mu^2\right) d\mu. \tag{2.15}$$

The results of the calculations based on formula (2.15) for different values of z and the action potential at the node of Ranvier V_{ap} are shown in figure 2.5. Figure 2.5 (A) shows the time dependence of the function $V(t, z)$, and figure 2.5(B) shows the dependence of the maximum voltage on the distance z from the active node of Ranvier. Assuming the threshold potential difference across the membrane $\Delta V_{th} = 20$ mV and the characteristic time interval required for the initiation of an action potential $\Delta t_{ex} = 0.1$ m s, we find in figure 2.5 that the length of the myelinated section cannot exceed $L_M \approx 6.5$ mm for the assumed values of the coefficients α and β determined by (2.3) and (2.4), respectively. If the length of the myelinated section exceeds ~7 mm, then propagation of the action potential in the axon becomes impossible and is completely blocked. This blockage can occur in certain diseases of the nervous system in which there is pathological overgrowth of the nodes of Ranvier.

Note that this estimate of the limiting length is ~3 times more than the length of a typical myelinated segment of the toad axon (~2 mm). This is likely due to a selective advantage of myelinated segment lengths with a large margin of safety, which ensures saltatory conduction of the action potential along the axon, notwithstanding significant variations in the parameters of the nerve fiber.

Thus, in the process of saltatory conduction of the action potential, the propagating impulse jumps from one node of Ranvier to the next. In each node of Ranvier (non-myelinated section), when the potential difference across the membrane exceeds the threshold, an action potential is initiated. This action potential charges the next myelinated section, which can be considered a long line with leakage.

Our chosen coefficients α and β in equation (2.2) correspond to the parameters of the nervous tissue of the Xenopus frog [3]. Let us show that the speed of propagation of the action potential does not greatly depend on the transverse conductivity of the myelin fiber, which determines the quality of the insulating coating. For certainty, we assume, as we did earlier in this section, that the threshold of action potential excitation at the node of Ranvier is 20 mV. Therefore, for the action potential to propagate along the myelinated fiber, the maximum potential at the end of the myelinated segment at the inactive node of Ranvier must be at least as high as the threshold, $V(L_M, t) \geqslant \Delta V_{\text{th}} \approx 20$ mV. Considering the parameter α fixed in equation (2.2), for any value of the parameter β, we can find the corresponding length of the myelinated segment L_M at which the potential in the nearest inactive node of Ranvier reaches the threshold value ΔV_{th} during the time of action potential development in the neighboring active node. In this case, if the threshold at the edge of the myelinated segment is reached at time t_M (the time that elapsed after the action potential was excited in the active node of Ranvier), then we can make the following estimate of the propagation velocity of the action potential in the myelinated fiber:

$$v_{\text{ap}} \sim L_M/(t_M + \Delta t_{\text{ex}}), \tag{2.16}$$

where Δt_{ex} is the time interval of action potential excitation at the node of Ranvier, which can be neglected compared with t_M. For fixed values of $\alpha = 0.052$ m^2 s^{-1} and $L_M \approx 6.5$ mm, our calculations of t_M for $\beta = 0.\ 21 \cdot 10^4 \text{s}^{-1}$ and $\beta = 0$ yield $v_{\text{ap}} = 6.9$ and 7.55 m s^{-1}, respectively, using estimation (2.16).

2.2 Key experiments in ephaptic coupling

During the initiation of an action potential in a node of Ranvier, the myelin segment is charged by currents flowing in the internal and external electrolytes. Since the currents in the external electrolyte are distributed over its volume, they can charge not only the myelin coating of the excited axon but also the membranes of the nodes of Ranvier and the myelin segments of the axons of neighboring neurons, and they can thus be the cause of action potential initiation in them. The transmission of signals from an active neuron to an inactive neuron through the external environment is called ephaptic coupling. The term 'ephaptic' comes from the Greek word αφή, which means 'to touch.' To a certain extent, saltatory transfer and ephaptic coupling can be considered to have a common nature. In both cases, the action potential is transferred from an excited membrane area to an unexcited one at some distance by currents induced in the electrolyte. It is clear that the ephaptic coupling effect occurs not only for nearby myelinated axons but also for non-myelinated axons. Note that in the literature, ephaptic coupling is sometimes referred to as the extrasynaptic transmission of excitation.

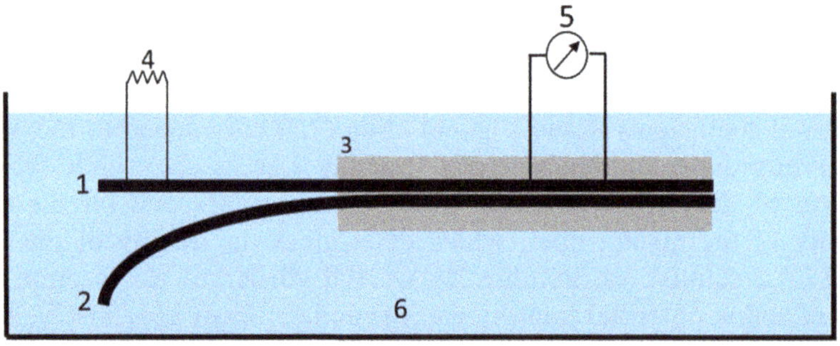

Figure 2.6. Schematic of the experiment in which the ephaptic connection of neighboring neurons was demonstrated for the first time [18]. 1—active non-myelinated axon in which the action potential was excited, 2—passive non-myelinated axon, 3—non-myelinated nerve in which non-myelinated axons were placed, 4—system of electrodes for the excitation of the action potential, 5—system of electrodes for the detection of the action potential in the first and second fibers, and 6—a vessel with a conductive physiological solution.

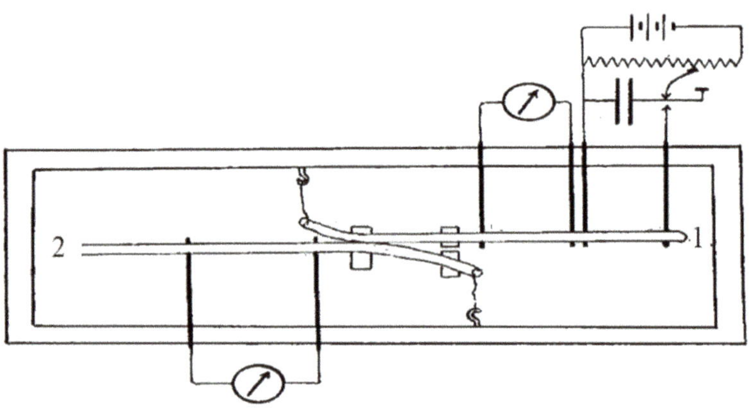

Figure 2.7. The ephaptic coupling measurement scheme used in the experiments [19]. 1—active (pre-ephaptic) non-myelinated axon, 2—initially unexcited (post-ephaptic) axon. Adopted with permission from [19].

The transmission of excitation between nearby neurons was first experimentally demonstrated by Katz[1] and Schmitt in 1940 [18]. In this experiment, the schematic of which is shown in figure 2.6, two unmyelinated axons 30 microns in diameter within the limb nerve of a crab (*Carcinus maenas*) were dissected so that they could be stimulated independently. The excitation of an action potential in one axon resulted in the excitation of the other. However, the spacing between axons in the experiments [18] was fixed, so it was not possible to determine up to what distance ephaptic coupling was possible.

Similar experiments were also performed by Arvanitaki [19] using giant axons of the common cuttlefish (*Sepia officinalis*) with diameters of 200 and 300 μm. The measurement scheme used in the experiments [19] is shown in figure 2.7.

[1] Sir Bernard Katz (March 26, 1911–April 20, 2003), born in Germany, was a distinguished British biophysicist and physiologist who was awarded the Nobel Prize for Physiology or Medicine in 1970.

These experiments showed that only when a voltage spike of sufficient amplitude is generated in axon 1 (pre-ephaptic axon) is an action potential also excited in the initially unexcited axon 2 (post-ephaptic axon). The measurements described in [19] showed that the delay in excitation of the action potential in the passive fiber is related to the time required to reach the excitation threshold in the post-ephaptic axon and to the time required for the action potential to develop. However, the experiments [19] did not investigate the dependence of action potential excitation on the distance between axons, although this was possible under the conditions of the experiments.

Studies of squid giant axons [19], crab motoneurons [20], the frog sciatic nerve [21], and algal strands [22] showed that when two axons were placed in a medium with reduced extracellular conductance, activity in one axon could depolarize the other (see also [23] and references therein). The reason that decreased extracellular conductance led to an increase in ephaptic coupling was not, however, explained in these or later papers. In the following sections of this chapter, we present a physical picture of the events that take place during ephaptic coupling and explain the effect of enhanced ephaptic coupling in a medium with reduced extracellular conductance.

In our opinion, the qualitative explanation for the effect of ephaptic coupling enhancement on decreasing extracellular conductance, that is, at lower intercellular fluid salinity, is as follows. In experiments [19–22], the distance between the axons was so small that they almost touched each other. Therefore, during the passage of an action potential, the pumping of sodium and potassium ions between the neuron and the external electrolyte changed their local densities in the external electrolyte. It is clear that if the equilibrium density of sodium and potassium ions in the intercellular electrolyte is lower, their relative change in the region of the propagating action potential near neurons is greater. Since the resting potential is mainly determined by the logarithm of the ratio of the potassium ion densities (see chapter 1, section 1.2), the release of potassium ions into the external electrolyte from an active axon during the action potential can significantly change the potassium ion density in the solution at a nearby passive axon, thus changing the resting potential at its membrane. In view of the data presented in table 2.1 [24], it follows that

Table 2.1. Ion distributions in model cells (in mmol l^{-1}) [24]. The cell membrane is impermeable to N_a^+ and the internal anion A^- and permeable to K^+ and Cl^-. $\tilde{v}$– relative volume. V_R—resting potential.

	Normal		High potassium		Low chloride	
	Extracellular	Intercellular	Extracellular	Intercellular	Extracellular	Intercellular
N_a^+	117	30	114	29	117	30.5
K^+	3	90	6	91	3	89.3
Cl^-	120	4	120	7.9	60	2.0
A^-	0	116	0	112.1	60	118
$\tilde{v}$		1.0		1.035		0.98
V_R		−85 mV		−68 mV		−85 mV

changing the density of potassium ions in the external electrolyte can dramatically change the resting potential of neurons. Therefore, we can expect that a local increase in the density of potassium ions in the external electrolyte should increase the resting potential in the nearby neuron by ~15 mV. Such a change in membrane potential may be sufficient to initiate an action potential in the neighboring neuron. Thus, ephaptic coupling can occur through two mechanisms: (i) currents induced in the intercellular medium charging the membranes of neighboring axons to a potential that exceeds the threshold; (ii) changes in the resting potential. Such changes are a result of changes in the concentration of potassium ions in the intercellular medium when neurons are close enough to each other and the salinity of the solution is relatively low.

If the volume of the external electrolyte is many times greater than the volume of the electrolyte inside the neuron, then pumping ions from the external electrolyte to the internal electrolyte and back does not affect ion densities in the external electrolyte.

A study [25] reported the appearance of synchronization spikes in four neurons located within 100 μm (the distance between initial segments did not exceed 10–15 microns). In that paper, it was suggested that a mechanism responsible for the observed synchronization of neurons could be the change in electric potential near the neuronal soma (initial segment) caused by spikes in one of the neurons.

A detailed study of ephaptic coupling in Purkinje cells[2] and other types of neurons was described in [26–31]. The experimental results of this study showed that during action potential propagation in axons, Purkinje cells generate extracellular potentials large enough to open sodium channels in nearby Purkinje cell axons. To prove that the synchronization of Purkinje cells is solely related to the generation of a potential in an external electrolyte by active neurons, chemical and electrical synapses were blocked during the experiments. The results convincingly showed that the size of the interaction correlation of individual Purkinje cells is on the order of 20–100 μm. Furthermore, they showed that the correlation of Purkinje cells depends only on the proximity of the initial segments of myelinated axons.

The large size of the interaction correlation of individual Purkinje cells in the experiments should not be surprising. If the volume of the external electrolyte is many times greater than the volume of the electrolyte inside the neuron, then pumping ions from the external electrolyte to the internal electrolyte and back should not affect the ion densities in the external electrolyte. However, since the volume of extracellular fluid is about 20% of the volume of all fluid [32, 33], it would be wrong to assume that the neurons in the body are immersed in an electrolyte of 'infinite' volume, as was the case in Hodgkin and Huxley's experiments. Therefore, during the passage of an action potential, the pumping of sodium and potassium

[2] Purkinje cells (Latin: neuronum piriforme) are pear-shaped neurons of the cerebellar cortex, the largest in the cerebellum. They were the first neurons to be discovered. They were named in honor of their discoverer (1.37), the Czech physician and physiologist Jan Evangelista Purkinje, who called them 'ganglion cells.'

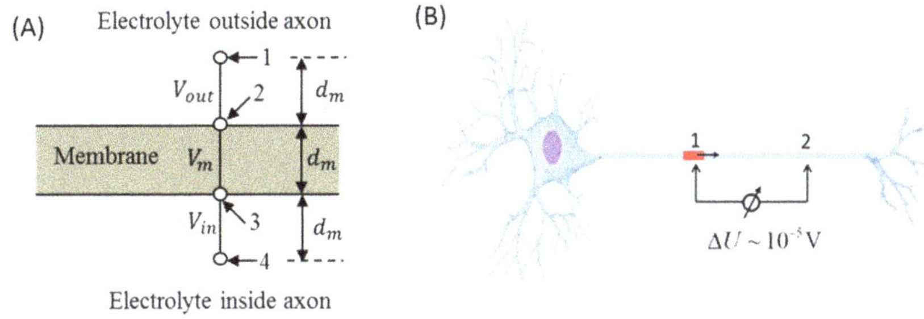

Figure 2.8. (A) Potential differences between selected points 1–2, 2–3, and 3–4 (equation (2.17)). (B) Action potential propagation along the axon, where 1 is the action potential, with the arrow indicating the direction of its propagation, 2 is the unperturbed area of the axon, and ΔU is the potential difference in the electrolyte near the axon. Reprinted with permission from [19], Copyright (1942) by the American Physical Society.

ions between the neuron and the external electrolyte should significantly change their local densities in a large volume of external electrolyte.

Among the large series of works devoted to the synchronization of action potentials in nearby neurons [34–39], the problem of interaction between two non-myelinated axons was considered on the basis of the Hodgkin–Huxley model. In these papers, the interactions of the axons were described by introducing cross terms determined by the product of the current in a parallel axon and the corresponding coupling coefficient. However, based on the results of [38, 39] and other similar works, it is difficult to estimate the characteristic scale of the correlation between two neurons, since the description of the relationship between axons in these studies is essentially phenomenological.

According to [40, 41], which are studies of the magnetic field generated by currents of the action potential, the propagating action potential causes a change of just a few microvolts in the potential on the outer surface of the membrane. Indeed, the potential difference between, for example, equidistant points 1–4 (figure 2.8 (A)) is equal to:

$$V_{\text{ap}} = V_4 - V_1 = V_{\text{in}} + V_m + V_{\text{out}} = I_m \rho_m d_m + I_m r_\| d_m + I_m \rho_\| d_m, \qquad (2.17)$$

where $\rho_m \approx \frac{1}{G_{\text{Na}} d_m} \approx 10^5\ \Omega \cdot \text{m}$ is the membrane-specific resistivity, $\rho_\| \approx 1\ \Omega \cdot \text{m}$ is the electrolyte-specific resistivity inside and outside the axon, and I_m [A m^{-2}] is the current passing through the membrane during action potential propagation. Since $\rho_\| \approx 10^{-5} \rho_m$, then $V_{\text{in}} \approx V_{\text{out}} \approx 10^{-5} V_{\text{ap}} \sim 10^{-6}$ V. Thus, the voltage drop in the near-axon electrolyte is several microvolts, while on the membrane, it is greater by five orders of magnitude (figure 2.8(B)).

It would not seem possible that such a small change in the surface potential of the axon's membrane could excite an action potential in neighboring neurons. For this reason, neuronal interaction is considered impossible for most mammalian nerve tissues [41–44]. However, the low voltages on the order of microvolts obtained in [40, 41] do not represent the potential difference between the outer and inner surfaces of the membrane; therefore, they are not related to the excitation of action potentials in neurons.

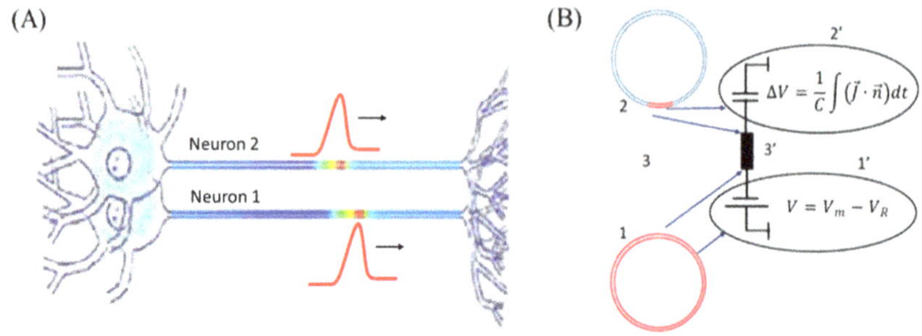

Figure 2.9. Schematic illustrating the interaction between neighboring neurons. (A) Propagation of the action potential along two correlated neurons. (B) Excitation of the action potential in the inactive axon by the active axon. 1—active axon and 2— inactive axon; red indicates the portion of the membrane being charged by currents induced in saline 3. 1′, 2′, 3′—an equivalent circuit diagram for the charging surface of the inactive axon's membrane; $\vec{j}$—local charging current of the inactive axon's membrane; $\vec{n}$—normal unit vector to the membrane surface; ΔV—local potential difference between the capacitor plates (outer and inner surfaces of the membrane); V– electromotive force source (potential difference between the surfaces of the axon membrane, along which the action potential propagates), V_m—potential on the membrane (action potential), and V_R—the resting potential of the axon.

In [14], the synchronization mechanism between nearby neurons (ephaptic coupling) was considered (figure 2.9), based on the fact that the propagating action potential along an axon is always accompanied by currents in physiological saline in the vicinity of the membrane (figure 2.2). These currents may cause neighboring neurons' axon membranes to be charged, leading to the appearance of a potential difference across the membrane greater than the threshold for action potential initiation. The estimations of the scale of the correlations between the myelinated neurons' initial parallel segments, obtained in [14, 15], are in agreement with the experimental data [25, 26]. Such an approach allows estimates of the synchronization areas (scale of correlation) of action potentials to be obtained, both for the case of myelinated and non-myelinated fibers.

2.3 Ephaptic coupling. A physical–mathematical model

In [14, 15], a simple theoretical model of ephaptic coupling was proposed, which we will consider in this chapter. Saline, the fluid in which the neurons are located in living organisms, is a highly conductive electrolyte, with $\sigma \sim 1 - 3\,\Omega^{-1}\,\text{m}^{-1}$. Therefore, the relaxation time of the volume charge perturbations in it (the Maxwell time) [46] is on the order of $\tau_M = \frac{\varepsilon_W \varepsilon_0}{\sigma} \sim 10^{-9}$ s, where ε_0 is the dielectric constant of the vacuum, and $\varepsilon_W \approx 80$ is the dielectric permittivity of water, which is several orders of magnitude smaller than the characteristic excitation and relaxation times of the action potential in axons.

The size of the quasi-neutrality violations in the electrolyte is determined by the Debye length:

$$\lambda_D = \left(\varepsilon_W \varepsilon_0 k_B T / \sum_{k=1}^{K} n_k q_k^2\right)^{1/2}, \tag{2.18}$$

where k_B is the Boltzmann constant, T is the temperature, and n_k and q_k are the density and charge of the ions, respectively. The density of the ions in the electrolyte outside and inside the cells is close to the ion density in saline: $n_k \approx 2 \cdot 10^{26}\ \text{m}^{-3}$ [47]. For typical parameters of interstitial fluid at $T \approx 300$ K, (2.18) yields $\lambda_D \approx 0.5$ nm; that is, λ_D is at least three orders of magnitude smaller than the typical axon radius (see table 1.2).

This means that the effects on action potential propagation associated with the violation of quasi-neutrality in the conducting fluid inside and outside the axon can be neglected. Accordingly, the current continuity equation can be used to find the potential distribution inside and outside the axon:

$$\nabla \cdot \vec{I} = 0, \tag{2.19}$$

where $\vec{I} = -\sigma \nabla \varphi$ is the current density.

Since σ $[\Omega^{-1}\,\text{m}^{-1}]$ is a constant in the electrolyte, equation (2.19) is reduced to the Laplace equation:

$$\Delta\varphi = 0, \tag{2.20}$$

with the Neumann boundary conditions on the membrane surface:

$$\left.\frac{\partial \varphi}{\partial r}\right|_{r=a} = -I_m/\sigma, \tag{2.21}$$

and the Dirichlet condition away from the surface of the membrane, which is

$$\varphi_{r\to\infty} = 0, \tag{2.22}$$

where $a = d_R/2$ is the radius of the node of Ranvier (see figure 1.35) and I_m is the density of the total radial current flowing through the axon membrane. In the non-myelinated parts of the axon (the nodes of Ranvier and the initial segment), the current I_m is composed of the ionic current, which is associated with the work done by voltage-gated ion channels and ionic pumps, and the capacitive current, which is associated with the charging of the membrane by currents flowing inside and outside the axon. These components of the total current density in the axon membrane during the passage of the action potential along the non-myelinated axon, calculated according to the equations of the Hodgkin–Huxley model [48], are shown in figure 2.10. We emphasize that in equation (2.21) and later in this chapter, it is assumed that I_m is equal to the total current passing through the membrane shown in figure 2.10. This is the case because we are considering the current in an intercellular electrolyte in which the displacement current is negligible compared to the total ionic current.

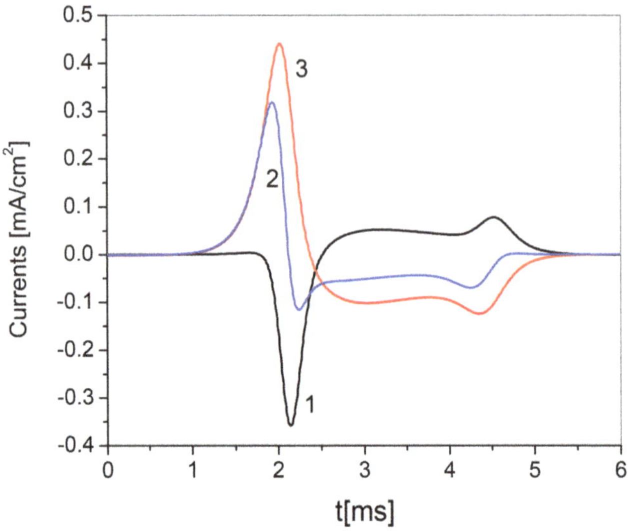

Figure 2.10. Time dependence of the radial currents in the membrane obtained on the basis of the Hodgkin–Huxley equations [45]. Line 1—ionic current, line 2—capacitive current, and line 3—total current.

2.3.1 Ephaptic coupling between neighboring squid axons

Within the body of the giant squid, axons are separated by a distance of a few tens of centimeters. Therefore, there cannot be a correlation between the action potentials of these axons. However, squid axons are a traditional and convenient object for experimental studies. Let us estimate the size of the correlation area for action potentials in squid axons that can be observed in a laboratory experiment.

Figure 2.11 shows the z-distribution of the total current passing through the squid axon membrane during action potential propagation and its Gaussian approximation:

$$I_m = I_0 \exp\left(-\left(\frac{z + v_{ap}\, t}{L}\right)^2\right), \tag{2.23}$$

where $v_{ap} \approx 15$ m s^{-1} is the propagation velocity of the action potential in the squid axon. The Fourier transform of I_m is given by:

$$I_{m,\,k} = \sqrt{\pi}\, I_0(t) L \cdot \exp\left(-\frac{L^2 k^2}{4} - ikv_{ap}\, t\right), \tag{2.24}$$

and radial and longitudinal currents outside the squid axon ($r > a = 0.24$ mm) have the form [48, 49]:

$$I_r(r,\, z,\, t) = \frac{I_0 L}{\sqrt{\pi} a} \int_0^{\infty} \frac{K_1\left(\xi \frac{r}{a}\right)}{K_1(\xi)} \exp\left(-\left(\frac{L}{2a}\xi\right)^2\right) \cos\left(\frac{\xi(z + v_{ap}\, t)}{a}\right) d\xi, \tag{2.25}$$

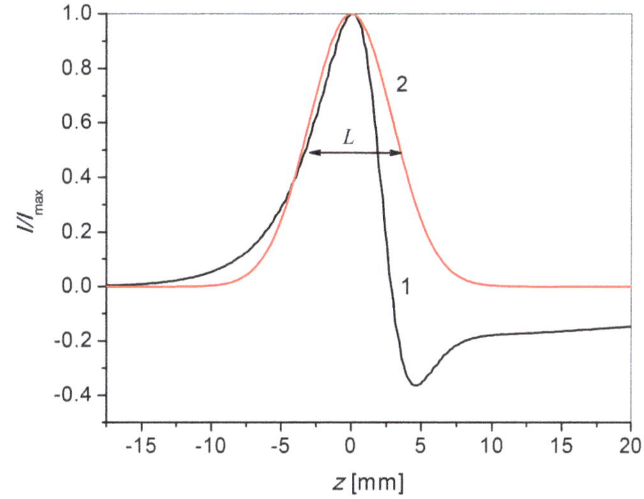

Figure 2.11. The z-distribution of the total current passing through the membrane of the squid axon (curve 1) and its approximation by a Gaussian distribution (curve 2) for the propagating action potential.

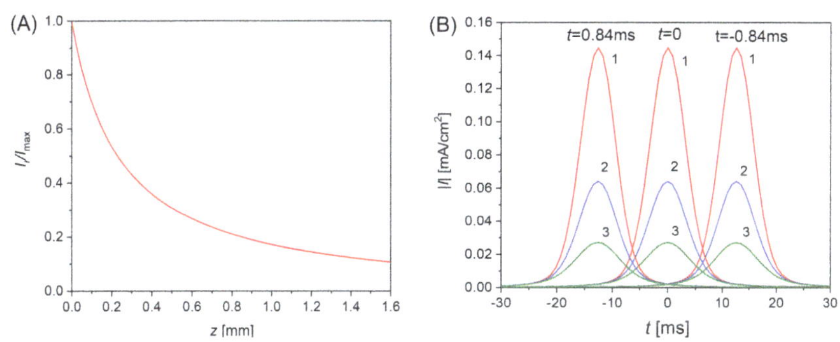

Figure 2.12. (A) The radial dependence of the current I_r at the point $z = 0$ in $t = 0$ for the case of a Gaussian distribution along z (curve 2 in figure 2.11). (B) Examples of the longitudinal distribution of the charging current $|I| = (I_r^2 + I_z^2)^{1/2}$, with curve 1 corresponding to the current at a distance $R_s = r - a = 0.27$ mm from the surface of the membrane at $\Delta V_{\text{th}} = 20$ mV, curve 2 to a distance $R_s = 0.84$ mm, and curve 3 to a distance $R_s = 1.96$ mm.

$$I_z(r, z, t) = \frac{I_0 L}{\sqrt{\pi} a} \int_0^\infty \frac{K_0\left(\xi \frac{r}{a}\right)}{K_1(\xi)} \exp\left(-\left(\frac{L}{2a}\xi\right)^2\right) \sin\left(\frac{\xi(z + v_{\text{ap}}\, t)}{a}\right) d\xi. \tag{2.26}$$

Since we are interested only in the 'charging' phase of the axon membrane, which is located in the field of currents initiated by the action potential propagation in adjacent axons, it is sufficient to restrict ourselves to the Gaussian approximation shown in figure 2.11. Figure 2.12(A) shows the radial distribution of the current J_r, normalized to the maximum current at the point $z = 0$ for the case of a Gaussian distribution along the z-axis (curve 2 in figure 2.11). Figure 2.12(B) shows examples of the longitudinal distribution of the charging current.

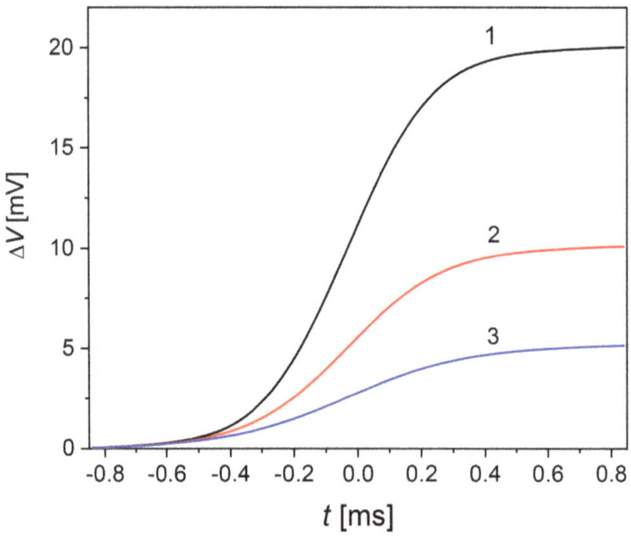

Figure 2.13. The time dependence of charging to the potential difference ΔV at the membrane of the inactive axon for different distances between the membranes of the active and inactive axons. Curve 1 corresponds to the current at a distance $R_s = 0.27$ mm from the membrane surface, curve 2 corresponds to a distance $R_s = 0.84$ mm, and curve 3 corresponds to a distance $R_s = 1.96$ mm.

The potential difference across the inactive membrane (see figure 2.9), without charge removal, was determined by the charge on its surface. Knowing the time dependence of the charge current and its spatial distribution makes it possible to estimate the potential difference across the membrane of the inactive axon initial segment as a function of its position:

$$\Delta V(r, z) \sim \frac{1}{C_m} \int_0^{\infty} (\vec{I}(r, z, t) \cdot \vec{n}) \mathrm{d}t. \tag{2.27}$$

Figure 2.13 shows the time dependence of charging to the potential difference ΔV at the inactive (post-ephaptic) axon membrane for different distances between the membranes of the active (pre-ephaptic) and inactive axons. In this case, the radii of synchronization are $R_s = r - a = 1.96$ mm at $\Delta V_{\text{th}} = 5$ mV, $R_s = r - a = 0.85$ mm at $\Delta V_{\text{th}} = 10$ mV, and $R_s = 0.27$ mm at $\Delta V_{\text{th}} = 20$ mV.

2.3.2 Ephaptic coupling between myelinated neurons

Consider the conditions for ephaptic coupling between myelinated neurons shown in figure 1.35. In principle, currents induced in any part of the axon during action potential propagation can cause excitation transmission between neighboring neurons. However, because the initial segment is the longest element of the excitable part of the myelinated axon, currents originating there are expected to transmit excitation to much more distant neurons than currents originating in nodes of Ranvier. Therefore, the maximum correlation length of the ephaptic connection is determined by the action potential in the initial segment.

Without loss of generality, we assume that the longitudinal distribution of the radial current passing through the membrane of the initial segment length L_{IS} is Gaussian:

$$I_m = I(t)\exp\left(-\frac{4z^2}{L_{IS}^2}\right). \tag{2.28}$$

In this case, the Fourier transform of I_m is given by:

$$I_{m,k} = \frac{\sqrt{\pi}}{2}I_0(t)L_{IS}\exp\left(-\frac{L_{IS}^2k^2}{16}\right), \tag{2.29}$$

and the radial current J_r and the longitudinal current J_z outside the axon ($r > a$) have the form [49, 50]:

$$I_r(r, z, t) = \frac{I_0(t)L_{IS}}{2\sqrt{\pi}a}\int_0^\infty \frac{K_1\left(\xi\frac{r}{a}\right)}{K_1(\xi)}\exp\left(-\left(\frac{L_{IS}}{4a}\xi\right)^2\right)\cos\left(\frac{\xi z}{a}\right)d\xi, \tag{2.30}$$

$$I_z(r, z, t) = \frac{I_0(t)L_{IS}}{2\sqrt{\pi}a}\int_0^\infty \frac{K_0\left(\xi\frac{r}{a}\right)}{K_1(\xi)}\exp\left(-\left(\frac{L_{IS}}{4a}\xi\right)^2\right)\sin\left(\frac{\xi z}{a}\right)d\xi, \tag{2.31}$$

where K_0 and K_1 are modified Bessel functions of the second kind corresponding to the zeroth order and the first order, respectively. The current J_0 in equations (2.30)–(2.31) corresponds to the total current, which is equal to the sum of the capacitive (displacement) and ion currents. Figure 2.14 shows the radial

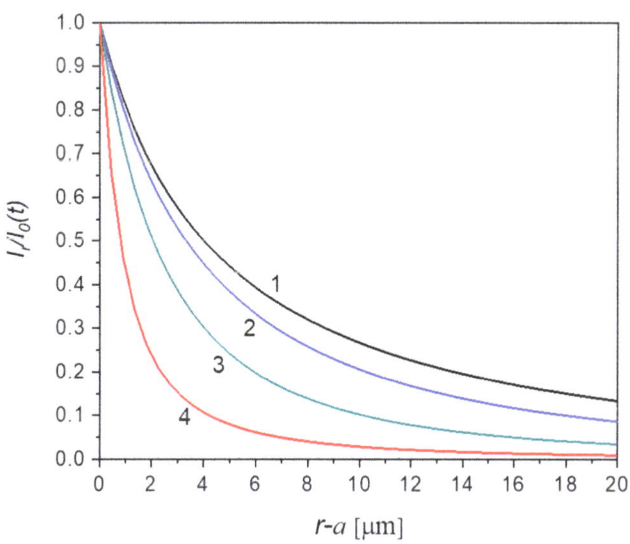

Figure 2.14. The radial dependence of the current at the point $z = 0$ for different lengths of the initial segment, with $a = 4.5$ μm. Line 1 corresponds to $L_{IS} = 70$ μm, line 2 to $L_{IS} = 30$ μm, line 3 to $L_{IS} = 10$ μm, and line 4 to $L_{IS} = 2.5$ μm (the length of the node of Ranvier).

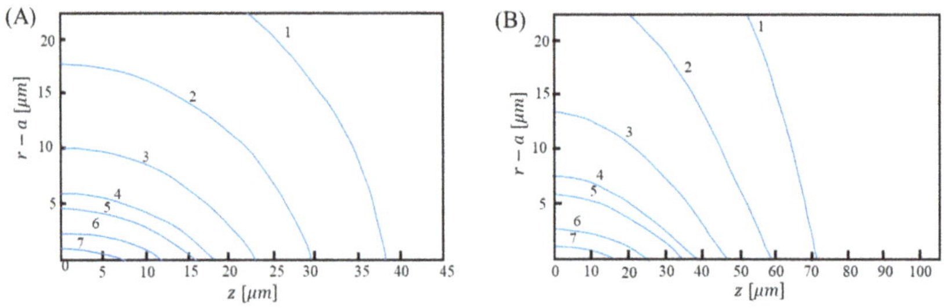

Figure 2.15. The instantaneous normalized amplitude distributions of the current density $I_N = (I_r^2 + I_z^2)^{1/2}/I_0(t)$ in the vicinity of the initial segment with lengths $L_{IS} = 30\ \mu m$—(A) and $L_{IS} = 70\ \mu m$—(B). Lines 1 on (A) and (B) correspond to $I_N = 0.05$, lines 2—0.1, lines 3—0.2, lines 4—0.33, lines 5—0.4, lines 6—0.6, lines 7—0.08.

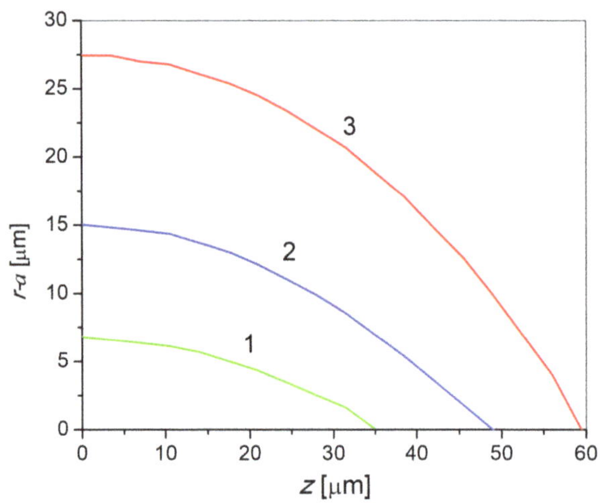

Figure 2.16. Areas of neuron synchronization at $L_{IS} = 70\ \mu m$, at an assumed initiation time $\Delta t_{ex} = 0.1$ ms with $C_m = 0.02\ F\ m^{-2}$, and at the assumed threshold initiation voltage. Line 1 corresponds to $V_{th} = 20$ mV, line 2 corresponds to $V_{th} = 10$ mV, and line 3 corresponds to $V_{th} = 5$ mV.

distribution of currents at $z = 0$ for the initial segment with radius $a = 4.5\ \mu m$. It can be seen that the shorter the initial segment of an excited neuron, the closer the neighboring neuron must be for the action potential to be initiated in the neighboring neuron.

The contours of the normalized instantaneous current amplitudes $I_N(r, z, t) = (I_r^2 + I_z^2)^{1/2}/I_0(t)$ for $L_{IS} = 30\ \mu m$ and $70\ \mu m$ are shown in figure 2.15.

Figure 2.16 shows the areas of action potential synchronization for the axons in the case $L_{IS} = 70\ \mu m$, assuming that the threshold potential differences across the membrane are $V_{th} = 5$, 10, and 20 mV; the initiation time interval is $\Delta t_{ex} = 0.1$ ms and $C_m = 0.02\ F \cdot m^{-2}$.

2.4 Physical model of electrical synapses in a neural network

In chapter 1, section 1.7, we briefly considered electrical synapses when discussing the synaptic transmission of nerve impulses between neurons. In our view, the operation of an electrical impulse has much in common with ephaptic coupling. This explains why we decided to consider a simple physical model of the electrical synapse in the chapter dealing with ephaptic coupling and its manifestations.

An electrical synapse (figure 2.17) is similar to the connection of wires in an electrical circuit, which, unlike a chemical synapse, allows an action potential to propagate in both directions, from one neuron to another, and in the opposite direction [50–55]. In works [51–55], it is assumed that the electrical connection between neurons is provided by the transport of ions and small molecules through the connexons. Various ways of connecting neurons by electrical synapses (more precisely, by connexons) that have been considered in the literature are shown in figure 2.17. The mathematical description of electrical synapses is usually reduced to an electrical circuit connecting two axons, along one of which an action potential propagates [36, 56–59]. However, the simplified equivalent circuit does not always reveal the physical mechanism underlying the operation of the electrical synapse and is phenomenological in nature.

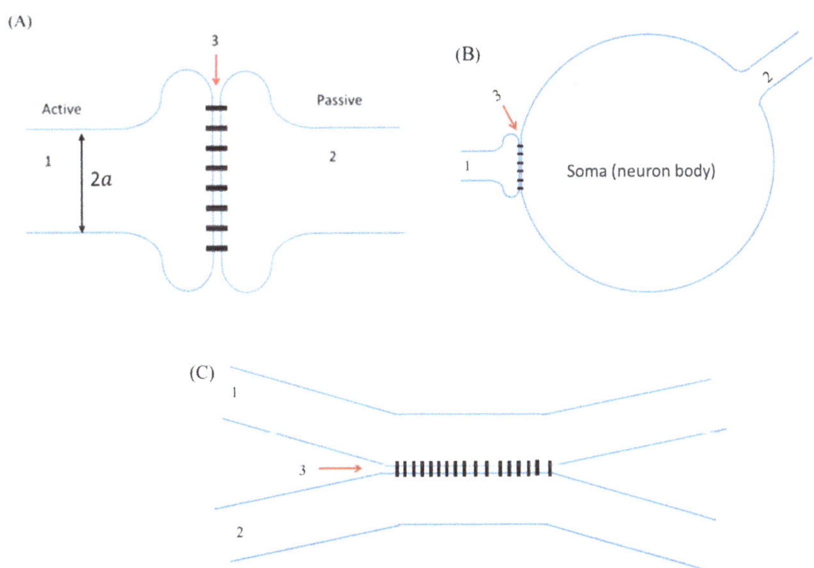

Figure 2.17. Electrical synapse. (A)—Connection of an axon to a dendrite (or another axon) by an electrical synapse: 1 is the active axon, 2 is the dendrite (or passive axon), and 3 is a system of connexons. An axon radius is denoted by a. The action potential propagating along axon 1 'jumps' through the electrical synapse to the dendrite (or axon 2) and then propagates in it. (B)—Electrical connection by connexons of the axon with the soma of the neighboring neuron. An action potential propagating along axon 1 through an electrical synapse excites an action potential on the body of a neighboring neuron, which in turn stimulates the propagation of an action potential in axon 2. (C)—Connection of non-myelinated regions of two axons 1 and 2 by connexons 3.

Earlier in this chapter, we discussed key experiments and simple theoretical models of ephaptic communication between neurons and concluded that 'communication between nearby neurons,' that is, the transfer of an action potential from an active neuron to an initially unexcited neuron, is realized very efficiently by currents induced in the external conducting intercellular medium. Moreover, the distances between ephaptically 'communicating' neurons are about 10–100 μm, which is three to four orders of magnitude larger than the size of the synaptic gap in electrical synapses $d_s \approx$ 2–4 nm. In this section, we consider a simple model of the electrical synapse [60] in which the connexons play the role of 'nails' holding non-myelinated regions of neurons at distance d_s. In this case, electrical coupling is provided by charging the membrane of the inactive neuron with currents generated in the intercellular electrolyte by the action potential in the active neuron, similar to the ephaptic coupling between neurons discussed earlier.

As in ephaptic coupling problems, the distribution of the potential in the external electrolyte associated with the propagation of the action potential in one of the neurons is determined by solving the Laplace equation (2.20) with the Neumann (2.21) and Dirichlet (2.22) boundary conditions.

For the sake of illustration, consider two cases of an electrical synapse. In the first case, an electrical synapse connects an axon to a dendrite (figure 2.18(A)–(C)), and in the second case, an electrical synapse connects an axon to a soma (figure 2.18(B)). Since the distance between the soma and the axon is about d_s=

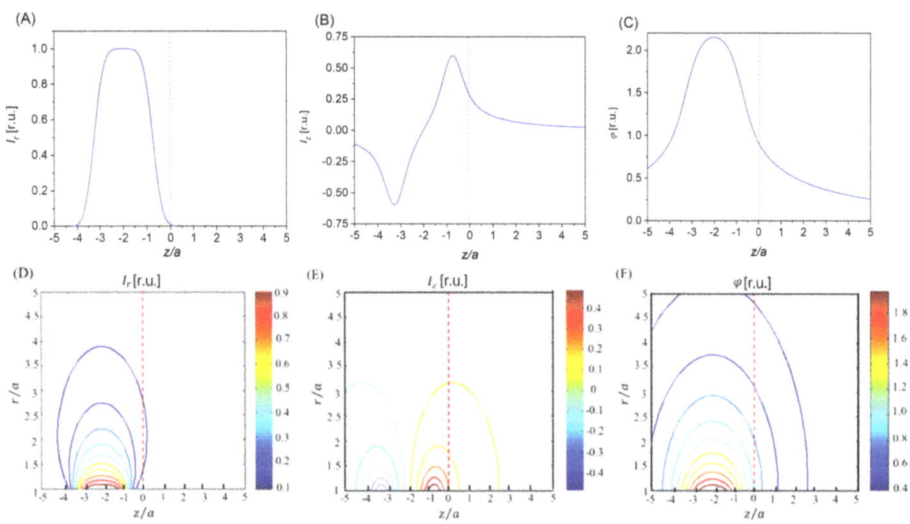

Figure 2.18. Current and potential distributions in relative units for a radial current pulse on contiguous axons: (A), (B), and (C)—Distributions of the radial current I_r, the longitudinal current I_z, and the potential φ^e on the membranes of contiguous neurons; (D), (E), and (F)—corresponding volumetric distributions of currents and potential in saline. The active axon corresponds to the line $r/a \geqslant 1$, $z < 0$, to the left of the dashed line, and the passive axon corresponds to $2r/a \geqslant 1$, $z > 0$, to the right of the dashed line. The currents I_r and I_z are normalized to the value of the radial current at the point $r/a = 1$, $z/a = -2$ (see (2.39)), and the potential φ is normalized to $\varphi_{\text{norm}} = I_m(z/a = -2)a/\sigma$.

3.5 nm, the radius of the axon is $a\sim$ 1–8 μm [61], and the radius of the neuron body (soma) R_b is several times larger than the radius of the non-myelinated region of the axon, so that $R_b \gg a \gg d_s$. In the case of electrical contact between an axon and a dendrite or soma, the axon can be considered a cylinder with a radius of a, directly connected to a cylindrical dendrite (axon) or to the soma of a neighboring neuron. Since $R_b \gg a$, then, without loss of generality, the body of the axon can be considered a plane.

An estimation of the charging time of a cylindrical capacitor with radius a and capacitance per unit area C_m in an electrolyte with conductivity σ is given by [62]:

$$t_{\mathrm{tr}} \sim 2\frac{C_m a}{\sigma}. \tag{2.32}$$

Since the membrane capacitance of the non-myelinated section of the axon per unit area is $C_m \approx 10^{-2}$ F m^{-2}, and the electrolyte conductivity $\sigma \sim 1$–$3\ \Omega^{-1}\,\mathrm{m}^{-1}$, then for an axon radius of 1.5–8 μm, τ_{tr} varies from 0.035 to 0.1 μs. The typical duration of the action potential impulse at the interface between the active axon and the passive dendrite (passive axon) is $t_{\mathrm{ap}} \sim$ 1 ms. Since $\tau_{\mathrm{tr}} \ll t_{\mathrm{ap}}$, we can assume that each value of the radial current on the active axon corresponds to the acquisition of an additional potential on the membrane of the passive axon. The same applies to the contact of the axon with the soma, since the radius of the neuron is only several times the radius of the axon [47]. Obviously, the statement about the linear connection of the potential on the inactive axon or on the body of the neuron from the radial current on the active axon is valid until the additional potential on the dendrite or soma of the neighboring neuron exceeds the threshold value required for the initiation of the action potential. In other words, until that time, the membrane of a dendrite, axon, or soma of a neighboring inactive neuron can be considered impermeable to ions.

Accordingly, the boundary condition that applies to an inactive dendrite (axon) (figure 2.17(A)) is:

$$I_n = -\sigma\frac{\partial\varphi}{\partial r}\bigg|_{r=a,\ z>0} = 0, \tag{2.33}$$

and the condition that applies to the soma of the neuron is (figure 2.17(B)):

$$I_n = -\sigma\frac{\partial\varphi}{\partial z}\bigg|_{r>a,\ z=0} = 0, \tag{2.34}$$

where I_n is the normal component of the current on the dendrite (axon) or soma of an inactive neuron.

If we assume that the radial current passing through the membrane in the activated axon has a Gaussian spatial distribution of the form

$$I_m(t, z) = I_0(t)\exp\left(-b^2(z - z_0)^2\right), \tag{2.35}$$

where $I_0(t)$ is the maximal density of the current passing through the membrane, then the distributions of the potential φ and currents outside the axon have the forms [14, 15]:

$$\varphi\left(\frac{r}{a} > 1, z\right) = \frac{I_0}{\sqrt{\pi}b\sigma}\int_0^\infty \frac{K_0(\xi r/a)}{\xi K_1(\xi)} \exp\left(-\xi^2/(2ba)^2\right)\cos\left(\xi\frac{z - z_0}{a}\right)d\xi, \quad (2.36)$$

$$I_r\left(\frac{r}{a} > 1, z\right) = \frac{I_0}{\sqrt{\pi}ba}\int_0^\infty \frac{K_1(\xi r/a)}{K_1(\xi)} \exp\left(-\xi^2/(2ba)^2\right)\cos\left(\xi\frac{z - z_0}{a}\right)d\xi, \quad (2.37)$$

$$I_z\left(\frac{r}{a} > 1, z\right) = \frac{I_0}{\sqrt{\pi}ba}\int_0^\infty \frac{K_0(\xi r/a)}{K_1(\xi)} \exp\left(-\xi^2/(2ba)^2\right)\sin\left(\xi\frac{z - z_0}{a}\right)d\xi. \quad (2.38)$$

We can say that formulas (2.36)–(2.38) determine the corresponding distributions of the potential and currents in the vicinity of the contacts of the electrical synapses shown in figure 2.17(A).

In general, any distribution of radial currents on the membrane of the active axon can be approximated by the sum of the Gaussian distributions:

$$I_m(t, z) = \sum_{i=1}^{I} I_i(t)\exp\left(-b_i^2(z - z_i)^2\right). \quad (2.39)$$

In this case, if (2.39) is substituted into (2.36)–(2.38), it is easy to obtain formulas describing the contact between an active axon and a dendrite.

Figure 2.18 shows the distributions of currents and potentials on the membranes of active and passive axons and in the electrolyte region for an active axon in contact with a passive dendrite or axon. The radial current at the membrane surface was given by formula (2.39), where $b_1 = b_2 = b_3 = b_4 = b_5 = 2/a$, $I_1 = I_2 = I_3 = I_4 = I_5 = 1$, $z_1/a = -1$, $z_2/a = -1.5$, $z_3/a = -2$, $z_4/a = -2.5$, and $z_5/a = -3$. To the left of the dashed line, $z < 0$ is an active axon; to the right, $z > 0$ is a passive axon.

The electrical contact between an active axon and the soma of a neighboring unexcited neuron can be described by a radial current density:

$$I_m(t, z) = I_0(t)\left(\exp\left(-b^2(z - z_0)^2\right) + \exp\left(-b^2(z + z_0)^2\right)\right). \quad (2.40)$$

Indeed, due to the symmetry of the radial current (2.40) with respect to the point $z = 0$, the normal current to the plane passing through $z = 0$—$I_z(z = 0) = 0$, which corresponds to the boundary condition (2.34).

The distributions of the potential and currents corresponding to the currents (2.40) in adjacent regions of the intercellular electrolyte have the following forms:

$$\varphi\left(t, \frac{r}{a} \geqslant 1, z \geqslant 0\right) = \frac{I_0(t)}{\sqrt{\pi}b\sigma}\int_0^\infty \frac{K_0(\xi r/a)}{\xi K_1(\xi)}\exp\left(-\left(\frac{\xi}{2ba}\right)^2\right) \left(\cos\left(\xi\frac{z - z_0}{a}\right) + \cos\left(\xi\frac{z + z_0}{a}\right)\right)d\xi, \quad (2.41)$$

$$I_r\left(t, \frac{r}{a} \geqslant 1, z \geqslant 0\right) = \frac{I_0(t)}{\sqrt{\pi}ba} \int_0^{\infty} \frac{K_1(\xi r/a)}{K_1(\xi)} \exp\left(-\left(\frac{\xi}{2ba}\right)^2\right) \left(\cos\left(\xi\frac{z - z_0}{a}\right) + \cos\left(\xi\frac{z + z_0}{a}\right)\right) d\xi, \tag{2.42}$$

$$I_z\left(t, \frac{r}{a} \geqslant 1, z \geqslant 0\right) = \frac{I_0(t)}{\sqrt{\pi}ba} \int_0^{\infty} \frac{K_0(\xi r/a)}{K_1(\xi)} \exp\left(-\left(\frac{\xi}{2ba}\right)^2\right) \left(\sin\left(\xi\frac{z - z_0}{a}\right) + \sin\left(\xi\frac{z + z_0}{a}\right)\right) d\xi. \tag{2.43}$$

In general, any distribution of radial currents on the membrane of the active axon can be approximated by the sum of the Gaussian distributions:

$$I_m(t, z) = \sum_{i=1}^{I} I_i(t) \exp\left(-b_i^2 (z - z_i)^2\right) + \exp\left(-b_i^2 (z + z_i)^2\right). \tag{2.44}$$

In this case, if (2.44) is substituted into (2.41)–(2.43), it is easy to obtain equations describing the electrical contact between an axon and a soma.

Figure 2.19 shows the distributions of currents and potential on the soma membrane and in the electrolyte region when the active axon is in contact with

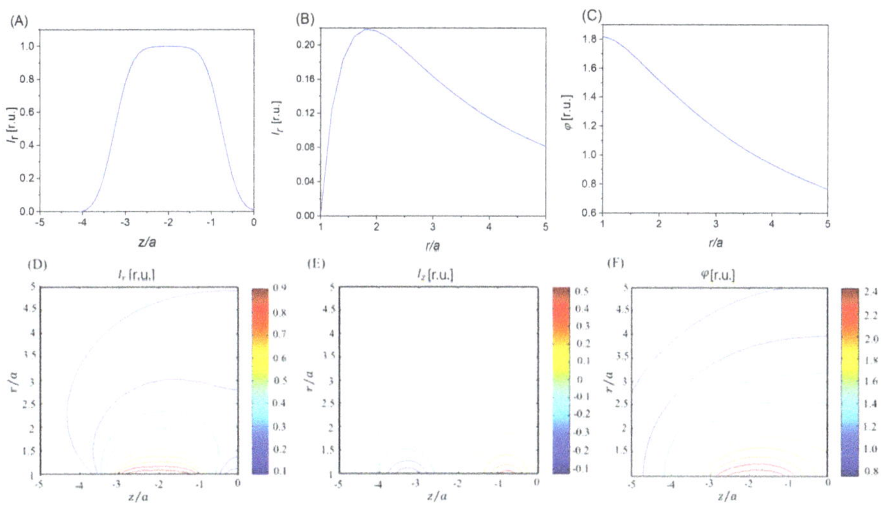

Figure 2.19. Current and potential distributions in relative units for a radial current pulse on an active axon in contact with a soma, as shown in figure 2.15(B). (A) Distribution of radial current I_r on the membrane of the active axon. (B) and (C) Distributions of radial current I_r and potential φ on the membrane of the soma ($z = 0$, r/a); the longitudinal current on the soma is equal to zero. (D), (E), and (F) Corresponding volumetric distributions of currents and potential in saline. The currents I_r and I_z are normalized to the value of the radial current at the point $r/a = 1, z/a = -2$, $I_{am} = I_m(z/a = -2)$ (see (2.44)), and the potential φ is normalized to $\varphi_{norm} = I_m(z/a = -2)a/\sigma$.

the passive soma. The radial current at the membrane surface was given by formula (2.43), where $b_1 = b_2 = b_3 = b_4 = b_5 = 2/a$, $I_1 = I_2 = I_3 = I_4 = I_5 = 1$, $z_1/a = -1$, $z_2/a = -1.5$, $z_3/a = -2$, $z_4/a = -2.5$, and $z_5/a = -3$.

According to the calculations, the characteristic size of the change in currents and potentials on the passive axon and the neuron body is on the order of two to three axon radii. Therefore, in our calculations, we can: (i) neglect the size of the gap between the active axon and the dendrite or soma and (ii) treat the soma as a plane. At the same time, the calculations show that the change in potential on the surface of the dendrite (axon) or the surface of the soma of an unexcited neuron is up to 30% of the maximum potential on the active axon. That is, the potential difference at the membrane surface (external and internal) in a passive dendrite (axon) or soma can be up to 20–30 mV. In principle, this should be sufficient to activate the action potential via the electrical synapse.

Note that the discussed mechanism by which the action potential 'jumps' from the active axon to the passive axon through the electrical synaptic gap is also applicable to the surface contact shown in figure 2.17(C). Thus, the role of connexons is reduced to keeping axons and dendrites close enough for the action potential to 'jump' from the active site to the initially inactive one.

To conclude this section, we note again that a model of the electrical synapse has been proposed in which connexons play the role of 'nails,' holding non-myelinated areas of neurons at a distance of several nanometers. In this case, the transmission of excitation in the electrical synapse is provided by charging the membrane of an inactive neuron with currents generated by the action potential in the saline of an active neuron. This model explains the transmission of excitation across the electrical synapse without the need to generate ion fluxes across connexons.

References

[1] Goldman L and Albus J S 1968 Computation of impulse conduction in myelinated fibers *J. Biophys.* **8** 596

[2] Shneider M N, Voronin A A and Zheltikov A M 2011 Modeling the action-potential-sensitive nonlinear-optical response of myelinated nerve fibers and short-term memory *J. Appl. Phys.* **110** 094702

[3] Frankenhaeuser B and Huxley A F 1964 The action potential in the myelinated nerve fiber of *Xenopus laevis* as computed on the basis of voltage clamp data *J. Physiol.* **171** 302

[4] Rushton W A H 1951 A theory of the effects of fibre size in medullated nerve *J. Physiol.* **115** 101

[5] Hursh J B 1939 Conduction velocity and diameter of nerve fibers *Amer. J. Physiol.* **127** 131

[6] Hursh J B 1939 The properties of growing nerve fibers *Amer. J. Physiol.* **127** 140

[7] Sanders F K 1948 The thickness of the myelin sheaths of normal and regenerating peripheral nerve fibres *Proc. Roy. Soc.* B **135** 323

[8] Sanders F K and Whitteridge D 1946 Conduction velocity and myelin thickness in regenerating nerve fibres *J. Physiol.* **105** 152

[9] Gasser H S 1935 Conduction in nerves in relation to fiber types *Proc. Assoc. Res. Nerv. Mental Dis.* **15** 35

[10] Gasser H S 1950 Unmedullated fibers originating in dorsal root ganglia *J. Gen. Physiol.* **33** 651

[11] Gasser H S and Grundfest H 1939 Axon diameters in relation to the spike dimensions and the conduction velocity in mammalian A fibers *Amer. J. Physiol.* **127** 393

[12] Grundfest H 1939 The properties of mammalian B fibers *Amer. J. Physiol.* **127** 252

[13] Tasaki I, Ishii K and Ito H 1943 On the relation between the conduction-rate, the fibre-diameter and the internodal distance of the medullated nerve fibre *Jpn J. Med. Sci. III, Biophysics* **9** 189

[14] Shneider M N and Pekker M 2015 Correlation of action potentials in adjacent neurons *Phys. Biol.* **12** 066009

[15] Shneider M N and Pekker M 2019 Stimulated activity in the neural tissue *J. Appl. Phys.* **125** 211101

[16] Carslaw H S and Jaeger J C 1986 *Conduction of Heat in Solids* (Oxford: Oxford Science Publications)

[17] Polyanin A 2001 *Handbook of Linear Partial Differential Equations for Engineers and Scientists* 1st edn (Boca Raton, FL: Chapman and Hall)

[18] Katz B and Schmitt O H 1940 Electric interaction between two adjacent nerve fibers *J. Physiol.* **97** 471

[19] Arvanitaki A 1942 Effects evoked in an axon by the activity of a contiguous one *J. Neurophysiol.* **5** 89

[20] Katz B and Schmitt O H 1942 A note on interaction between nerve fibers *J. Physiol.* **100** 369

[21] Kocsis J D, Ruiz J A and Cummins K L 1982 Modulation of axonal excitability mediated by surround electrical activity: an intraaxonal study *Exp. Brain Res.* **47** 151

[22] Tabata T 1990 Ephaptic transmission and conduction velocity of an action potential in Chara internodal cells placed in parallel and in contact with one another *Plant Cell Physiol.* **31** 575

[23] Bullock T H 1965 Comparative neurology of transmission ed T H Bullock and G A Horridge *Structure and Function in the Nervous Systems of Invertebrates* **vol I** (San Francisco, CA: WH Freeman) 181

[24] Nicholls J G, Martin A R, Fuchs P A, Brown D A, Diamond M E and Weisblat D A 2012 *From Neuron to Brain* 5th edn (Sunderland, MA: Sinauer Associate, Inc. Publishers)

[25] Anastassiou C A, Perin R, Markram H and Koch C 2011 Ephaptic coupling of cortical neurons *Nat. Neurosci.* **14** 217

[26] Han K - S, Guo C, Chen C H, Witter L, Osorno T and Regehr W G 2018 Ephaptic coupling promotes synchronous firing of cerebellar Purkinje cells *Neuron* **100** 564

[27] Anastassiou C A and Koch C 2015 Ephaptic coupling to endogenous electric field activity: why bother? *Curr. Opin. Neurobiol.* **31** 95

[28] Dudek F E, Yasumura T and Rash J E 1998 Non-synaptic' mechanisms in seizures and epileptogenesis *Cell Biol. Int.* **22** 793

[29] Jefferys J G 1995 Nonsynaptic modulation of neuronal activity in the brain: electric currents and extracellular ions *Physiol. Rev.* **75** 689

[30] Jefferys J G and Haas H L 1982 Synchronized bursting of CA1 hippocampal pyramidal cells in the absence of synaptic transmission *Nature* **300** 448

[31] Wise A K, Cerminara N L, Marple-Horvat D E and Apps R 2010 Mechanisms of synchronous activity in cerebellar Purkinje cells *J. Physiol.* **588** 2373

Chapter 3

On the criteria of nonthermal interaction of cell membranes exposed to microwave radiation

This chapter examines how nonthermal reversible external stimuli, such as microwave radiation, influence the lipid membranes of cells and thus stimulate activity in nervous tissues. Phase transitions in biological lipid membranes during their heating are also considered.

In the following chapters, we examine the effects of microwave radiation in stimulating and blocking action potentials in neurons. Since any effect of an electromagnetic field on nervous tissue is accompanied by energy absorption and heating (depending on the intensity, frequency of the electromagnetic field, exposure time, and thermal conductivity properties), a natural question arises: Under what conditions can electromagnetic radiation and its effects on nervous tissue be considered nonthermal and reversible? A similar question arises regarding the control of neural tissue activity by current pulses generated by an external source in the intercellular medium.

Interaction with electromagnetic fields acts directly or indirectly on the nervous system, causing morphologic, chemical, or electrical changes in the nervous system that can lead to neurophysiologic effects, such as changes in excitation thresholds and action potential propagation velocity or blockage, and leading to anesthesia. Even a small degree of heating or cooling of nerve tissue can noticeably change the rate of physiological processes in neurons. However, it is necessary to separate the thermal and nonthermal effects caused by electromagnetic radiation in nerve tissue. Nonthermal effects are not directly related to changes in the temperature of the intercellular medium and neurons. The current understanding of thermal and nonthermal effects in nervous tissue interacting with electromagnetic fields in different frequency ranges and relevant literature references are presented in reviews [1–4].

doi:10.1088/978-0-7503-6034-0ch3

3.1 Phase transition in cell membranes during heating

In what follows, we determine the upper limit of energy absorption under the condition that the heating of cell membranes does not lead to irreversible consequences or their destruction.

The work of the internal systems of an organism aims to maintain homeostasis, one of the parameters of which, for warm-blooded creatures, is body temperature. Thus, for example, the normal temperature of internal organs is in the range of 36 °C–37.5 °C in humans, 38.7 °C–39.8 °C in pigs, and 40.6 °C–43 °C in chickens. Fish and amphibians have no thermoregulatory mechanism, so their temperature is the same as the ambient temperature and can vary from 0 °C to 40 °C, depending on the species. As for insects, they have a partial thermoregulatory mechanism that allows them to maintain an acceptable temperature in certain parts of the body. Since all species of living beings possess a nervous system, it is reasonable to say that the nervous system is quite stable in the temperature range of 0 °C–40 °C. Let us then ask the question of how much local heating of the nervous tissue of an organism is acceptable and what can be related to it. For this purpose, we need to consider the properties of the phospholipid membrane in which the ion channels are embedded.

In biological membranes, the lipid layer is a liquid with a viscosity similar to that of sunflower oil. When the temperature drops, the lipid layer of the membrane 'freezes' and essentially turns into a two-dimensional crystal, as shown in figure 3.1.

Figure 3.2 shows the heat capacity profile of porcine spinal cord membranes [5]. The gray peak corresponds to lipid melting, and the dashed line represents the body temperature of pigs (~39.3 °C). Two additional peaks above the body temperature correspond to the transformation of proteins embedded in the membrane.

It should be noted that, unlike water, where the ice–liquid temperature difference is a fraction of a degree, in a lipid membrane, part of the membrane can be crystalline and part can be in a liquid state over a wide temperature range. The presence of two additional peaks shown in figure 3.1 is due to protein unfolding at 56.5 °C and 79 °C. At the same time, if the membrane is heated to 85 °C–90 °C and then cooled, only one of the three peaks remains, which is associated with the

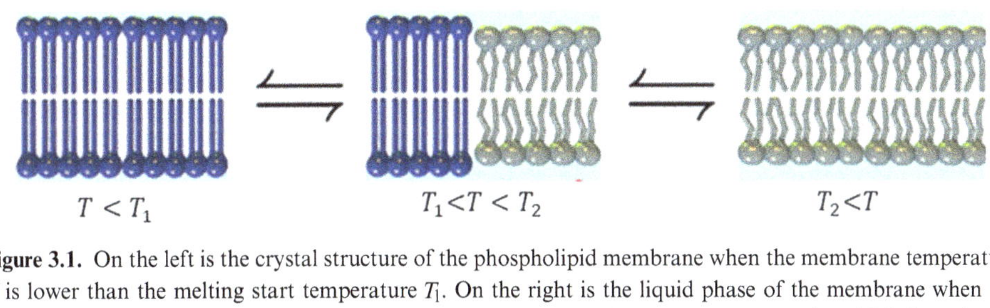

Figure 3.1. On the left is the crystal structure of the phospholipid membrane when the membrane temperature T is lower than the melting start temperature T_1. On the right is the liquid phase of the membrane when the membrane temperature T is higher than the membrane melting end temperature T_2. In the middle is a mixture of liquid and crystalline phases of the membrane when $T_1 < T < T_2$.

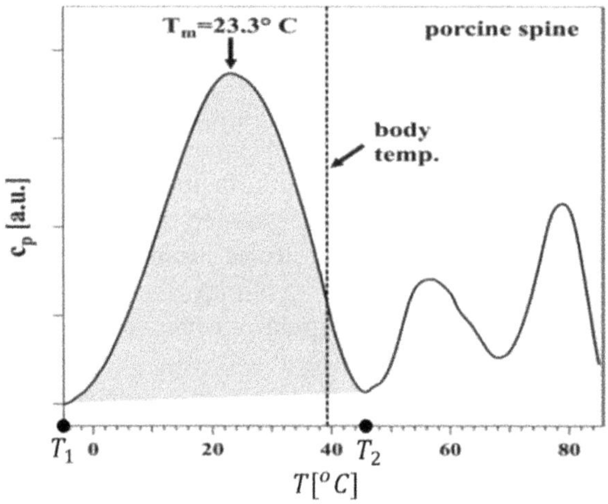

Figure 3.2. Temperature dependence of the specific heat capacity of the porcine spinal cord membrane. The gray-shaded peak represents lipid melting. The dashed line represents the body temperature of pigs (~39.3 °C). The peaks above the body temperature indicate protein unfolding (the transformation of proteins embedded in the membrane). Point T_1 corresponds to the beginning of the melting process of the membrane, and T_2 corresponds to the end. To the left of point T_1, the membrane is in the crystalline state, and to the right of point T_2, it is in the liquid state. Reprinted from [5], Copyright (2018), with permission from Elsevier.

melting of the phospholipid membrane. In other words, heating the membrane to a temperature close to the transformation temperature of the proteins embedded in it leads to irreversible processes; after cooling, the transformed protein remains in its changed configuration and cannot perform the functions it performed previously. This statement is true for all membranes in which proteins are embedded (see e.g., [6, 7]).

Since the melting peak is quite broad, a natural question is: What part of the phospholipid membrane at a given temperature is in crystalline form, and what part is in liquid form? The answer is quite simple. If we consider that the heat capacity of the crystalline structure up to the melting point T_1 is almost the same as that of the liquid structure above the melting point T_2 (see figure 3.2), we can determine that the total energy required for the formation of the liquid phase of the membrane is:

$$q_{\text{crystalline}\rightarrow\text{liquid}} = \int_{T_1}^{T_2} (c_p - c_{0,\,p})\mathrm{d}T, \tag{3.1}$$

where $c_{0,\,p}$ is the value of the heat capacity at the temperature T_1 at which melting begins. Accordingly, the ratio of the mass of the membrane in the liquid state m_l to the total membrane mass $m_l + m_c$ (m_c is the mass of the membrane in the crystalline form) at a fixed temperature $T(T_1 \leq T \leq T_2)$ is as follows:

$$\alpha_l = \frac{m_l}{m_l + m_c} = \frac{\int_{T_1}^{T} (c_p - c_{0,\,p})\mathrm{d}T}{\int_{T_1}^{T_2} (c_p - c_{0,\,p})\mathrm{d}T}. \tag{3.2}$$

Temperature dependencies of the specific heat capacity similar to those shown in figure 3.2 have also been obtained for lung surfactants [5, 6, 8], membranes of *Escherichia coli* [8], membranes of *Bacillus subtilis* [8], and various types of cancer cells [7]. Surprisingly, the melting temperature of all biological membranes is 10–20 degrees below body temperature [5, 8]; that is, the temperature at which part of the membrane is in the crystalline phase and part in the liquid phase is normal for the vital activity of a living organism. Therefore, a shift in the membrane melting temperature is a deviation from normal homeostasis and necessarily affects the vital activity of the organism. Accordingly, the heating (or cooling) of membranes under the influence of external factors should not significantly disturb the balance between the liquid and crystalline phases of the phospholipid membrane and should not lead to irreversible changes in the conformation of the proteins embedded in the membrane.

Warm-blooded animals maintain an almost constant temperature due to their metabolism, and the heat capacity of their membranes corresponds to this temperature. As for the membranes of fish, reptiles, microbes, and bacteria, whose temperature is equal to the ambient temperature, the question naturally arises of whether the heat capacity of their membranes changes when the ambient temperature changes. As an example, figure 3.3 shows plots of the specific heat capacity of *E. coli* grown at 37 °C and 15 °C. It can be seen that in both cases, the positions of the peaks corresponding to the transformation of the proteins embedded in the

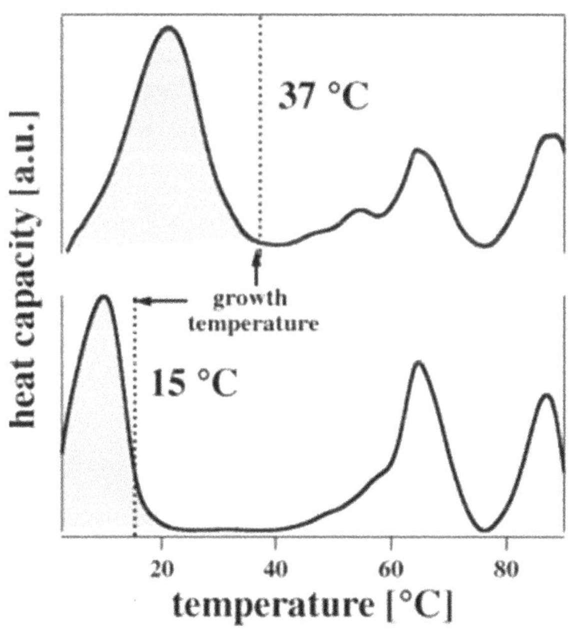

Figure 3.3. Temperature dependencies of heat capacity profiles of *E. coli* membranes grown at 37 °C (top) and 15 °C (bottom). The dashed lines represent growth temperature. The lipid melting peak (shaded gray) adapts to growth temperature, whereas the protein unfolding peaks remain unaltered. Reprinted from [9].

membrane (to the right of the temperature at which cell growth occurred) coincide. It can be concluded from figure 3.3 that the adaptation of cold-blooded organisms to ambient temperature occurs at the level of cell membranes.

The 'freezing' point depends on many factors: lipid composition, ion concentration, hydrostatic pressure, pH, and anesthetic concentration. Below, we will consider the influence of anesthetics and pH on the position of the melting point.

3.2 Influence of anesthetic drugs and pH on membrane phase transitions

Anesthetics are a class of drugs that block the propagation of action potentials in nerve tissue, resulting in the loss of the sensation of pain. Anesthetics can be molecules with completely different chemical compositions. Anesthetics include the noble gas xenon (Xe), laughing gas (N_2O), diethyl ether ($(C_2H_5)_2O$), and many other alcohols, as well as more complex molecules, such as propofol ($C_{12}H_{18}O$) or thiopental ($C_{11}H_{18}N_2O_2S$). As the consideration of the mechanisms of anesthetic effects on action potential propagation is beyond the scope of our book, we will only consider their effect on the state of the phospholipid membrane.

Figure 3.4 shows the changes in the specific heat capacity of artificial membranes as a function of the concentration of different anesthetics [10]. It can be seen that the melting point shifts to the left with increasing anesthetic concentration. This is probably due to the fact that anesthetics embedded in the membrane alter the phospholipid bonds, unlike ion channels and other proteins embedded in the membrane.

Figure 3.5 shows the dependence of the specific heat capacity of the *E. coli* membrane at different pH values. As the pH increases, the peak of the specific heat capacity shifts to the left.

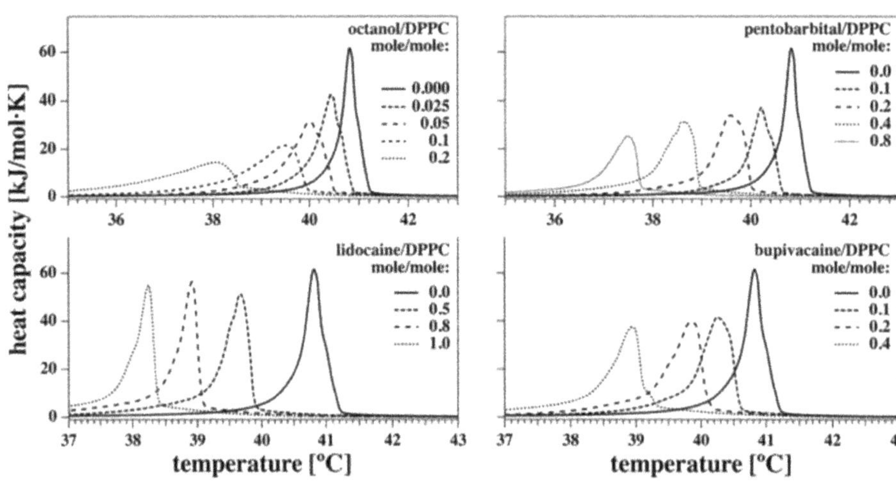

Figure 3.4. Decrease in melting point for four different anesthetics at different concentrations. The alcohol octanol and the barbiturate pentobarbital are general anesthetics, while lidocaine and bupivacaine are local anesthetics. Reprinted from [10], Copyright (2014), with permission from Elsevier.

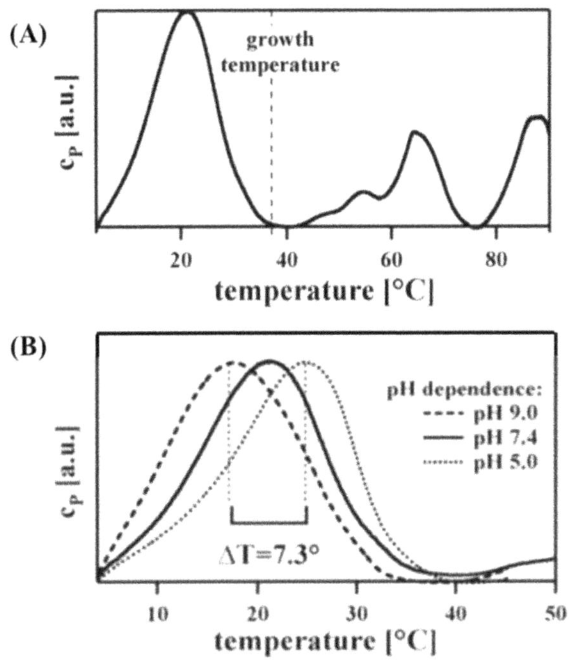

Figure 3.5. (A) Melting profile of *E. coli* membranes. (B) pH dependence of the lipid melting peak of *E. coli* membranes. Reprinted from [11], Copyright (2007), with permission from Elsevier.

3.3 Conclusions

Based on the material presented in this chapter, in the rest of this book, we will consider effects to be nonthermal if they meet the following criteria: (i) they occur in the phospholipid membrane of nerve tissue; (ii) they cause only insignificant changes in the local temperature of the membrane; (iii) such temperature changes do not lead to any physiological consequences; and (iv) the membrane remains in the same phase (i.e. liquid, crystalline, or a mixed phase).

References

[1] Azizi M S N, Aris N A, Salleh A, Othman A and Mohamad N R 2015 Non-ionizing electromagnetic radiation effect on nerve fiber action potential of human body—a review *J. Teknologi* **77** 31

[2] 2019 *Biological and Medical Aspects of Electromagnetic Fields* 4th edn ed B Greenebaum and F Barnes (Boca Raton FL: CRC Press)

[3] Zhao X, Dong G and Wang C 2021 The non-thermal biological effects and mechanisms of microwave exposure *Int. J. Radiat. Res.* **19** 483

[4] Mumtaz S, Rana J N, Choi E H and Han I 2022 Microwave radiation and the brain: mechanisms, current status, and future prospects *Int. J. Mol. Sci.* **23** 9288

[5] Wang T, Mužić T, Jackson A D and Heimburg T 2018 The free energy of biomembrane and nerve excitation and the role of anesthetics *Biochim. Biophys. Acta* **1860** 2145

[6] Ebel H, Grabitz P and Heimburg T 2001 Enthalpy and volume changes in lipid membranes I. The proportionality of heat and volume changes in the lipid melting transition and its implication for the elastic constants *J. Phys. Chem.* B **105** 7353
[7] Højholt K L, Mužić T, Jensen S D, Bilgin M, Nylandsted J, Heimburg T, Frandsen S K and Gehl J 2019 Calcium electroporation and electrochemotherapy for cancer treatment: importance of cell membrane composition investigated by lipidomics, calorimetry and *in vitro* efficacy *Sci. Rep.* **9** 4758
[8] Heimburg T and Jackson A D 2005 On soliton propagation in biomembranes and nerves *Proc. Natl. Acad. Sci.* **102** 9790
[9] Heimburg T 2009 *Physical Properties of Biological Membranes* arXiv:0902.2454 [physics.bio-ph]
[10] Græsbøll K, Sasse-Middelhoff H and Heimburg T 2014 The thermodynamics of general and local anesthesia *Biophys. J.* **106** 2143
[11] Heimburg T and Jackson A D 2007 The thermodynamics of general anesthesia *Biophys. J.* **92** 3159

IOP Publishing

Low-Intensity Control of Nerve Tissue Activity

Mikhail N Shneider and Mikhail Pekker

Chapter 4

Nonthermal weak microwave field impact on nerve fiber activity

In this chapter, we consider the experimental evidence and theoretical basis for the effects of microwave radiation on neuronal action potential thresholds. We discuss how these effects can result from the redistribution of transmembrane protein ion channels caused by the forced acoustic vibrations of the axon membrane under the influence of microwave radiation. In addition, we explain that the excitation of longitudinal membrane oscillations has a resonant character, with the lowest harmonics in the range of 30–100 GHz. The possibility of initiating or blocking action potentials in nervous tissue is also discussed.

4.1 Brief introductory overview

Studies of the effects of weak (nonthermal) microwave radiation on cellular structures began in the 1960s and 1970s with the pioneering work of Devyatkov *et al* in the Soviet Union [1–3] and Fröhlich in the West [4–6]. These early studies clearly demonstrated that the response of cells to microwave radiation is highly selective. At certain frequencies, the cellular response becomes extremely strong. Although different investigators reported different values of resonant frequencies obtained in experiments, all of these frequencies were in the range of tens of gigahertz [7, 8] (see, for example, figure 4.1, taken from [8]).

The reason for the resonant interaction of the microwave with the cells has been explained either by natural oscillations inherent to the cells themselves or by separate molecular structures or individual molecules [1–6]. However, a clear understanding of the mechanism of microwave interaction with cells has not yet been achieved. As an example, we offer this quote from a relatively recent review [9]: 'The energy of MiliMeterWave radiation is too low to directly disrupt any

doi:10.1088/978-0-7503-6034-0ch4

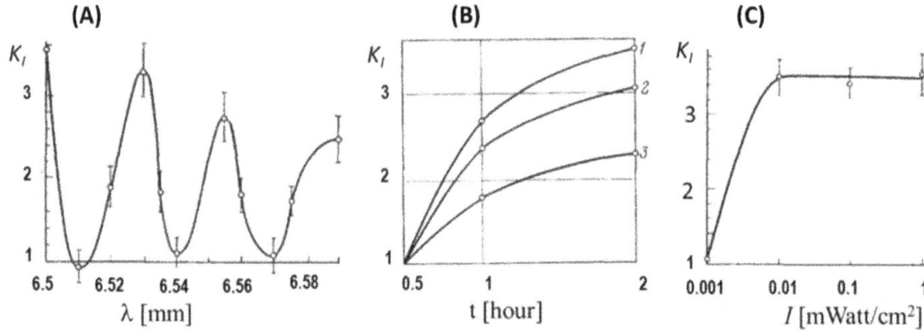

Figure 4.1. Dependencies of K_I colicin synthesis induction in *E. coli* C600(E1) under microwave radiation: (A) on the wavelength, (B) on the exposure time, and (C) on the microwave intensity. Reproduced with permission from [8]. © Uspekhi Fizicheskikh Nauk 1973.

biochemical interaction, such as van der Waals or hydrogen bonds. Only a resonance-type interaction might lead to an appreciable biological effect. However, the existence of such a resonance at the cellular level remains unknown. According to the literature, cell membranes represent a promising potential target and this topic requires further experimental investigations in the coming years.'

It should be noted that many experiments have revealed the threshold character of microwave influence [8, 10, 11]. An example of stimulated cell activity was presented in [8], which studied the effect of microwave radiation on the synthesis of colicin in *Escherichia coli* C600(E1). The dependencies of the measured induction coefficient K_I (K_I is the ratio of the number of cells that synthesize colicin when exposed to microwaves to the number of cells that synthesize colicin without being affected by microwaves) on the wavelength, exposure time, and intensity of radiation are shown in figure 4.1. It can be seen that the effect of microwave radiation has a pronounced threshold and resonant nature and that it depends on the exposure time. At a certain minimum intensity, saturation was reached: the effect of radiation on the organism did not change, even if the intensity was increased $\sim$1000 times.

Apparently, Fröhlich was the first to point out the coincidence of the resonant frequencies of microwave radiation with the frequencies of the natural transverse vibrations of the cell membrane [4–6]. Indeed, if we consider the cell membrane as a thin plate of thickness $d_m = 9$ nm (the thickness of the membrane is in the range of 7–10 nm [14–16]), and assume, as in [12, 13], that the speed of sound in membranes is close to the speed of sound in water $c_s \approx 1500$ m s^{-1}, then the frequency of the pth acoustic harmonic in it is equal to:

$$f_{r,p} \approx \frac{c_s}{4d_m}(2p - 1) = 41.6(2p - 1)\ [\text{GHz}]. \tag{4.1}$$

Note that based on the data on Young's modulus in the lipid membrane given in [17, 18], the estimated speed of sound in the membrane is much slower than the speed of sound in water, with an approximate value of $c_s \sim 300$ m s^{-1} [19]. Therefore, according to (4.1), the minimum resonant frequency is $f_{r,\,1} \approx 8.3$ GHz, which is more than four times slower than that observed in experiments. Note that in section 4.8 of this chapter, we show that the resonant frequency resulting from electromagnetic oscillations of the membrane is equal to $f_{r,\,p} = \frac{c_S}{d_m}p$, which gives $f_{r,\,1} = 34.7$ GHz for $d_m = 9$ nm.

In his works, Fröhlich assumed that the relationship between the natural oscillations of the membrane and microwave radiation is due to proteins 'floating' in the membrane that have a dipole moment. He proposed a hypothesis of Bose condensation of sound waves in the membrane [4], which has not been confirmed experimentally, since free vibrations at ultrasonic frequencies are strongly damped. However, Fröhlich's theoretical work drew the attention of physicists to the problem of the interaction of microwaves with the membrane and stimulated the search for the mechanisms of this interaction.

Another mechanism of microwave interaction with cell membranes is the interaction of the microwave electric field with the charges on the membrane surface. Therefore, the question of the charge on the membrane surface is key to understanding the interaction of cells with electromagnetic fields. If the membrane is electrically neutral, the electromagnetic field can have only a negligible effect on the membrane due to its interaction with the dipole heads of the phospholipids and proteins in the membrane, which have a dipole moment. If the membrane is charged and ions are bound to its surface strongly enough, the electric component of the electromagnetic field causes the membrane to deform. If the ions bound to the surface are relatively weak, the ions on the membrane surface move freely along its surface without having any effect on it. The question of the value of the surface charge of cell membranes has been studied in many experimental works. We will not go into all the papers; we refer only to [20, 21], where experimental data for the surface charges of cell membranes are obtained by different methods. The range of values obtained for the surface charge density is quite broad: $\sigma_m = 0.002 - 0.3\ \mathrm{C\,m^{-2}}$. In the next chapter, we discuss the surface charge of the lipid membrane, which can interact with the electric field of the microwave radiation and give rise to longitudinal mechanical oscillations.

In [13, 22, 23], Krasil'nikov considered several model problems related to the oscillations of a charged thin shell that mimics the cell membrane located in a liquid electrolyte under the influence of a periodic electric field. The resonant frequency and Q-factor corresponding to the natural oscillations of the membrane of spherical vesicles are found in [22, 23]. The obtained results were used to evaluate the displacement of the free ions in the vicinity of the shell. However, major questions remained unanswered: what is the value of the surface charge of the membrane (it was assumed to be given), how strongly is the surface charge bound to the membrane, and what is the mechanism of action of weak electromagnetic fields on cellular processes?

The effect of millimeter waves on nerves has been studied experimentally in many works. The results obtained were quite contradictory. In some studies, an increase in nerve activity was observed under the influence of millimeter waves, while in others, the suppression of activity (stimulation of the action potential) was noted, and in others, the effect was not observed to any notable degree. The most systematic study of the effect of millimeter waves on nerve tissue was first conducted in [24]. After 20 min of nerve irradiation with microwave radiation at an intensity of 2–3 mW cm^{-2}, the frequency of action potential excitation only increased by 2%–3%. Based on these measurements, the authors of [24] concluded that millimeter microwave (MMW) radiation has practically no effect on the excitation thresholds of action potentials in nervous tissue. However, the authors of another paper [25] came to the opposite conclusion, namely that MMW radiation can significantly affect the excitation of nerve tissue. In the experiments reported in [25], the hind leg of an anesthetized mouse was irradiated with microwave radiation at a frequency of 42 GHz. After irradiation, the excitation of the sural sensory nerve was monitored for 1 min. At irradiation intensities of 45–220 mW cm^{-2}, skin temperature increased by 1.7 °C–4.5 °C, and calf nerve excitation was suppressed by 44%. In the control experiment, the same calf nerve sample was irradiated with an infrared radiation source so that the temperature of the sample was also increased by 4.5 °C, and the excitation of the calf nerve was suppressed by 40%. However, while nerve stimulation was observed for 20–40 s when MMW radiation was turned on, followed by stimulation suppression, no excitation phase was observed when an infrared heat source was used. The possibility of the opposite effect on the sensory sural nerve—its stimulation and suppression—was considered unexpected by the authors of [25]. However, the effects of MMWs on neural tissue in [24, 25] and others have been studied only in whole nerve preparations. In [26], the effect of millimeter radiation on separate groups of neurons was investigated for the first time. The authors used slices of cortical tissue to evaluate the effects of MMW on individual pyramidal neurons under conditions that mimic their *in vivo* environment.

Experiments have shown that relatively weak microwave radiation at intensities of 0.01–0.1 W m^{-2} in the range of 50–100 GHz leads to spontaneous excitation of neuronal activity [26]. The experimental scheme is shown in figure 4.2. The

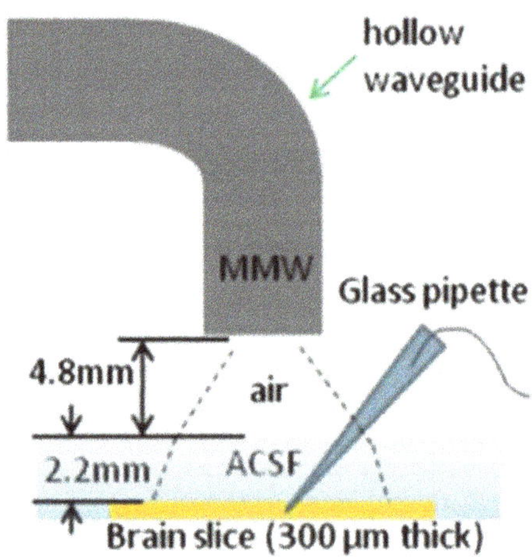

Figure 4.2. Schematic showing the probe geometry and spacing used to calculate the beam profile and power distribution at the tissue slice. ACSF: artificial cerebrospinal fluid. Reproduced from [26]. © 2010 IOP Publishing Ltd.

interaction of microwave radiation with a nerve fiber was studied in [26] using a mouse cerebral cortex placed in artificial cerebrospinal fluid and irradiated with plane-polarized microwaves at a frequency of 60.125 GHz. At that frequency, the attenuation length of the microwave radiation was ~ 0.02 cm (figure 4.11(C)), so the effective power of microwave radiation directly affecting nerve tissue in the experiments [26] varied from several tens of nW cm^{-2} to 1000 nW cm^{-2}, according to the authors' calculations.

Let us briefly describe the scheme of the experiments conducted in [26]. The duration of an experiment was usually 25–30 min. To ensure the stability of neuronal excitation during the entire measurement time, the depolarizing current was intracellularly injected at a duty cycle of 25% (figure 4.3(A)). Various MMW power levels were applied to the slice in a randomized order to eliminate any possible effects of cumulative exposure. Each exposure lasted 60 s (or three 20 s cycles). In some experiments, microwave irradiation led to an increase in the excitation frequency of the action potential (lowering the excitation threshold), while in others, it led to suppression of the action potential (raising the excitation threshold). The aforementioned figure shows a sample recording of neuronal activity (membrane voltage, V_m) and injected membrane current (I_m) versus time at three applied power levels.

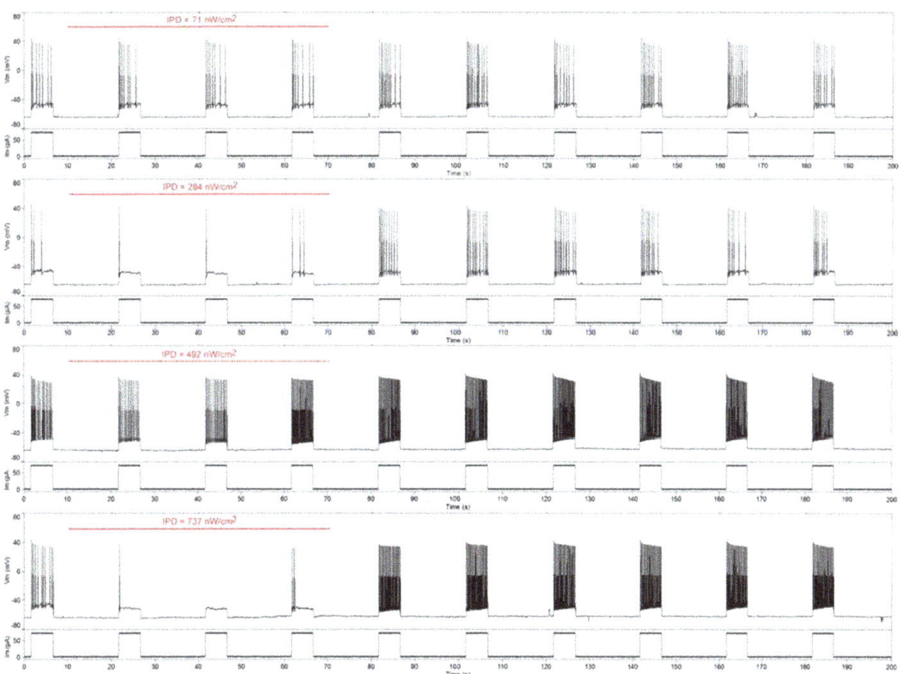

Figure 4.3(A). Sample recording of neuronal activity (membrane voltage, V_m) and injected membrane current (I_m) against time at three power levels applied for 1 min. The red bars indicate the time and duration of exposure. For each sequence above, the neuron was stimulated for 5 s and allowed to rest for 20 s. As the power was increased, strong inhibition of the neuron action potential firing rate was seen during the exposure. Excitation was also observed. In all cases, the neuron returned to pre-exposure firing rates within 6 min. Reproduced from [26]. © 2010 IOP Publishing Ltd.

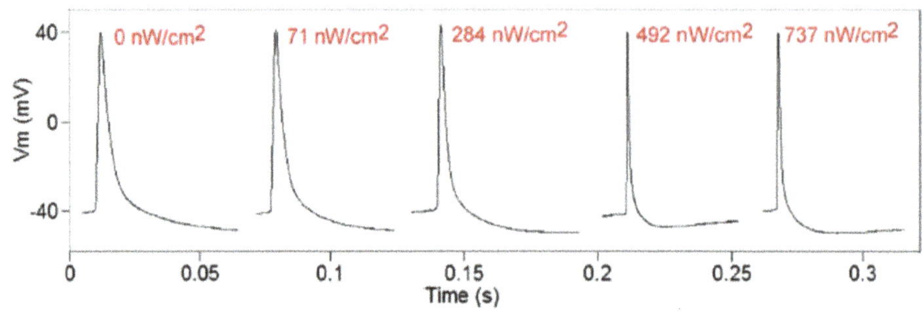

Figure 4.3(B). Typical action potential shapes versus microwave radiation intensity. Reproduced from [26]. © 2010 IOP Publishing Ltd.

Figure 4.3(A) also shows an example measurement for three microwave power values. With increasing microwave irradiation intensity, a significant increase in the frequency of membrane self-excitation after microwave irradiation (figure 4.3(A)) and a shortening of the recovery time of the resting membrane potential (figure 4.3(B)) were observed in the experiments. The results obtained in [26] seem surprising. For example, figure 4.3(A) shows that at a microwave intensity of 492 nW cm^{-2}, the frequency of action potential self-excitation is higher than at an intensity of 71 nW cm^{-2} and increases toward the end of the exposure. However, at an intensity of 737 nW cm^{-2}, the action potential is not excited at all. In other words, as the intensity of microwave radiation increases, the threshold for action potential excitation decreases, but at a certain critical value of microwave intensity, the action potential is blocked. However, it is noteworthy that after switching off the microwave radiation, the frequency of action potential excitation in the cases of 71 and 492 nW cm^{-2} does not change for quite a long time. In the third case, at an intensity of 737 nW cm^{-2}, the action potential is excited after switching off the microwave radiation, which completely blocks the action potential excitation. According to the authors of [26], the results obtained cannot be explained by the thermal effect, since the microwave intensities are too low to change the temperature of the membrane and the cerebrospinal fluid (CSF) solution. Note that, as will be shown below, the frequency of the microwave source selected in [22] is close to the resonant frequency of the natural oscillations of the membrane.

A natural question arises as to the exact mechanism of forced excitation of the action potential in the experiment reported in [26]. In fact, the intensity of the microwave radiation in [25] was so low that it could not noticeably change the membrane temperature. Moreover, the forced oscillations of the charged membrane mentioned in [13, 22, 23], for example, cannot by themselves cause the initiation of the action potential or be the reason for the continued excitation of the action potential after the microwave source is turned off.

As noted in chapter 1, section 1.4, transmembrane ion channels (and some other proteins) are not fixed at specific locations on the membrane and can be moved by lateral diffusion (the corresponding lateral diffusion coefficients are in the range $D_L = 10^{-13}$–10^{-14} s^{-2} [27–29]). Changes in the local surface density of sodium ion channels affect the action potential excitation thresholds (see figure 1.34). Therefore, it can be assumed that microwave radiation somehow redistributes ion channels in the region of the initial segments where the action potential is initiated, which explains the results of the experiments reported in [26].

Before proceeding to a qualitative picture of the effect of microwave radiation on the excitability of the action potential, it is important to note that the experiments [26] were performed with plane-polarized microwave radiation at a frequency of 60.125 GHz. Two important conclusions follow:

1. The microwave frequency at which the experiments were performed was in the range of the resonant frequencies determined by formula (4.1).
2. Since the experiments used a mouse cerebral cortex immersed in CSF [26], the electric field of plane-polarized radiation was directed along the axons of at least some of the neurons.

This section is reproduced with permission from [33].

4.2 Effect of low-intensity microwave radiation on the neuron: qualitative picture

A schematic representation of a neuron interacting with microwave radiation is shown in figure 4.4. The arrow indicates the direction of microwave incidence. Assume that the microwave is polarized so that the electric field is directed along the axon. The myelinated segment of the axon is also shown. The thickness of the membrane, as mentioned above, is in the range of 7–10 nm [14–16], while the typical size of the axon initial segment (AIS) is in the range of 20–60 μm [30]. The other parameters of the myelinated axon can be found in chapter 1, section 1.6.

Typical dimensions of the AIS for all types of axons are much smaller than microwave wavelengths corresponding to frequencies ranging from tens to hundreds

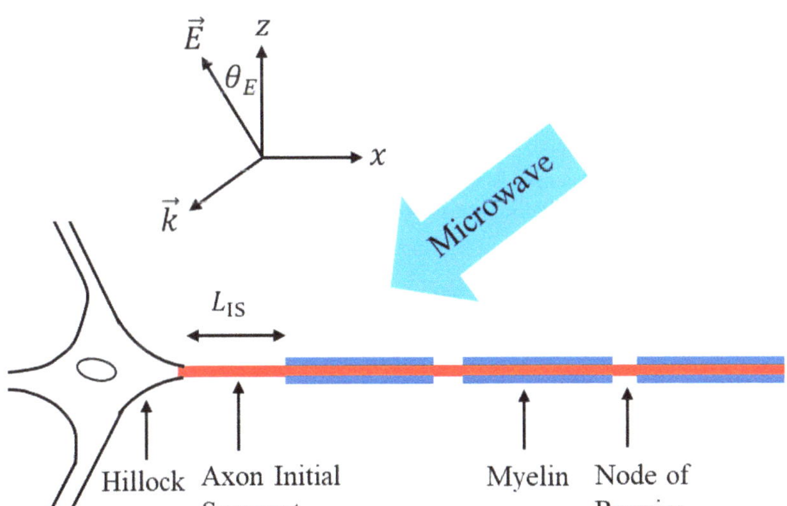

Figure 4.4. Scheme of a neuron, showing the characteristic segments of the myelinated axon interacting with an arbitrarily directed plane-polarized microwave field (see also figure 1.35).

of gigahertz, so we can assume that the electric field acting on the charged surface of the AIS membrane is uniform in space and varies only in time. Since the AIS is bounded at one end by a hillock and at the other by a myelin sheath (figure 4.4), we can think of the charged AIS membrane as a plate clamped at the ends (figure 4.5). This is because the membrane thickness is several orders of magnitude thinner than the diameter of the thinnest neuron. Displacements of the membrane in the case where the charges on the inner and outer sides of the membrane have different signs are shown in figure 4.5(A), and displacements in the case where the charges of the surfaces have the same sign are shown in figure 4.5(B). Forced oscillations of a charged elastic plate in an alternating electric field have pronounced resonances. The corresponding characteristic resonant frequencies are $\omega_{r,\,p} \approx \pi p c_s/d_m$, where c_s is the longitudinal velocity of sound in the membrane $p = 1,\ 2,\ \ldots$ (section 4.8 of this chapter, [19, 31–34]).

Forced longitudinal vibrations of the plate membrane lead to a redistribution of transmembrane proteins (ion channels) due to acoustic radiation pressure (see section 4.3 of this chapter [30–35]). In the case of excitation of a longitudinal standing acoustic wave in the membrane, ion channels are shifted to the edges, and either a rarefied area is formed in the center or condensation occurs in the center, forming a rarefied area at the edges (figure 4.6). The density of ion channels at the edges or in the center depends on the ratio of phospholipid membrane density ρ_m to the ion channel density ρ_p. If $\varsigma = \rho_m/\rho_p < 5/2$, the channels in the standing-wave

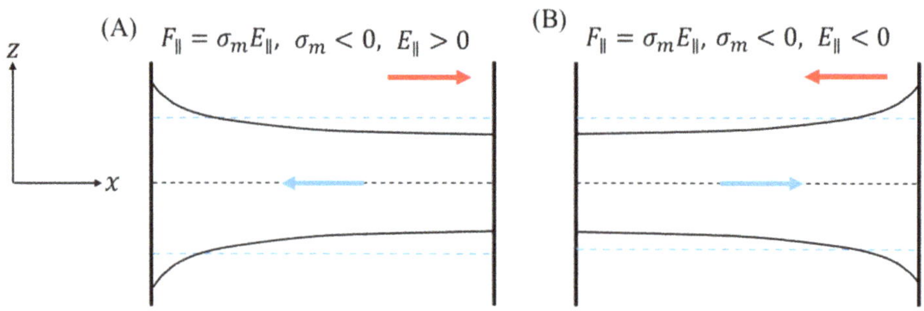

Figure 4.5. Membrane deformations caused by a microwave electric field. The edges of the membrane (unlimited in the y-direction) are clamped. Blue arrows indicate elastic displacements inside the membrane, red arrows the direction of the electric field. (A) corresponds to $E_{\|} > 0$, (B)—to $E_{\|} < 0$.

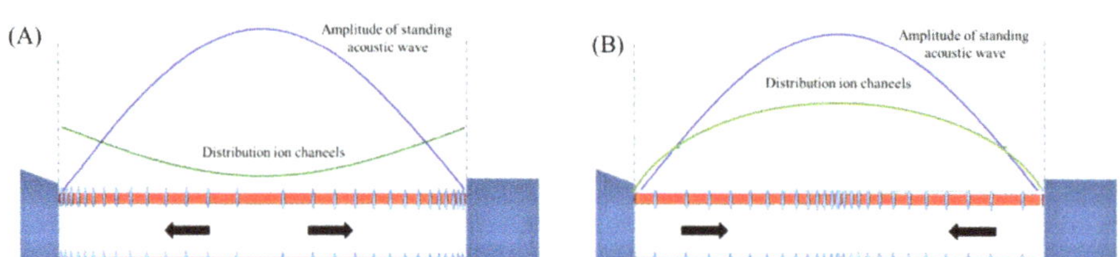

Figure 4.6. An example of the redistribution of transmembrane ion channels under the influence of acoustic radiation pressure. Arrows indicate the direction of the forces acting on the ion channel protein. (A) corresponds to $\varsigma = \rho_m/\rho_p \approx 1$, (B) – to $\varsigma > 5/2$.

field are densified at the edges, whereas if $\varsigma > 5/2$, they are densified in the center (see section 4.3 of this chapter, or [31–35]).

The redistribution of sodium transmembrane channels caused by longitudinal acoustic vibrations leads to a decrease in the excitation threshold of the action potential (or spike) in the areas of increased surface density of ion channels. With significant rarefaction and a sufficiently long rarefied region, it is possible to block action potential propagation (see section 4.4 of this chapter).

Note that the vibrations of the membrane in the electromagnetic wave field are forced. Although they are similar to the oscillations of a sound wave, they cannot be called acoustic, because the frequency of the oscillations and the wavelength are not related by the dispersion relation that is valid for a sound wave $\lambda_s f_s = c_s$, where λ_s is the wavelength, f_s is the frequency of the wave, and c_s is the speed of sound. The wavelength of the considered forced oscillations of the membrane is determined by the size of the initial segment, and the frequency is determined by the frequency of the incident microwave wave.

4.3 Lateral diffusion and drift of transmembrane proteins in an acoustic field

In this section, we answer questions about the reason for the redistribution of transmembrane channels and how long it takes [31–34].

It is a well-known fact in acoustics that suspended particles in the field of a traveling wave are displaced either to the region of maximum intensity of acoustic oscillations or to the region of minimum intensity. In the field of a standing wave, suspended particles are collected in antinodes in the nodal regions [35, 36]. The direction of displacement of the suspended particles is determined by their density relative to the density of the medium.

For simplicity, we assume that the sodium channel is not a cylinder but an incompressible sphere with a radius of $r_p = d_m/2 \ll \lambda_s$, where λ_s is the ultrasonic wavelength. For numerical estimates, we use a simple analytical formula derived for spherical particles in an ultrasonic field. We expect that for real channels (of cylindrical shape), the results would not be very different.

The acoustic radiation force acting on the incompressible sphere of radius $r_p \ll \lambda_s$ due to the traveling sound wave is [37]:

$$F_{\text{tr}} = 4\pi r_p{}^6 k_s{}^4 \overline{E}_s \frac{1 + \frac{2}{9}(1 - \varsigma)^2}{(2 + \varsigma)^2}, \tag{4.2}$$

or, in a plane standing sound wave, it is:

$$F_{\text{st}} = 2\pi r_p{}^3 k_s \overline{E}_s \sin(2k_s x) \frac{1 + \frac{2}{3}(1 - \varsigma)}{2 + \varsigma}, \tag{4.3}$$

where

$$\overline{E}_s = \frac{1}{2}\rho_0 \omega_s^2 A_s^2 \tag{4.4}$$

is the energy density in the sound wave; $\omega_s = 2\pi f_s$ is the angular frequency of the ultrasound; A_s is the amplitude of the oscillatory displacements in the wave; $k_s = \frac{2\pi}{\lambda_S} = \frac{c_S}{\omega_S}$ is the wave number; $\varsigma = \frac{\rho_0}{\rho_p}$, where ρ_0 and ρ_p are the densities of the medium and the particles, respectively; x is the position of a particle in the standing wave; $k_s = \frac{\pi n}{l}$, where $n = 1, 2, 3, \ldots$; and l is the length scale of the region in which the standing wave exists.

Note that the average density of the membrane depends on many factors, such as the temperature of the medium and the content of water molecules in its hydrophobic part. The value of the average density of the channel also differs from the average density of the protein due to the presence of the empty channel itself. Therefore, determining the exact value of the parameter ς is a separate problem that is beyond the scope of our considerations. However, all qualitative conclusions of this chapter and the obtained quantitative estimates remain valid for all possible values of the parameter ς.

It is easy to see that in a traveling wave, the force always acts on a suspended particle in one direction, regardless of its density, while in a standing wave, the force is positive if $\varsigma < 5/2$ and negative if $\varsigma > 5/2$. In other words, heavy particles in standing-wave fields move to the nodes of the standing wave, and light particles move to the wave's amplitude maxima (wave antinodes).

For the case of $\varsigma \approx 1$, equations (4.2) and (4.3) respectively reduce to:

$$F_{\mathrm{tr}} \approx \frac{4\pi}{9} r_p^6 k_s^4 \overline{E}_s, \tag{4.5}$$

$$F_{\mathrm{st}} \approx \frac{2\pi}{3} r_p^3 k_s \overline{E}_s \sin(2k_s x). \tag{4.6}$$

Taking, for example, the value $\varsigma \approx 3$, equations (4.2) and (4.3) have the form:

$$F_{\mathrm{tr}} \approx F_t = \frac{68}{225} \pi r_p{}^6 k_s^4 \overline{E}_s, \tag{4.7}$$

$$F_{\mathrm{st}} \approx \frac{2\pi}{15} r_p{}^3 k_s \overline{E}_s \sin(2k_s x). \tag{4.8}$$

The initial homogeneous distribution of transmembrane proteins is disturbed in the acoustic wave field. The transmembrane proteins drift under the influence of the acoustic radiation pressure until their forced drift is no longer compensated by the reverse diffusion flux. The continuity equation for the density of proteins per unit membrane area in the acoustic wave field is:

$$\frac{\partial n_{\mathrm{ch}}}{\partial t} + \mathrm{div}\vec{\Gamma} = 0;\ \vec{\Gamma} = \mu_L \vec{F} n_{\mathrm{ch}} - D_L \vec{\nabla} n_{\mathrm{ch}}. \tag{4.9}$$

Here, n_{ch} is the density of the protein channels per unit membrane area, D_L is the lateral diffusion coefficient, and μ_L is the lateral mobility of the transmembrane protein channels, which is related to the lateral diffusion coefficient and the local temperature by the Einstein relation:

$$\mu_L = D_L/k_B T. \tag{4.10}$$

We assume that the external force $\vec{F}$ associated with the pressure of a plane ultrasound wave on the transmembrane channels is directed only along the axis of the axon. Since the thickness of the membrane is much smaller than the radius of the axon, the membrane can be considered a flat plate, unbounded in a direction perpendicular to the wave propagation. In this case, equation (4.9) can be rewritten as follows:

$$\frac{\partial n_{\text{ch}}}{\partial t} = D_L \frac{\partial}{\partial x}\left(\frac{\partial n_{\text{ch}}}{\partial x} - \frac{F}{k_B T} n_{\text{ch}}\right). \tag{4.11}$$

4.4 Redistribution of transmembrane channels in a standing acoustic wave

Let us consider the possibility of a stimulated redistribution of transmembrane protein channels in the field of a standing ultrasound wave maintained in the initial segment of the axon. A standing wave can be obtained through the addition of two waves moving toward each other. In such a case, one of the waves can be formed by the reflection of the primary wave from an obstacle. Without going into the mechanism of excitation of acoustic oscillations in the axon membrane, which is discussed later in section 4.8 of this chapter, let us consider longitudinal standing sound waves excited in the membrane of the initial segment of the axon bounded by the hillock and the first myelinated segment shown in figure 4.7. The corresponding wave numbers for the harmonics of longitudinal standing waves are as follows:

$$k_n = \frac{\pi n}{L_{\text{IS}}}, \quad n = 1, 2, 3, \ldots. \tag{4.12}$$

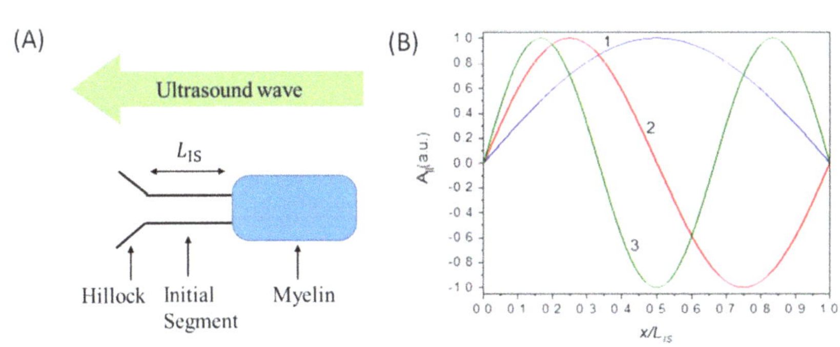

Figure 4.7. (A) Schematic view of ultrasonic waves acting on the initial segment. (B) Longitudinal displacement amplitude in the membrane. Line 1 corresponds to $k_1 = \frac{\pi}{L_{\text{IS}}}$, line 2 to $k_2 = \frac{2\pi}{L_{\text{IS}}}$, and line 3 to $k_3 = \frac{3\pi}{L_{\text{IS}}}$.

Under the influence of acoustic forces, the initially homogeneously distributed free protein ion channels are redistributed in the membrane of the initial segment. This continues until an equilibrium distribution is reached, where lateral diffusion compensates for the drift flux of the protein transmembrane channels:

$$\frac{\partial n_{\mathrm{ch}}}{\partial x} - \frac{F}{k_B T} n_{\mathrm{ch}} = 0. \tag{4.13}$$

Thus, the steady-state distribution of the protein channel density satisfies the Boltzmann distribution:

$$n_{\mathrm{ch}}(x) = n_0 \exp\left(-U(x)/k_B T\right) \tag{4.14}$$

with the potential

$$U(x) = -\int_0^x F(x)\mathrm{d}x. \tag{4.15}$$

The factor n_0 can be found from the conservation law for the total number of sodium channels along the length of the membrane:

$$n_{\mathrm{ch}}(x) = \frac{\exp\left(-\frac{U(x)}{k_B T}\right)}{\frac{1}{L_{\mathrm{IS}}}\int_0^{L_{\mathrm{IS}}} \exp\left(-\frac{U(x)}{k_B T}\right)\mathrm{d}x} n_{\mathrm{ch},\,0}, \tag{4.16}$$

where $n_{\mathrm{ch},\,0}$ is the undisturbed density of sodium channels per unit membrane area before the onset of acoustic forces.

For example, in the case of the ratio of membrane and protein channel densities of $\varsigma \approx 1$, it follows from equation (4.16) that:

$$\frac{n_{s,\,\mathrm{ch}}(x)}{n_{\mathrm{ch},\,0}} = \frac{\exp\left(-\frac{\frac{\pi}{3} r_p^3 \overline{E}_s (1-\cos(2k_n x))}{k_B T}\right)}{\frac{1}{L_{\mathrm{IS}}}\int_0^{L_{\mathrm{IS}}} \exp\left(-\frac{\frac{\pi}{3} r_p^3 \overline{E}_s (1-\cos(2k_n x))}{k_B T}\right) dx} = \frac{\exp\left(\xi_s \cos(2k_n x)\right)}{I_0(\xi_s)},\ \xi_s = \frac{\pi}{3}\frac{r_p^3 \overline{E}_s}{k_B T}, \tag{4.17}$$

where $n_{s,\,\mathrm{ch}}(x)$ is the longitudinal density distribution of sodium channels, $\overline{E}_s = \frac{1}{2}\rho_m \omega^2 A_s^2$ is the energy density of the standing ultrasound wave, ρ_m is the mean membrane density, and $I_0(\xi_s)$ is the modified Bessel function [38].

The difference between the maximum and minimum channel densities is:

$$\frac{\Delta n_{s,\,\mathrm{ch}}}{n_{\mathrm{ch},\,0}} = \frac{2\sinh(\xi_s)}{I_0(\xi_s)}. \tag{4.18}$$

Another example, taking a density ratio of $\varsigma \approx 3$, gives a similar expression:

$$\frac{\tilde{n}_{s,\mathrm{ch}}(x)}{\tilde{n}_{\mathrm{ch},0}} = \frac{\exp\left(\frac{\frac{\pi}{15}r_p^3\overline{E}_s(1-\cos(2k_n x))}{k_B T}\right)}{\frac{1}{L_{\mathrm{IS}}}\int_0^{L_{\mathrm{IS}}}\exp\left(\frac{\frac{\pi}{15}r_p^3\overline{E}_s(1-\cos(2k_n z))}{k_B T}\right)\left(1-\cos(2k_n x)\right)\mathrm{d}x} = \frac{\exp\left(-\tilde{\xi}_s\cos(2k_n x)\right)}{I_0\left(\tilde{\xi}_s\right)},\ \tilde{\xi}_s = \frac{\pi}{15}\frac{\pi r_p^3\overline{E}_s}{k_B T}. \tag{4.19}$$

The difference between the maximum and minimum channel densities is:

$$\frac{\Delta\tilde{n}_{s,\,\mathrm{ch}}}{n_{\mathrm{ch},\,0}} = \frac{2\sinh(\tilde{\xi}_s)}{I_0(\tilde{\xi}_s)}. \tag{4.20}$$

Figure 4.8 shows the dependencies of the equilibrium longitudinal distributions of sodium channels along the initial segment for the first harmonic ($n = 1$) of standing acoustic waves of different intensities.

Note that for the case $\varsigma \approx 1$ with $\xi_s > 1$, the sodium channels are almost completely shifted to the edges of the initial segment, while for $\varsigma \approx 3$ with $\tilde{\xi}_s > 1$, all channels are gathered in the central part of the initial segment. On the one hand, this can lower the excitation threshold of the action potential, since there are areas where the channel density is higher than in the unperturbed equilibrium. On the other hand, this can lead to a drastic increase in the action potential threshold and thus block the action potential due to the formation of regions with highly depleted transmembrane channel density.

Let us estimate the time Δt_s necessary to establish the equilibrium distribution (4.17) under the influence of an ultrasound acoustic pressure force F. It follows from equation (4.11) that the drift velocity of the ion channels is given by:

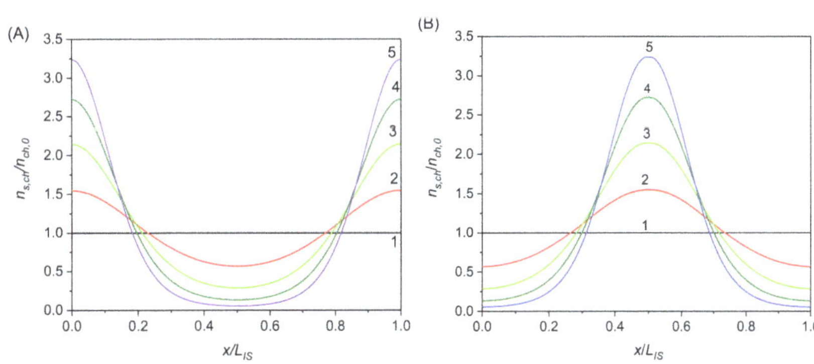

Figure 4.8. The relative densities of sodium channels along the initial segment interacting with the main mode of an ultrasonic standing wave ($n = 1$) for different values of the parameter ξ_s. In (A), $\varsigma \approx 1$. Line 1 relates to $\xi_s = 0$; line 2 to $\xi_s = 0.5$; line 3 to $\xi_s = 1$; line 4 to $\xi_s = 1.5$; and line 5 to $\xi_s = 2$. In (B), $\varsigma \approx 3$. Line 1 relates to $\tilde{\xi}_s = 0$; line 2 to $\tilde{\xi}_s = 0.5$; line 3 to $\tilde{\xi}_s = 1$; line 4 to $\tilde{\xi}_s = 1.5$; and line 5 to $\tilde{\xi}_s = 2$.

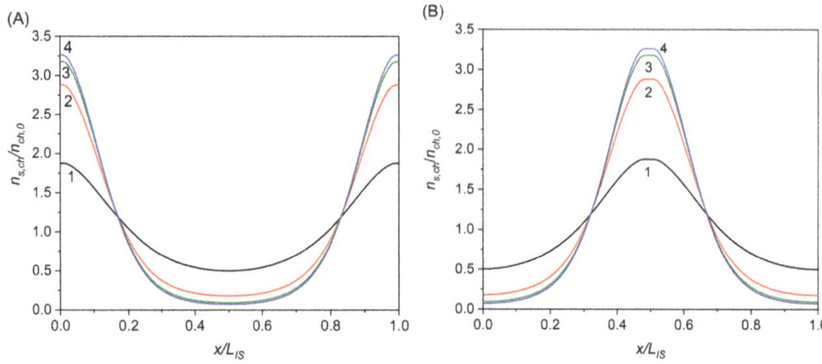

Figure 4.9. The relative densities of sodium channels along the initial segment interacting with the main mode of the ultrasound standing wave ($n = 1$) at different times. (A) corresponds to $\varsigma = 1$ and $\xi_s = 2$. (B) corresponds to $\varsigma = 3$ and $\tilde{\xi}_s = 2$. Lines labeled 1 relate to $t/t_D = 0.01$; lines 2, to $t/t_D = 0.03$; lines 3, to $t/t_D = 0.05$; and lines 4, to $t/t_D = 0.07$, where $t_D = L_{\rm IS}^2/D_L$.

$$V_d = \frac{D_L}{k_B T} F. \tag{4.21}$$

Thus, for the case of $\varsigma \approx 1$, we have:

$$t_s \approx \frac{L_{IS}}{2V_d} = \frac{L_{IS} \cdot k_B T}{2D_L F_s} = \frac{L_{IS}^2}{4\pi D_L \xi_s}, \tag{4.22}$$

and for $\varsigma \approx 3$, we have:

$$\tilde{t}_s \approx \frac{L_{IS}^2}{4\pi D_L \tilde{\xi}_s}. \tag{4.23}$$

Figure 4.9 shows the density of sodium channels at different moments in time obtained through the numerical solution of equation (4.7). It follows from figure 4.9 that, for $\xi_s = 2$ and $\tilde{\xi}_s = 2$, the formation of a new equilibrium distribution of ion channels happens very quickly, taking approximately $\frac{1}{4\pi\xi_s}$ of the characteristic time for lateral diffusion, $t_D = L_{\rm IS}^2/D_L$. In other words, the time required for the formation of regions of reduced or increased ion channel density is much shorter than the time required for channel density restoration after ultrasound exposure ends.

4.5 Ultrasound absorption during ion channel redistribution

A standing wave is formed by the superposition of two traveling waves. Each of these waves is absorbed by the medium as it propagates. Therefore, it is reasonable to assume that a standing wave is also an attenuator of ultrasound, with an absorption length that corresponds to the length of the traveling waves forming the standing wave. In the case of a traveling wave, the energy density of the acoustic waves decays due to viscosity as follows:

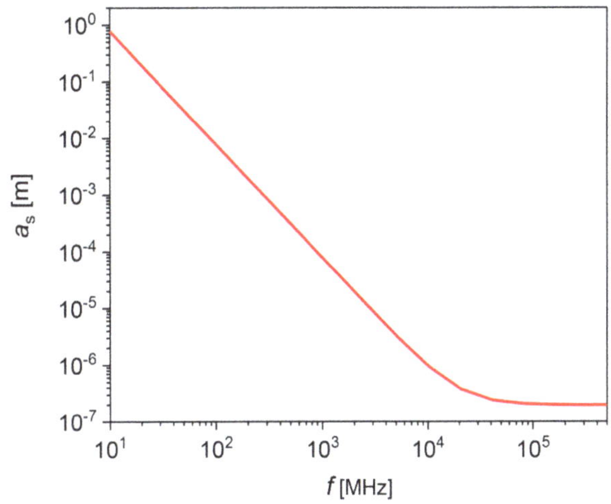

Figure 4.10. Sound attenuation length versus frequency in water.

$$\overline{E}(x) = \overline{E}_0 e^{-2x/a_s}, \tag{4.24}$$

where $a_s \approx c_s^3/\omega^2\nu$ is the attenuation length of sound waves,

$$\nu \approx \nu_0/(1 + \omega^2\tau^2) \tag{4.25}$$

is the kinematic viscosity in water [39, 40], $\nu_0 \approx 10^{-6}\,\mathrm{s}^{-1}$, $\tau \approx 8 \cdot 10^{-12}\,\mathrm{s}$ [41], and $c_s \approx 1450\,\mathrm{m\,s}^{-1}$ is the speed of sound in water. Figure 4.10 shows the dependency of the attenuation length a_s on the sound frequency in water.

To simplify the analysis and estimation in this section, we will limit ourselves to a consideration of ultrasound absorption in water, without considering the specific properties of lipid membranes. This is justified because the ultrasound source must be located at some distance from the nerve tissue and the scale of ultrasound absorption is much larger than the characteristic size of the initial segment of the axon. According to (4.17), the energy density in the standing wave of ultrasound leading to the redistribution of ion channels at $\varsigma \approx 1$ is:

$$\overline{E}_s = \frac{1}{2}\rho_0\omega^2 A_s^2 = \xi_s \frac{3k_B T}{\pi r_p^3}. \tag{4.26}$$

The corresponding sound intensity is:

$$P_s = \overline{E}_s c_s = \xi_s \frac{3k_B T c_s}{\pi r_p^3}, \tag{4.27}$$

and, according to (4.22), the energy absorbed by a unit volume of the medium per unit time is:

$$W_s \approx \frac{2P_s}{a_s} = \xi_s \frac{3k_B T c_s}{\pi r_p^3 a_s}. \tag{4.28}$$

The time required for channel redistribution depends on the ultrasonic intensity, which, as we have seen, can be reduced to a dependence on the dimensionless parameter ξ_s (figure 4.9). Taking $\xi_s = 2$ for certainty, we obtain from (4.22) that the redistribution time of the ion channels is of the order of $t_s \approx 0.04 L_{IS}^2/D_L$. Accordingly, the energy absorbed in a unit volume during this time and the corresponding temperature change are equal:

$$\Delta E_s = W_s t_s \approx 0.24 \frac{k_B T c_s}{\pi r_p^3 a_s} \frac{L_{IS}^2}{D_L}, \tag{4.29}$$

$$\Delta T_s = \frac{\Delta E_s}{\rho_0 c_p} = 0.24 \frac{k_B T c_s}{\pi r_p^3 \rho_0 a_s} \frac{L_{IS}^2}{D_L c_p}. \tag{4.30}$$

Suppose that the standing ultrasonic wave is maintained in the initial segment of the axon, with length $L_{IS} = 50$ μm. Thus, the frequency of the first harmonic of the standing wave $f_s = \frac{2c_s}{L_{IS}} \approx 60$ MHz, for which the characteristic absorption length is $a_s \approx 0.02$ m, as shown in figure 4.10. Substituting $T = 300\ K$, $r_p = 3 \cdot 10^{-9}$ m, and $D_L = 10^{-13}\ \mathrm{m^2\,s^{-1}}$ into (4.29) and (4.30), and taking into account the specific heat capacity of water, $c_p = 4200$ J/(kg·K), we get unrealistically high values for the absorbed energy density and temperature change: $\Delta E_a \approx 2.12 \cdot 10^{13}\ \mathrm{J\,m^{-3}}$ and $\Delta T_s \approx 5 \cdot 10^6$ K.

In these estimates, we do not consider phase transitions and heat removal due to heat conductivity. However, it is clear that the use of ultrasound to stimulate the redistribution of transmembrane channels leads to irreversible consequences and the destruction of the cell membrane at much lower values of sound intensity than those required. A similar pessimistic conclusion can be drawn from the consideration of traveling ultrasound waves. However, as mentioned in section 4.2 of this chapter, external microwave radiation can be used as a source of ultrasonic vibrations in the axonal membranes of nerve tissue. A possible example of the realization of such an interaction is the experiment [26] described earlier in section 4.1 of this chapter.

4.6 Microwave radiation in water and weak electrolytes

The penetration depth of microwave radiation is determined by its absorption in an aqueous solution and the skin effect in the intercellular medium, which is an electrolyte with relatively good conductivity. The dielectric constant of water depends on the microwave frequency and is a complex function: $\varepsilon_W = \varepsilon' + i\varepsilon''$. The following expressions determine the corresponding values of the refractive index n, the attenuation coefficient κ, and the attenuation length a_{MW} [42]:

$$n = \left(\left(\sqrt{\varepsilon'^2 + \varepsilon''^2} + \varepsilon'\right)/2\right)^{1/2}, \quad \kappa = \left(\left(\sqrt{\varepsilon'^2 + \varepsilon''^2} - \varepsilon'\right)/2\right)^{1/2}, \tag{4.31}$$

$$a_{\mathrm{MW}} = c/2\pi f \kappa, f = \omega/2\pi. \tag{4.32}$$

Table 4.1. Parameters of the complex permittivity of water used in formula (4.32) [43].

T [°C]	ε_1	τ_1[ps]	ε_2	τ_2[ps]	ε_3
0.2	87.57	17.67	6.69	0.9	3.92
5	85.89	14.92	6.76	1.0	4.10
10	83.93	12.70	6.57	0.9	4.08
15	82.24	11.00	6.64	1.0	4.34
20	80.31	9.60	6.53	1.2	4.42
25	78.32	8.38	6.32	1.1	4.57
30	76.39	7.39	5.75	0.9	4.60
35	74.91	6.69	6.22	1.5	4.74

The dielectric constant of water at different microwave frequencies can be approximated as follows:

$$\varepsilon(f) = \frac{\varepsilon_1 - \varepsilon_2}{1 + i\omega\tau_1} + \frac{\varepsilon_2 - \varepsilon_3}{1 + i\omega\tau_2} + \varepsilon_3, \tag{4.33}$$

up to frequencies f of several hundred gigahertz [43]. Table 4.1 shows the values of ε_1, ε_2, ε_3, τ_1, and τ_2 at different temperatures [43].

The corresponding microwave wavelength in a medium is $\lambda = \lambda_0/n$ ($\lambda_0 = c/f$ is the wavelength in a vacuum). The amplitude of the electric field in a medium is attenuated as $E(x) \propto \exp(-x/\alpha_{\rm MW})$, where x is the depth of penetration of an incident plane microwave that is normal to the surface. Examples of microwave frequency dependencies of the real and imaginary parts of the dielectric constant and refractive index in water at a temperature of $T = 25$ °C are shown in figure 4.11. The calculations are based on data given in [43]. Figure 4.12 shows the corresponding attenuation length values.

The skin layer thickness for microwave radiation of cyclic frequency ω in an aqueous electrolyte solution with conductivity σ is $\delta_s = \sqrt{2/\mu_0\sigma\omega}$, where $\mu_0 = 4\pi \cdot 10^{-7}\,\mathrm{m}^{-1}$ is the permeability of free space [44]. Considering that typical values of the intercellular medium's conductivity are $\sigma \sim 1\,\Omega^{-1}\,\mathrm{m}^{-1}$, the corresponding thickness of the skin layer in the frequency range of microwave radiation $f \sim 20 - 100$ GHz is $\delta_s \sim 3.5 - 1.5$ mm. The comparison between the obtained estimates of the skin layer and the characteristic absorption depth in figure 4.12 shows that the main mechanism limiting the penetration of microwave radiation into the extracellular medium is its absorption in water. Thus, it is possible to observe the nonthermal physiological effects of microwave radiation on the activity of the nervous tissue only when the nervous tissue is covered by a very shallow layer of an aqueous solution. This was the case, for example, in the experiments reported in [26], where the thickness of the aqueous solution on top of the microwave-irradiated nerve tissue did not exceed 2.5 mm.

This section is reproduced from [34], with the permission of AIP Publishing.

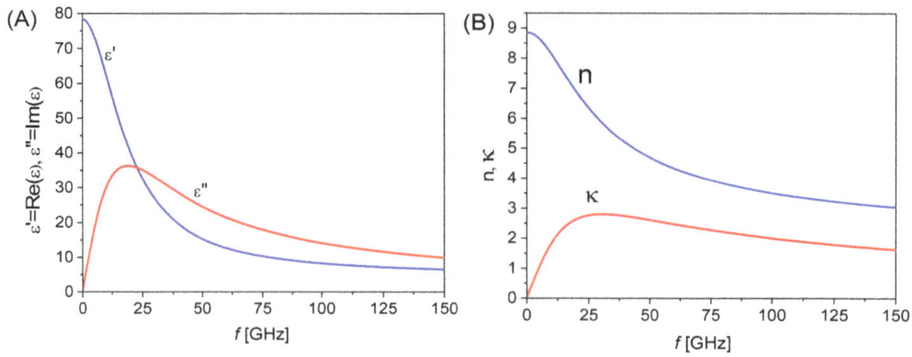

Figure 4.11. The microwave frequency dependences for (A) the real and imaginary dielectric constants of water, (B) the refractive index n and the attenuation κ at a water temperature of $T = 25$ °C.

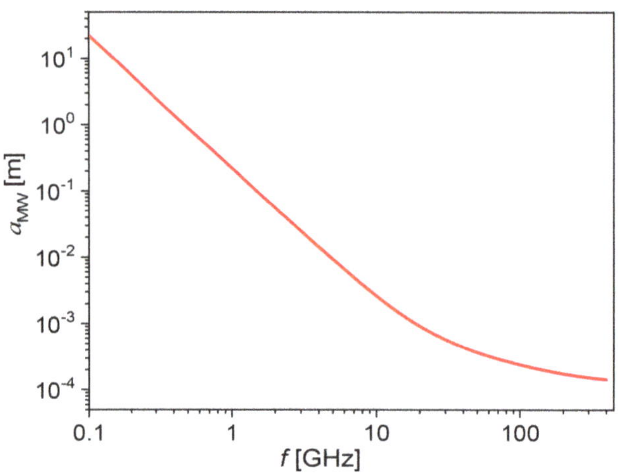

Figure 4.12. The attenuation length of microwaves in water at temperature $T = 25$ °C.

4.7 Forced vibrations of the membrane in a microwave field

Consider a microwave wave incident on the membrane. For the sake of clarity, let us assume that an electromagnetic wave is plane polarized, so that the electric field has normal and tangential projections with respect to the membrane surface (figure 4.12). We consider three characteristic sections of the myelin nerve fibers (see, e.g. [29, 30]): the initial segment, the parts covered by the myelin sheath, and the sections separated by the nodes of Ranvier; we call these zones 1, 2, and 3, respectively, as shown in figure 4.4.

The geometrical and mechanical properties of the nodes of Ranvier and the initial segment are very different from those of the terminal region and the areas covered by myelin (figure 1.35). Therefore, their vibrations (longitudinal and transverse), arising due to the action of the electric component of the electromagnetic field, can be treated independently, assuming that the ends of the vibrating areas are fixed. Since the thickness of the axon membrane in the nerve fiber is much smaller than its radius, we consider each part of the axon to be a plate that is unlimited in the y-direction with a uniformly distributed surface charge σ_m [m^{-2}] that is firmly fixed to the membrane surface. The key questions are as follows: How rigidly are ions fixed to the membrane surface? What is the value of the surface charge? In chapter 5, it is shown that, since the dipole heads of the phospholipid molecules forming the cell membranes face outward with a positive charge, they form local potential wells for the negative ions of the intercellular electrolyte. Additionally, the corresponding binding energy of the trapped ions is several $k_B T$. Therefore, the electric part of the electromagnetic wave acting on the charges can shift the membrane surface.

In general, the direction of the electric field with respect to the axon may be arbitrary. Due to the linearity of the problem, for an arbitrary direction of the wave vector of a plane-polarized microwave field, the mechanical vibrations arising in the membrane are the result of the superposition of the vibrations caused by the longitudinal and transverse components of the electric field. Thus, the problem of the impact of microwave radiation on the membrane of the nerve fibers is reduced to the excitation caused by ultrasonic standing waves in a plate fixed at the edges with the given surface charge density. The geometric, mechanical, and physical properties of the plate depend on the considered segment of the myelinated axon. The corresponding formulas for the case of a cylindrical membrane and an arbitrary circularly polarized microwave field are shown in the next chapter.

The wavelength of an electromagnetic wave in a medium is $\lambda(f) = c/fn(f)$, where c is the speed of light in a vacuum and n is the refractive index. In the frequency range $f \sim 20-100$ GHz, $n \sim 8-4$, as shown in figure 4.11(B), and correspondingly, $\lambda(f)$ is in the range of a few millimeters. That is, the microwave wavelength is much greater than the length of any element of the myelinated nerve fiber ($L_{IS} \sim 20 - 60$ µm, $L_R \sim 1-2.5$ µm, figure 1.35). Therefore, we can assume that the electric field acting on the charged membrane is spatially uniform and varies only in time. The force acting per unit area of the membrane's charged surface is:

$$\vec{F} = \sigma_m \vec{E}, \tag{4.34}$$

where $\vec{E}$ is the electric field of the microwave acting on the surface charges and σ_m is the surface charge density. For an electromagnetic wave of intensity I_{MW}, the amplitude of the electric field in the medium [44] is:

$$|\vec{E}| = \sqrt{\frac{2I_{\text{MW}}}{\varepsilon_0 \varepsilon^{1/2} c}}. \tag{4.35}$$

In (4.17), we considered that the intensity remains constant during the transition from vacuum to a dielectric medium, that is,

$$I_{\text{MW}} = \frac{\varepsilon_0 \varepsilon E_a^2}{2} c_\varepsilon = \frac{\varepsilon_0 E_{0,a}^2}{2} c, \tag{4.36}$$

where the phase velocity of light in a medium with the dielectric permittivity ε is equal to $c_\varepsilon = c/\sqrt{\varepsilon}$, and $E_{0,a}$ is the amplitude of the electromagnetic wave in a vacuum. If the ions associated with the surface charge of the resting potential are 'below' the

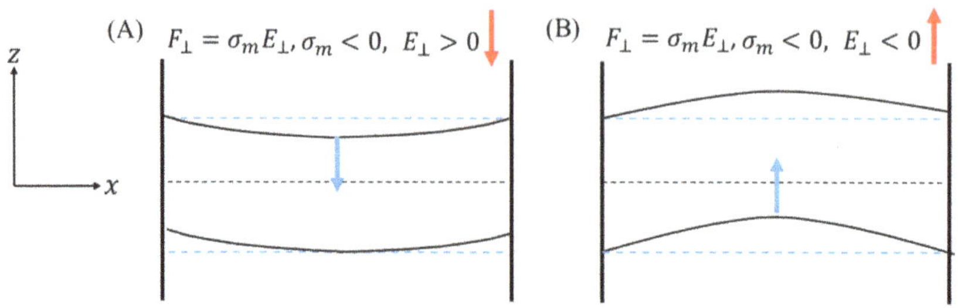

Figure 4.13. Membrane deformations caused by the electric field of microwave radiation perpendicular to the membrane surface. The charges at the edges of the membrane are equal in absolute magnitude but different in sign. The edges of the membrane (unlimited in the y-direction) are clamped. The blue arrows indicate the direction of elastic displacements of the membrane, while red arrows indicate the direction of force.

membrane surface, then ε in expressions (4.35) and (4.36) should be set equal to the dielectric permittivity of the membrane, $\varepsilon = \varepsilon_m = 2$. However, if the bound ions are 'above' the surface of the membrane, then $\varepsilon = \varepsilon_W(\omega)$. For microwave radiation in water in the frequency range of 50–300 GHz, $\varepsilon_W(\omega) \approx 5$ [43]. Taking into account the dependence of the field amplitude on the dielectric permittivity (4.35), $E_a \sim \varepsilon^{-1/4}$, all the results and conclusions remain essentially unchanged.

In the microwave range from hundreds of megahertz to hundreds of gigahertz, the wavelength of the electromagnetic radiation is considerably larger than any of our areas of interest in the myelinated nerve fiber. Therefore, the external electric field interacting with these regions can be considered uniform and only dependent on time. The direction of the electric field relative to the axon is not fixed; it may be arbitrary.

So, as we have already noted, we will consider two possible cases. Figure 4.5 shows the case where the electric field is directed parallel to the surface and figure 4.13 where it is normal to the membrane.

Reproduced with permission from [34], with the permission of AIP Publishing.

4.8 Model of membrane vibrations in the electromagnetic field of microwave radiation

The equations describing the longitudinal and transverse vibrations of a membrane, such an elastic bar, under the influence of external driving forces have the form [45]:

$$\frac{\partial^2 \vec{u}}{\partial t^2} = c_t^2 \Delta \vec{u} + \left(c_l^2 - c_t^2\right) \vec{\nabla} \left(\vec{\nabla} \cdot \vec{u}\right) \tag{4.37}$$

$$\vec{u} = \vec{i}_x u_x + \vec{i}_y u_y + \vec{i}_z u_z.$$

Here, $\vec{u}$ is the displacement vector, and c_l and c_t are the sound velocities in the longitudinal (along the x-axis) and transverse (along the z-axis) directions. In our model, we assume that $c_l \approx c_t$. For a planar plate of infinite extent in the y- direction, equation (4.37), written for the displacement projections, takes the form:

$$\begin{aligned}\frac{\partial^2 u_x}{\partial t^2} &= c_l^2\frac{\partial^2 u_x}{\partial x^2} + c_t^2\frac{\partial^2 u_x}{\partial z^2} + \nu\frac{\partial}{\partial t}\left(\frac{\partial^2 u_x}{\partial x^2}\right) + \left(c_l^2 - c_t^2\right)\frac{\partial^2 u_z}{\partial x \partial z}\\ \frac{\partial^2 u_z}{\partial t^2} &= c_t^2\frac{\partial^2 u_z}{\partial x^2} + c_l^2\frac{\partial^2 u_z}{\partial z^2} + \nu\frac{\partial}{\partial t}\left(\frac{\partial^2 u_z}{\partial x^2}\right) + \left(c_l^2 - c_t^2\right)\frac{\partial^2 u_x}{\partial x \partial z}\end{aligned}, \tag{4.38}$$

where u_x and u_z are displacements along the x and z axes, c_l and c_t are the longitudinal (along the x-axis) and transverse (along the z-axis) sound velocities, and ν is the effective kinematic viscosity associated with the dissipation of the induced vibrations of the membrane due to the friction of the membrane surface with intercellular saline (water). In general, the longitudinal and transverse sound velocities in membranes may be different. In our model, for simplicity of analysis, we assume that $c_l \approx c_t$.

The boundary conditions corresponding to the electric field perpendicular to the surface of the membrane (figure 4.13(A) and (B)) are:

$$\left.\frac{\partial u_z}{\partial z}\right|_{d_m/2} = \frac{F_z}{c_l^2 \rho_m}, \tag{4.39}$$

$$\left.\frac{\partial u_z}{\partial z}\right|_{-d_m/2} = \frac{F_z}{c_l^2 \rho_m}, \tag{4.40}$$

$$u_z|_{x=0,\ x=L_{IS}} = 0, \tag{4.41}$$

where ρ_m is the density of the membrane. In accordance with equations (4.39) and (4.40),

$$F_z = \sigma_m E_z = \sigma_m\sqrt{\frac{2I_{\mathrm{MW}}}{\varepsilon_0\varepsilon_m^{1/2}c}}\,e^{i\omega t}\cos\left(\theta_E\right), \tag{4.42}$$

where θ_E is the angle between the direction of the electric field and the z-axis shown in figure 4.12.

When the surface charges on the inner and outer surfaces of the membrane σ_m are of the same sign, the boundary conditions corresponding to the longitudinal electric field (figure 4.13(A) and (B)) are:

$$\left.\frac{\partial u_x}{\partial z}\right|_{z=d_m/2} = \frac{F_x}{c_l^2 \rho_m}, \tag{4.43}$$

$$\left.\frac{\partial u_x}{\partial z}\right|_{z=-d_m/2} = \frac{F_x}{c_l^2 \rho_m}, \tag{4.44}$$

$$u_x|_{z=0,\ L_{IS}} = 0. \tag{4.45}$$

$$F_x = \sigma_m E_x = \sigma_m\sqrt{\frac{2I_{\mathrm{MW}}}{\varepsilon_0\varepsilon_m^{1/2}c}}\,e^{i\omega t}\,\sin(\theta_E). \tag{4.46}$$

Recall that the longitudinal and transverse vibrations described by the system of equation (4.38) and boundary conditions (4.39)–(4.41) and (4.43)–(4.45) are forced and are therefore not related by the sound dispersion relation.

4.8.1 The electric field perpendicular to the membrane surface

We will look for a solution of equation (4.37) with the boundary conditions in equation (4.38) in the following form:

$$u_x = A_\parallel e^{i\omega t}\cos(k_n x)\sin(\xi z),\quad u_z = A_\perp e^{i\omega t}\sin(k_n x)\cos(\xi z),\quad k_n = \frac{\pi n}{L_{IS}}. \tag{4.47}$$

Substituting equation (4.47) into equations (4.38)–(4.40) and (4.42), we obtain:

$$\left(\omega^2 - k_n^2 c_l^2 - i\omega\nu k_n^2 - c_t^2\xi^2\right)A_\parallel + k_n\left(c_l^2 - c_t^2\right)\xi A_\perp = 0, \tag{4.48}$$

$$\left(\omega^2 - k_n^2 c_t^2 - i\omega\nu k_n^2 - c_l^2\xi^2\right)A_\perp + k_n\left(c_l^2 - c_t^2\right)\xi A_\parallel = 0, \tag{4.49}$$

$$A_\perp = -\frac{F_{n,z}}{c_l^2\rho_m\xi\sin\left(\frac{\xi d m}{2}\right)}, \tag{4.50}$$

where $F_{n,z} = \frac{2}{L_{IS}}\int_0^{L_{IS}} F_z\sin(k_n x)\mathrm{d}x$ is the Fourier component of the amplitude of external force F_z. If the wavelength of the external force is much greater than the length of the initial gap L_{IS}, then:

$$F_{n,z} = \frac{2}{L_{IS}}\int_0^{L_{IS}} F_{0,z}\sin(k_n x)\mathrm{d}x = \frac{4}{\pi n}F_{0,z} = \frac{4}{\pi n}\sigma_m E_{0,z} = \frac{4}{\pi n}\sigma_m\sqrt{\frac{2I_{MW}}{\varepsilon_0\varepsilon^{1/2}c}}, \quad n = 1, 3, 5, \ldots . \tag{4.51}$$

Note that although the driving force $F_{n,z}$ is a real function, the amplitudes $A_\perp$ and $A_\parallel$ are complex quantities.

Looking at (4.50), we can see that as ξ approaches $2\pi p/d_m$, where p is an integer, the amplitude of the transverse oscillations $A_\perp$ grows without bounds. In other words, when $\xi = 2\pi p/d_m$, resonance occurs. Since the values of ξ must satisfy equations (4.48) and (4.49), ξ is a complex quantity whose imaginary part determines the width of the resonances.

Since we are interested in the frequency range $\omega \gg k_n c_l,\ k_n c_t, \nu k_n^2$, then it follows from (4.49) that:

$$\xi^2 \approx \frac{\omega^2 - i\omega\nu k_n^2}{c_l^2},\ \xi \approx \frac{\omega}{c_l} - i\frac{\nu k_n^2}{2c_l}. \tag{4.52}$$

Substituting the value of ξ^2 (4.52) into (4.48), we get:

$$A_{\|} = -\frac{\left(c_l^2 - c_t^2\right)\xi k_n}{\left(\omega^2 - k_n^2 c_l^2 - i\omega\nu k_n^2 - c_t^2\xi^2\right)} A_{\perp} \approx -\frac{\xi k_n c_l^2}{\omega^2} A_{\perp} \approx -\frac{k_n c_l}{\omega} A_{\perp}. \quad (4.53)$$

It follows from equation (4.53) that the displacement amplitude of the membrane along the z-axis is much greater than the displacement along the x-axis, that is, $|A_{\|}| \approx \frac{k_n c_l}{\omega} |A_{\perp}| \ll |A_{\perp}|$.

Since $|A_{\perp}| \propto \frac{1}{|\sin(\frac{\xi dm}{2})|}$, the maximum of $|A_{\perp}|$ is determined by the values of ξ at which $|\sin(\frac{\xi dm}{2})|$ takes the minimum value. From relation (4.52), it follows that:

$$\left|\sin\left(\frac{\xi d_m}{2}\right)\right| = \left|\sin\left(\frac{\omega d_m}{2c_l} - i\frac{\nu d_m k_n^2}{4c_l}\right)\right| = \left(\sin^2\left(\frac{\omega d_m}{2c_l}\right) + \mathrm{sh}^2\left(\frac{\nu k_n^2 d_m}{4c_l}\right)\right)^{1/2}. \quad (4.54)$$

Since $\frac{\nu k_n^2 dm}{4c_l} \ll 1$, then:

$$\left|\sin\left(\frac{\xi d_m}{2}\right)\right| \approx \left(\sin^2\left(\frac{\omega d_m}{2c_l}\right) + \left(\frac{\nu k_n^2 d_m}{4c_l}\right)^2\right)^{1/2}. \quad (4.55)$$

It follows from (4.55) that the maximum value of $|A_{\perp}|$ is reached at values of ω at which $\sin(\frac{\omega dm}{2c_l}) = 0$. Accordingly, the cyclic resonant frequencies are:

$$\omega_{r,\,p} = 2\pi p\frac{c_t}{d_m}, \quad p = 1, 2, \dots. \quad (4.56)$$

In this case, at the points of resonance:

$$\left|A_{\perp}(\omega_{r,\,p})\right| \approx \frac{4}{\omega_{r,\,p}\nu k_n^2 d_m}\frac{F_{n,\,z}}{\rho_m}, \quad (4.58)$$

and the width of the resonance at half height is determined by viscous dissipation:

$$\delta\omega \sim 2\nu k_n^2. \quad (4.59)$$

For example, let us estimate the characteristic resonant width $\Delta f = \delta\omega/2\pi$ for $k_1 = \pi/L_{\mathrm{IS}}$. It follows from (4.52) that for the resonant frequency at $p = 1$, $f_{r,\,1} \sim 40$ GHz, the kinematic viscosity is $\nu \approx 1.4 \cdot 10^{-7}\ \mathrm{m^2\,s^{-1}}$. Assuming the length of the initial segment $L_{\mathrm{IS}} \approx 50\ \mu\mathrm{m}$, we obtain from (4.59) an estimate of $\Delta f \approx 200$ Hz. That is, the resonance is pronounced and very narrow. In fact, the resonance should be noticeably broader due to unaccounted-for dissipative processes within the vibrating membrane.

4.8.2 The electric field parallel to the membrane surface

Consider the case where the electric field is parallel to the membrane surfaces, as shown in figure 4.14. For simplicity, let us assume that the outer and inner surfaces of the membrane have the same surface charge σ_m. We are seeking the solution of equation (4.38) in the form:

$$u_x = A_{\|} e^{i\omega t} \sin (k_n x) \cos (\xi z), \quad u_z = A_{\perp} e^{i\omega t} \cos (k_n x) \sin (\xi z). \quad k_n = \frac{\pi n}{L_{\mathrm{IS}}} \tag{4.60}$$

Substituting (4.60) into (4.43) and (4.44), we get:

$$A_{\|} = -\frac{F_{n,x}}{c_l^2 \rho_m \xi \sin\left(\frac{\xi d_m}{2}\right)}, \tag{4.61}$$

where $F_{n,x} = \frac{2}{L_{IS}} \int_0^{L_{IS}} F_x \sin (k_n x) dx$ is the Fourier component of the amplitude of external force F_x. If the wavelength of the external force is much greater than the length of the initial segment L_{IS}, then:

$$F_{n,x} = \frac{2}{L_{\mathrm{IS}}} \int_0^{L_{\mathrm{IS}}} F_{0,x} \sin(k_n x) dx = \frac{4}{\pi n} F_{0,x} = \frac{4}{\pi n} \sigma_m E_{0,x} = \frac{4}{\pi n} \sigma_m \sqrt{\frac{2 I_{\mathrm{MW}}}{\varepsilon_0 \varepsilon^{1/2} c}}, \quad n = 1, 3, 5, \ldots . \tag{4.62}$$

As in the case of the transverse electric field, we now consider the case where $\omega \gg k_n c_l$, $k_n c_t$, and νk_n^2. Then, according to (4.48):

$$\xi^2 \approx \frac{\omega^2 - i\omega\nu k_n^2}{c_t^2}, \ \xi \approx \frac{\omega}{c_t} - i\frac{\nu k_n^2}{2c_t}, \tag{4.63}$$

and consequently, from (4.49),

$$A_{\perp} = -\frac{\left(c_l^2 - c_t^2\right)\xi}{\omega^2 - k_n^2 c_t^2 - i\omega\nu k_n^2 - c_l^2 \xi^2} A_{\|} \approx -\frac{k_n c_t}{\omega} A_{\|}, \tag{4.64}$$

while in the case of the transverse electric field, $|A_{\perp}| \gg |A_{\|}|$, and in the case of the longitudinal electric field, $|A_{\perp}| = \frac{k_n c_l}{\omega} |A_{\|}| \ll |A_{\|}|$. In other words, the lateral drift of the ion channels along the membrane is influenced by forced mechanical vibrations whose amplitude is much larger when the electric field is parallel to the membrane surface than when it is perpendicular.

As in the case of an electric field perpendicular to the membrane, a resonance of the field frequencies exists for forced oscillations of the membrane in a parallel electric field:

$$\omega_{r,p} = \frac{2\pi c_l}{d_m} p, \ p = 1, 2, 3, \ldots \tag{4.65}$$

$$A_{r,\|} \approx \frac{4}{\omega_{r,p} \nu k_n^2 d_m} \frac{F_{n,x}}{\rho_m} = \frac{16}{\omega_{r,p} \nu k_n^2 d_m} \frac{1}{\rho_m} \frac{1}{\pi n} \sigma_m \sqrt{\frac{2 I_{\mathrm{MW}}}{\varepsilon_0 \varepsilon_m^{1/2} c}}. \tag{4.66}$$

In the following, to simplify the analysis, we assume that the longitudinal sound velocity in the membrane is equal to the transverse sound velocity, that is, $c_l = c_t = c_s$. Substituting the estimate of the speed of sound in a lipid membrane $c_s \sim 300$ m s^{-1} [19] into equation (4.65) and assuming the width of the membrane to be $d_m \sim 7-10$ nm, we obtain the lowest resonant frequency: $f_{r,1} \sim 30-45$ GHz. Many works (see section 4.1 of this chapter) have experimentally demonstrated that the effects of low-intensity microwave exposure on living organisms have a resonant character and that the measured resonant frequencies are close to 40 GHz, as obtained above. Note that resonant frequencies are different for different membranes. This explains the contradictory experimental results obtained by different groups that investigated the influences of weak microwave radiation on cells. In our opinion, the success of the experiments in [26] is associated with the chosen frequency of 61.125 GHz for microwave radiation, which is apparently close to one of the mechanical resonances of the nerve membrane.

Substituting the value of $A_{r,\parallel}$ from (4.66) into the expression for the energy density in the effective ultrasonic wave $\overline{E} = \frac{1}{2}\rho_m \omega^2 A^2$ for harmonics $n = 1$, and $p = 1$, from formulas (4.17) for $\varsigma \approx 1$ and (4.19) for $\varsigma \approx 3$, we obtain the values of ξ_s and $\tilde{\xi}_s$, respectively:

$$\xi_s = \frac{32}{3\pi^5 k_B T}\frac{d_m L_{\mathrm{IS}}^4}{\rho_m \nu^2}\frac{\sigma_m^2 I_{\mathrm{MW}}}{\varepsilon_0 \varepsilon_m^{1/2} c}, \tag{4.67}$$

$$\tilde{\xi}_s = \frac{32}{15\pi^5 k_B T}\frac{d_m L_{\mathrm{IS}}^4}{\rho_m \nu^2}\frac{\sigma_m^2 I_{\mathrm{MW}}}{\varepsilon_0 \varepsilon_m^{1/2} c}. \tag{4.68}$$

Note that, in equations (4.67) and (4.68), the previously accepted approximation for the shape and size of transmembrane channels, $r_p = d_m/2$, was taken into account.

Substituting (4.67) into (4.18) and (4.22), we calculate the difference between the maximum and minimum of the channel density in the initial segment of the neuron $\Delta n_{\mathrm{ch}}/n_{\mathrm{ch},0}$ and the characteristic time required for transmembrane channel redis tribution t_s when $\varsigma = 1$. Similar values of $\Delta\tilde{n}_{\mathrm{ch}}/n_{\mathrm{ch},0}$, $\tilde{t}_s$ are determined for another model case, $\varsigma = 3$, by substituting (4.68) into (4.20) and (4.23). These values are given in table 4.2 for different membrane surface charges σ_m and microwave

Table 4.2. Calculated values of $\Delta n_{s,\mathrm{ch}}/\langle n_{\mathrm{ch},0}\rangle$ and Δt_s at different values of I_{MW}.

σ_m[C/m^2]	I_{MW}[W/m^2]	t_s [s] ($\varsigma = 1$)	$\Delta n_{\mathrm{ch}}/n_{\mathrm{ch},0}$ ($\varsigma = 1$)	$\tilde{t}_s$ [s] ($\varsigma = 3$)	$\Delta\tilde{n}_{\mathrm{ch}}/n_{\mathrm{ch},0}$ ($\varsigma = 3$)
0.05	0.0025	91.2	12	456	5
0.01	0.0025	2280	1.6	11 400	0.35
0.05	0.005	45.6	16	228	7.3
0.01	0.005	1140	2.9	5700	0.69
0.05	0.01	22.8	23	114	10
0.01	0.01	570	4.5	2850	1.3

radiation intensities I_{MW}. Values of $L_{IS} = 50\ \mu m$, $d_m = 10$ nm, and $\varepsilon_m = 2$ are assumed for the parameters of the initial segment of the neuron. The kinematic viscosity at the membrane–electrolyte interface is determined using formula (4.25), which at the frequency of the first resonance is of the order of 40 GHz: $\nu = 2 \cdot 10^{-7}\ s^{-1}$.

The values of the membrane charge σ_m that we chose fall within the values published in the research literature [20, 21], while the microwave intensities are close to those used in the experiments described in [26]. For the chosen membrane surface charge of $\sigma_m = 0.05\ C\,m^{-2}$, the calculated times required for a substantial redistribution of the transmembrane channels are in good agreement with the measured values [26].

4.9 Elastic cylindrical membrane

We have considered a model membrane as a flat elastic bar with clamped edges under the influence of longitudinal or normal forces. The actual nerve fiber is more like a tube formed by the lipid membrane (figure 4.14). We will show that all the above qualitative and quantitative results remain valid.

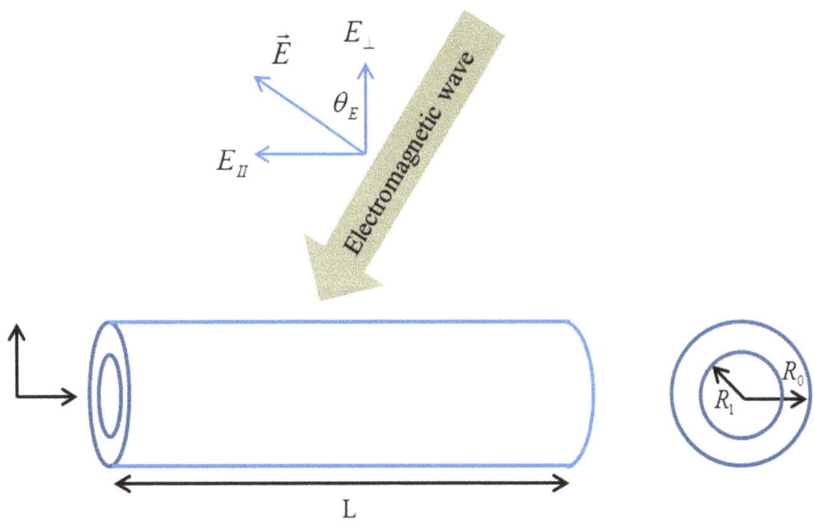

Figure 4.14. Elastic cylindrical membrane of the nerve fibers in the microwave field.

Since the main contribution to the redistribution of channels along myelinated axons results from forces directed along the fiber, we will limit our discussion to this case. The equations of elasticity theory (4.37) in a cylindrical coordinate system, taking into account the friction of the surface membrane on the water, have the form [45]:

$$\frac{\partial^2 u_r}{\partial t^2} = c_t^2\left(\frac{\partial^2 u_r}{\partial z^2} - \frac{\partial^2 u_r}{\partial r \partial z}\right) + c_l^2\left(\frac{\partial^2 u_r}{\partial r^2} + \frac{1}{r}\frac{\partial u_r}{\partial r} - \frac{u_r}{r^2} + \frac{\partial^2 u_r}{\partial r \partial z}\right) + \nu\frac{\partial}{\partial t}\frac{\partial^2 u_r}{\partial z^2}, \quad (4.69)$$

$$\frac{\partial^2 u_z}{\partial t^2} = c_t^2\left(\frac{1}{r}\frac{\partial u_z}{\partial r} + \frac{\partial^2 u_z}{\partial r^2} - \frac{\partial^2 u_r}{\partial r \partial z} - \frac{1}{r}\frac{\partial u_r}{\partial r}\right) + c_l^2\left(\frac{\partial^2 u_r}{\partial r \partial z} + \frac{1}{r}\frac{\partial u_r}{\partial z} + \frac{\partial^2 u_z}{\partial z^2}\right) + \nu\frac{\partial}{\partial t}\frac{\partial^2 u_z}{\partial z^2}. \quad (4.70)$$

For a cylinder with clamped edges, when the surface forces are oscillating at a frequency of ω, the solutions of equations (4.69)–(4.70) have the form:

$$u_r = U_{n,\,r} e^{i\omega t}\cos(k_n z), \quad (4.71)$$

$$u_z = U_{n,\,z} e^{i\omega t}\sin(k_n z). \quad (4.72)$$

The corresponding boundary conditions [45] are:

$$c_t^2\rho\left(\frac{\partial U_{n,\,r}}{\partial z} + \frac{\partial U_{n,\,z}}{\partial r}\right)_{r=R_0} = F_{z,\,n,\,R_0}, \quad (4.73)$$

$$c_t^2\rho\left(\frac{\partial U_{n,\,r}}{\partial z} + \frac{\partial U_{n,\,z}}{\partial r}\right)_{r=R_1} = F_{z,\,n,\,R_1}, \quad (4.74)$$

where

$$U_{n,\,r} = A_{n.r,\,J} J_1(\xi r) + A_{n,\,r,\,Y} Y_1(\xi r), \quad (4.75)$$

$$U_{n,\,z} = A_{n,\,z,\,J} J_0(\xi r) + A_{n,\,z,\,Y} Y_0(\xi r). \quad (4.76)$$

Here, J_0, J_1, Y_0, and Y_1 are the Bessel functions; $k_n = \pi n/L$; R_0 and R_1 are the outer and inner radii of the cylinder; and $F_{\parallel,\,n,\,R_0}$ and $F_{\parallel,\,n,\,R_1}$ are the amplitudes of the surface forces. Let us assume that the inner and outer surfaces of the membrane have the same surface charge. Thus, for a microwave field whose electric field is parallel to the cylinder axis, $F_{\parallel,\,n,\,R_1} = F_{\parallel,\,n,\,R_0}$.

Substituting expressions (4.75) for $U_{n,\,r}$ and (4.76) for $U_{n,\,z}$ into (4.69) and (4.70), we obtain:

$$\left(\left(\omega^2 - c_t^2 k_n^2 - i\omega\nu k_n^2\right) - c_l^2\xi^2\right) A_{n,\,r,\,J} + \left(c_t^2 - c_l^2\right)k_n\xi A_{n,\,z,\,J} = 0, \quad (4.77)$$

$$\left(\left(\omega^2 - c_t^2 k_n^2 - i\omega\nu k_n^2\right) - c_l^2\xi^2\right) A_{n,\,z,\,J} + \left(c_t^2 - c_l^2\right)k_n\xi A_{n,\,r,\,J} = 0, \quad (4.78)$$

$$\left(\left(\omega^2 - c_t^2 k_n^2 - i\omega\nu k_n^2\right) - c_l^2\xi^2\right) A_{n,\,r,\,Y} + \left(c_t^2 - c_l^2\right)k_n\xi A_{n,\,z,\,Y} = 0, \quad (4.79)$$

$$\left(\left(\omega^2 - c_t^2 k_n^2 - i\omega\nu k_n^2\right) - c_l^2\xi^2\right) A_{n,\,z,\,Y} + \left(c_t^2 - c_l^2\right)k_n\xi A_{n,\,r,\,Y} = 0. \quad (4.80)$$

The boundary conditions (4.73) and (4.74) are reduced to:

$$-(k_n A_{n,\,r,\,J} + \xi A_{n,\,z,\,J})J_1(\xi R_0) - (k_n A_{n,\,r,\,Y} + \xi A_{n,\,z,\,Y})Y_1(\xi R_0) = \frac{F_{\parallel,\,n,\,R_0}}{c_t^2\rho} \quad (4.81)$$

$$-(k_n A_{n,r,J} + \xi A_{n,z,J}) J_1(\xi R_1) - (k_n A_{n,r,Y} + \xi A_{n,z,Y}) Y_1(\xi R_1) = \frac{F_{\parallel,n,R_1}}{c_t^2 \rho}. \quad (4.82)$$

Here, we have used known relations for Bessel functions [38]:

$$J_1(\xi x) = -\frac{1}{\xi}\frac{\mathrm{d}J_0(\xi x)}{\mathrm{d}x} \quad (4.83)$$

$$J_0(\xi x) = \frac{1}{\xi x} J_1(\xi x) + \frac{1}{\xi} J_1(\xi x) \frac{\mathrm{d}J_1(\xi x)}{\mathrm{d}x}. \quad (4.84)$$

It is easy to see that the pairs of equations (4.77)–(4.78) and (4.79)–(4.80) coincide with equations (4.48)–(4.49). The system of equations consisting of (4.77)–(4.80) and (4.81)–(4.82) gives the complete solution to the problem of cylinder (membrane) vibrations under periodic axial-symmetric forces in the longitudinal direction of the surface. For a thin-walled cylinder $d_m = R_1 - R_0 \ll R_0 \ll L$ with clamped edges, the problem of elastic vibrations under the action of the longitudinal forces coincides with the problem of the plain plate vibrations considered in section 4.8.

4.10 Electromagnetic pollution of the human environment

At present, studies of the impact of microwave radiation on living organisms are very important due to the increasing level of electromagnetic pollution of the human environment (associated with the development of mobile communications, computers, radio, television, etc). The allowable standards for the power radiated by electronic devices, depending on their frequency, were developed through the joint efforts of scientists, engineers, and physicians. Figure 4.15 shows an example of U.S. standard limits on allowable radiated power at different frequencies [46]. Reference data are given in [46] for two limit cases: for the upper tier (humans in controlled environments) and for the lower tier (when no microwave safety program is available). These standards are based on calculations of the thermal effects of microwave radiation on the human body. The allowable power of microwave radiation increases linearly in the range from 20 MHz to 20 GHz and then remains constant, as can be seen in figure 4.15. A plateau occurs at frequencies above 20 GHz because at these frequencies, microwave penetration drops to the level of hundreds of microns and the radiation is almost completely absorbed by the skin [2].

A few years ago, there was a proposal to increase the frequency of the electromagnetic radiation used for telecommunications up to 30–300 GHz [47, 48]. This is based on the fact that at such frequencies, it is possible to transmit signals at a rate higher than 2 $\mathrm{Gb\,s^{-1}}$, which has enormous potential both for civilian purposes and for the military. On the other hand, such an increase in frequency also makes it possible to use low-power energy sources that essentially reduce the electromagnetic radiation flux down to lower than 1 $\mathrm{W\,m^{-2}}$. At that power of incident radiation, the thermal effect on the nerve fiber is insignificant and cannot affect the vital functions

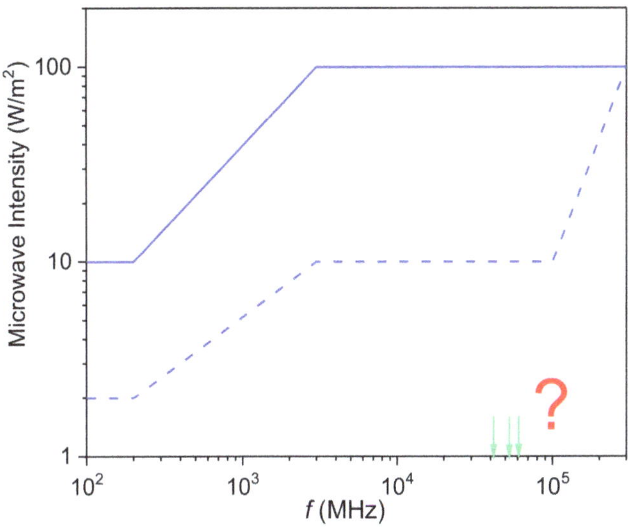

Figure 4.15. Standard upper and lower limits on the maximal allowable power radiated by electronic devices for environmental safety as a function of frequency [46], shown as solid and dashed blue lines, respectively. The green arrows indicate examples of resonant frequencies observed in experiments: 42.3, 53.8, and 61.2 GHz [51, 52]. In the regions of these resonant frequencies, nonthermal effects on neural tissue activity are possible at much lower intensities than the permitted maximum values for these frequencies.

of the human brain and the nervous system. In 2013, the first Wi-Fi routers operating at a frequency of 60–80 GHz appeared on the market [49, 50].

However, as noted above, in addition to the thermal effect associated with the microwave absorption by tissues of the body, there are resonant effects (the nature of which, until recently, remained unclear) that can lead to physiological implications at much lower intensities than the permitted safe range. These resonances are shown schematically in figure 4.15 and emphasized with a question mark. Resonant frequencies differ for different types of nerve tissue.

This section is reproduced with permission from [33].

4.11 Discussion

As shown above, the redistribution of transmembrane channels caused by standing ultrasonic waves in the membrane of the initial segment initially leads to a decrease in the excitation threshold of nerve impulses and then, with increasing amplitude of the channel density perturbations, to the possibility of spontaneous excitation of the action potential. However, the effect of purely mechanical ultrasonic vibrations is not as effective as the effect of forced electromechanical oscillation at resonant frequencies, excited by the interaction of charged membranes with microwaves. A further increase in the amplitude of transmembrane channel density perturbations can block the propagation of a pulse in areas with rarefied channel density. This effect was probably observed in experiments [26] in which frog nerves were irradiated for 70 s with a microwave pulse at a frequency of 60.125 GHz and a very low intensity of 70–770 nW cm^{-2}. At the minimum microwave power, spontaneous excitation of the action potential was observed. As the microwave power increased, the spontaneous excitation stopped and reappeared after the power was turned off. These results are in full qualitative agreement with our model. In [26], a change in the shape of the action potential and a shortening of the duration of the refractory period with increasing microwave power were also observed. All these experimental effects may be related to the ultrasound-induced change in transmembrane ion channel density [19, 31]. It should be noted that the microwave frequency of 60.125 GHz used in [26] is probably close to the resonant frequencies of the longitudinal vibrations of the axon membrane [6, 19].

The effect observed in [26], namely stimulation of action potential excitation (lowering of the excitation threshold) at a power of 492 nW cm^{-2} and subsequent blocking at a power of 737 nW cm^{-2}, is shown in figure 4.3(A). This effect is explained within the framework of our model of ion channel rearrangement and consequent lowering of the action potential excitability threshold (chapter 1). However, with increasing irradiation power, the stimulated redistribution of transmembrane channels can lead to such a strong rarefaction in a substantial part of the initial segment that the propagation of the action potential becomes impossible, meaning that it becomes blocked. When the microwave source is turned off, the channel distribution returns to its unperturbed equilibrium due to lateral diffusion, and the action potential blocking is removed. Of course, we are talking about the nonthermal reversible effect of microwaves on nerve tissue.

This raises the question: how can a weak microwave radiation field induce ultrasonic membrane vibrations that lead to a marked redistribution of transmembrane ion channels? Regardless of the magnitude of the field, energy and momentum are transferred from the field to the charged particles. Thus, the random thermal motion is superimposed on a small, ordered motion. This occurs, for example, in an electrolyte (plasma) when the drift velocity of the charged particles is a million times smaller than their average thermal velocity. The microwave field interacts with the ions rigidly bound to the membrane and forming a surface charge (see chapter 5), transferring momentum to them, which in turn is transferred to the membrane, causing forced oscillations. The same is true for weak ultrasound vibrations interacting with suspended particles (protein channels). The result is an acoustic drift superimposed on the average thermal motion, even for ultrasound of very low intensity. In this case, the potential of the acoustic force acting on the particles can be much lower than the potential of the thermal energy, as in the case of hydrodynamic or gaseous flows where the directional velocity is much lower than the average thermal velocity and the corresponding pressure drop is much lower than the unperturbed static pressure.

It should be noted that the resonant frequencies [53, 54], at which the displacement of the membrane is maximal, are proportional to the speed of sound in the membrane. It is difficult to know the exact value of the longitudinal speed of sound in the membrane at high frequencies, which, as mentioned above, can be much lower than the speed of sound in water or oil [17–19]. Since the resonance is very narrow [26], experimental measurement of the frequencies at which blocking or self-excitation of the action potential occurs allows the speed of sound in the membrane to be determined. It seems that the best experimental methods with which to observe the effect of transmembrane channel redistribution described in this chapter correspond to measurements of the spatial distribution of sodium channels along the axon membrane, including electro-optical measurements (see [55, 56]), since they allow one to directly measure the transmembrane channel density distribution before and immediately after the ultrasound (or microwave) pulse. An indirect confirmation of transmembrane channel redistribution could be obtained by observing the dependence of action potential excitation and propagation (or its blockage) on ultrasound amplitude. This can be done using conventional probe techniques [57] as well as nonintrusive optical methods, such as observing the dynamics of the generation of second-harmonic laser radiation scattered by the nerve fibers [58, 59].

Let us formulate the primary experimental tasks that arise in light of the possible mechanism of interaction of low-intensity microwaves with nerve fiber membranes considered in this chapter:

(1) **The redistribution of channels.** It is necessary to obtain data about the redistribution of transmembrane ion channels in the AIS when exposed to low-intensity microwave radiation. For example, fluorescently marked proteins [60–62] can be used for this purpose.
(2) **Measurement of the sound velocity in the membrane.** From the observation of the resonant frequencies of the microwave interaction with the membrane, the speed of sound can be determined, since $\omega_r \propto c_l$.

This section is reproduced with permission from [33].

4.12 Conclusions

Low-intensity microwave radiation, which does not cause thermal effects, can induce ultrasonic mechanical vibrations in the membranes of nerve tissue cells.

The interaction with the ultrasound vibrations could change the density of transmembrane protein sodium channels. As a result, it could also change the resting potential in the nerve fibers, and therefore, it may induce or, conversely, suppress the excitation of action potentials.

The presence of resonances in the range of tens of gigahertz is in good agreement with known experimental data. Resonant frequencies are different for different membranes. This explains the contradictory experimental results obtained by different groups that investigated the influences of weak microwave radiation on cells. In our opinion, the success of the experiments described in [26] is associated with the chosen frequency of microwave radiation, 61.125 GHz, which is apparently close to one of the mechanical resonances of the nerve membrane.

The most effective component of the microwave electric field is the component tangential to the membrane surface, and the most effective region in the myelinated axon is the initial segment.

Despite the encouraging results, our analysis is preliminary and requires further in-depth experimental and theoretical studies. First of all, this analysis deals with issues related to the density of surface charges, longitudinal and transverse sound velocities in the membrane and the surrounding fluid, and viscous losses in the gigahertz frequency range. A more advanced theory of forced lateral drift should also consider the more realistic cylindrical shape of transmembrane ion channels and their volume-averaged density.

We have only considered the influence of ultrasonic vibrations excited by microwave radiation on the distribution of Na^+ transmembrane protein channels. However, similar effects should be expected for other types of membrane proteins (such as transmembrane ion channels and peripheral surface proteins) that are affected by lateral diffusion. This could, in principle, significantly enhance the effects induced in nerve fibers by low-level microwave radiation.

References

[1] Devyatkov N D and Golant M B 1983 On the mechanism of the effect of electromagnetic radiation in the millimeter range of the nonthermal intensity on the vital activity of the body *The Effects of Non-thermal Effects of Millimeter Wave Radiation on Biological Objects* ed N D Devyatkov (Moscow: IRE Academy of Science USSR) 18

[2] Betski O V, Golant M B and Devyatkov N D 1988 *Millimeter Waves in Biology* (Moscow: Physica, Znanie)

[3] Devyatkov N D, Golant M B and Betski O V 1991 Millimeter waves and their role *Vital Processes* (Moscow: Radio and Communications)

[4] Fröhlich H 1968 Bose condensation of strongly excited longitudinal electric modes *Phys. Lett.* A **26** 402

[5] Fröhlich H 1968 Long-range coherence and energy storage in biological systems *Int. J. Quant. Chem.* **11** 641

[6] Fröhlich H 1980 The biological effects of microwaves and related questions *Adv. Electron. Electron. Phys.* **53** 85

[7] Betski O V 1999 Microwave radiation passage through the barriers: the interaction of microwaves with the human body *Radio* **10** 47

[8] Smolyanskaya F Z and Vilenskaya R L 1974 Effects of millimeter-band electromagnetic radiation on the functional activity of certain genetic elements of bacterial cells *Sov. Phys. Usp.* **16** 571

[9] Le Drean Y, Mahamoud Y S, Le Page Y, Habauzit D, Le Quement C, Zhadobov M and Sauleau R 2013 State of knowledge on biological effects at 40–60 GHz *C. R. Phys.* **14** 402

[10] Grundler W and Keilmann F 1983 Sharp resonances in yeast growth prove nonthermal sensitivity in microwaves *Phys. Rev. Lett.* **51** 1214

[11] Webb S J 1979 Factors affecting the induction of lambda prophages by milli-millimeter microwaves *Phys. Lett.* A **73** 145

[12] Norris A N and Rebinsky D A 1994 Acoustic coupling to membrane waves on elastic shells *J. Acoustic Soc. Am.* **95** 1809

[13] Krasil'nikov P M and and Fisun O I 1994 Natural oscillations of a charged spherical membranes *Biofizika* **39** 876

[14] Volkenstein M V 1983 *General Biophysics* **1** (Amsterdam: Elsevier Science & Technology Books)

[15] Nagle J F and Nagle S T 2000 Structure of lipid bilayers *Biochim. Biophys. Acta* **1469** 159

[16] Saiz L and Klein M L 2001 Electrostatic interactions in a neutral model phospholipid bilayer by molecular dynamics simulations *J. Chem. Phys.* **116** 3052
[17] Sugar I P 1979 A theory of the electric field-induced phase transition of phospholipid bilayers *Biochim. Biophys. Acta* **556** 72
[18] Passechnik V I, Hianik T, Karagodin V P and Kagan V E 1984 Elasticity, strength and stability of bilayer lipid membranes and their changes due to phospholipid modification *Gen. Physiol. Biophys.* **3** 475 http://www.gpb.sav.sk/1984.htm
[19] Pekker M and Shneider M N 2016 Comment on 'Non-thermal mechanism of weak microwave fields influence on neurons' [J. Appl. Phys. **119** 104701 (2.13)] *J. Appl. Phys.* **119** 086101
[20] Lakshminarayanaiah N and Murayama K 1975 Estimation of surface charges in some biological membrane *J. Membr. Biol.* **23** 279
[21] Heimburg T 2009 *Physical Properties of Biological Membranes* arXiv:0902.2454v2 [physics.bio-ph]
[22] Krasil'nikov P M 1999 Resonance interactions of surface charged lipid vesicles with the microwave electromagnetic field *Biofizika* **44** 1078 (in Russian)
[23] Krasil'nikov P M 2001 The relationship between charged surface and deformation of lipid membranes *Biofizika (Russia)* **46** 460
[24] Pakhomov A G, Prol H K, Mathur S P, Akyel Y and Campbell C B 1997 Search for frequency-specific effects of millimeter-wave radiation on isolated nerve function *Bioelectromagnetics* **18** 324
[25] Alekseev S I, Gordiienko O V, Radzievsky A A and Ziskin M C 2010 Millimeter wave effects on electrical responses of the sural nerve *in vivo Bioelectromagnetics* **31** 180
[26] Pikov V, Arakai X, Harrington M, Fraser S E and Siegal P H 2010 Modulation of neuronal activity and plasma membrane properties with low-power millimeter waves in organotypic cortical slices *J. Neural Eng.* **7** 0450
[27] Jacobson K, Ishihara A and Inman R 1987 Lateral diffusion of proteins in membranes *Ann. Rev. Physiol* **49** 163
[28] Almeida P F F and Vaz W L C 1995 Lateral diffusion in membranes *Handbook of Biological Physics* **vol 1** ed R Lipowsky and E Sackmann (Amsterdam: Elsevier) 6 305
[29] Ramadurai S, Holt A, Krasnikov V, van den Bogaart G, Killian J A and Poolman B 2009 Lateral diffusion of membrane proteins *J. Am. Chem. Soc.* **131** 12650
[30] Kole M H P and Stuart G J 2012 Signal processing in the axon initial segment *Neuron* **73** 235
[31] Shneider M N and Pekker M 2013 Non-thermal mechanism of weak microwave fields influence on nerve fiber *J. Appl. Phys.* **114** 104701
[32] Shneider M N and Pekker M 2014 Initiation and blocking of the action potential in an axon in weak ultrasonic or microwave fields *Phys. Rev.* E **89** 052713
[33] Shneider M N and Pekker M 2014 Non-thermal influence of a weak microwave on nerve fiber activity *Phys. Chem. Biophys* **4** 6
[34] Shneider M N and Pekker M 2019 Stimulated activity in the neural tissue *J. Appl. Phys.* **125** 211101
[35] Mednikov E P 1966 *Acoustic Coagulation and Precipitation of Aerosols* (New York: Consultation Bureau)
[36] Fuch N A 1964 *The Mechanics of Aerosols* (Oxford: Pergamon Press)
[37] King L V 1934 On the acoustic radiation pressure on spheres *Proc. R. Soc. Lond.* A **147** 212

[38] Korn G A and Korn T M 1968 *Mathematical Handbook for Scientists and Engineers: Definitions, Theorems, and Formulas for Reference and Review* 2nd edn (New York: McGraw-Hill)
[39] Mandelshtam L I and Leontovich M A 1937 On the Theory of Sound Absorption in Liquids *Zh. Eksp. Teor. Fiz. [Sov Phys JETP]* **7** 438
[40] Mikhailov I G and Gurevich S B 1948 Ultrasonic wave absorption in liquids *Usp. Fiz. Nauk* **35** 1
[41] Nimtz G and Weiss W 1987 Relaxation time and viscosity of water near hydrophilic surfaces *Z. Phys. B Cond. Mat* **67** 483
[42] Landau L D and Lifshitz E M 1960 *Electrodynamics of Continuous Media v. 8: Course of Theoretical Physics* (Oxford: Pergamon Press)
[43] Buchner R, Barthel J and Stauber J 1999 The dielectric relaxation of water between 0°C and 35°C *Chem. Phys. Lett.* **306** 57
[44] Panofsky W K H and Phillips M 1962 *Classical Electricity and Magnetism* (Reading, MA: Addison-Wesley)
[45] Landau L D and Lifshitz E M 1970 *Theory of Elasticity v.7: Course of Theoretical Physics* 2nd edn (Oxford: Pergamon Press)
[46] *IEEE standard for safety levels with respect to human exposure to radio frequency electromagnetic fields, 3 kHz to 300 GHz* in IEEE Std C95.1-2005 (Revision of IEEE Std C95.1-1991)
[47] Marcus M and Pattan B 2005 Millimeter wave propagation *IEEE Micro* **6** 54
[48] Lawton G 2008 Wireless HD video heats up *Computer* **41** 18
[49] Brown M 2013 Meet 60GHz Wi-Fi, the insanely fast future of wireless networking https://www.pcworld.com/article/457045/meet-60ghz-wi-fi-the-insanely-fast-future-of-wireless-networking.html
[50] http://www.e-band.com/70-80-GHz-Overview
[51] Pakhomov A G, Akyel Y, Pakhomova O N, Stuck B E and Murphy M R 1998 Current state and implications of research on biological effects of millimeter waves: a review of the literature *Bioelectromagnetics* **19** 393
[52] Rojavin M A and Ziskin M C 1998 Medical application of millimetre waves *QJM* **91** 57
[53] D'Andrea J A, Ziriax J M and Adair E R 2007 Radio frequency electromagnetic fields: mild hyperthermia and safety standards *Prog. Brain. Res.* **162** 107
[54] Marcus M and Pattan B 2005 Millimeter wave propagation *IEEE Micro.* **6** 54
[55] Angelides K J, Elmer L W, Loftus D and Elson E 1988 Distribution and lateral mobility of voltage-dependent sodium channels in neurons *J. Cell Biol.* **106** 1911
[56] England J D, Gamboni F, Levinson S R and Finger T E 1990 Changed distribution of sodium channels along demyelinated axons *Proc. Natl. Acad. Sci. USA* **87** 6777
[57] Malmivuo J and Plonsey R 1995 *Bioelectromagnetism: Principles and Applications of Bioelectric and Biomagnetic Fields* (New York: Oxford University Press)
[58] Shneider M N, Voronin A A and Zheltikov A M 2010 Action-potential-encoded second-harmonic generation as an ultrafast local probe for nonintrusive membrane diagnostics *Phys. Rev.* E **81** 031926
[59] Shneider M N, Voronin A A and Zheltikov A M 2011 Modeling the action-potential-sensitive nonlinear-optical response of myelinated nerve fibers and short-term memory *J. Appl. Phys.* **110** 094702

[60] Angelides K J, Elmer L W, Loftus D and Elson E 1988 Distribution and lateral mobility of voltage-dependent sodium channels in neurons *J. Cell Biol.* **106** 1911
[61] Chen Y, Lagerholm B C, Yang B and Jacobson K 2006 Methods to measure the lateral diffusion of membrane lipids and proteins *Methods* **39** 147
[62] Bannai H, Le'vi S, Schweizer C, Dahan M and Triller A 2006 Imaging the lateral diffusion of membrane molecules with quantum dots *Nat. Protoc.* **1** 2628

Mikhail N Shneider and Mikhail Pekker

Chapter 5

Interaction between electrolyte ions and the surface of a cell lipid membrane

This chapter addresses the interaction between electrolyte ions and the surface of the cell membrane. It is shown that both sides of the bilayer phospholipid membrane surface are negatively charged and that the ions in direct contact with the membrane surface are in relatively deep (compared with the thermal energy of the ions' translational motion) potential wells localized near the dipole heads of the phospholipid membrane. This makes it impossible for ions to slip along the membrane surface. We can say that the ions located on the axon membrane are strongly bound to the surface and essentially represent the Stern layer in the theory of the double layer formed at the membrane surface in the electrolyte. These are the ions that, when interacting with the electrical component of the microwave field during the microwave irradiation of cells discussed in chapter 4, transfer energy and momentum directly to the membrane and cause its forced mechanical vibrations, resulting in the redistribution of transmembrane protein ion channels.

5.1 Introduction

Electric charge distribution near cell membranes is a key factor in many problems related to the interaction between cells and external electromagnetic fields [1–6]. For example, if ions are not strongly bound to the membrane and can move freely along it, then the electromagnetic field can only have a weak influence on the membrane. On the other hand, if ions are tightly bound to the membrane, the electric component of the electromagnetic fields can lead to membrane deformation [7, 8]. The surface charge of the cell membrane has been studied in many experimental works. We will not consider all the works and refer only to [9, 10], which provide

doi:10.1088/978-0-7503-6034-0ch5

experimental data on the surface charge of cell membranes obtained by different methods. The range of results is quite broad: $\sigma_m \sim 0.002 - 0.3\ \mathrm{C\,m^{-2}}$.

The problem of the spatial distribution of the charge near the surface of biological membranes has been considered in many theoretical works (see, e.g. [1–5]). In all these works, the near-surface potential of the membrane has been considered within the framework of the Gouy–Chapman theory [11, 12] or its later modification by Stern [13], where the charge on the membrane surfaces is assumed to be given. In these theories, the membrane is considered a continuous dielectric without taking into account its fine structure, and the surface charge is determined based on the electrochemical properties of the dielectric surface (see e.g. [14, 15]).

Modern theories tend to distinguish two layers in the surface charge structure on the phospholipid membrane: a dense layer (the Stern layer), in which dehydrated electrolyte ions adhere to the membrane surface at the phospholipid heads, and a diffuse layer (the Gouy–Chapman layer), in which hydrated (solvated) ions can move freely (figure 5.1). The Stern layer is a monolayer, so its thickness is approximately equal to the diameter of the dehydrated ions adsorbed on a given surface. The plane separating the Stern layer from the Gouy–Chapman diffusion layer is called the slipping plane because ions on it can move freely, unlike ions in the Stern layer. The potential of the slipping plane is commonly called the zeta potential and is designated by ζ, as shown in figure 5.1. In this chapter, only the non-quasi-neutral Stern layer will be addressed, since it is the layer responsible for the momentum transfer to the membrane and the forced mechanical vibrations

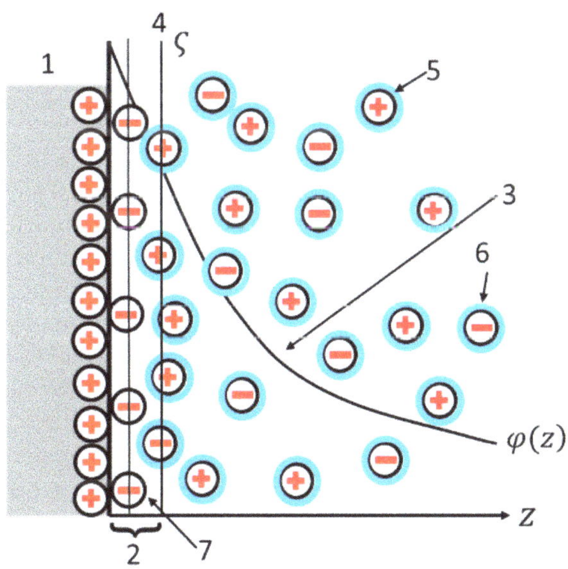

Figure 5.1. Double electrical layer at the membrane and electrolyte interface: 1—dielectric with a positive charge on the surface; 2—Stern layer, where electrolyte ions are dehydrated and bound to the membrane surface; 3—diffusion layer, where electrolyte ions are hydrated; and 4—slipping plane. The potential at the slip plane is called the electrokinetic potential or ς-potential.

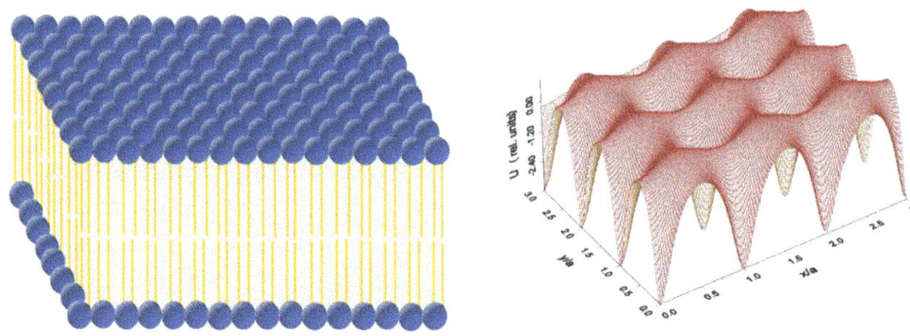

Figure 5.2. (A) Simplified mosaic model of a phospholipid membrane [16]. The spheres represent dipole heads on the inside and the outside of the membrane. (B) A fragment of a two-dimensional potential distribution pattern along the membrane surface at a distance equal to 0.15 of the lattice period (a description of the computational model is given in section 5.2).

stimulated by the electrical component of the microwave radiation considered in chapter 4.

In the phospholipid membrane, the electrolyte ions interact with phospholipid dipoles, which form a mosaic (lattice) structure, schematically shown in figure 5.2(A) [16]. As a result, the dehydrated electrolyte ions at the membrane boundary are exposed to a periodic potential, as shown in figure 5.2(B); that is, their free sliding along the membrane surface is suppressed. These are the ions that form the Stern layer in the double layer at the membrane–electrolyte interface. As already mentioned, this fact is crucial to the theory of the interaction between the weak microwave field and cell membranes proposed in [17] (see also review [18]). It was also essential in chapter 4, where it was assumed that the longitudinal electric field of the microwave acting on the surface charge causes forced longitudinal vibrations of the membrane, since the surface charge ions are rigidly bound to the surface and therefore cannot slip.

Considering the presence of a double layer at the interface between the cell membrane and the surrounding electrolyte, as well as the trapped ions sitting on the surface (Stern layer), the modern view of the potential distribution outside and inside the membrane has the form shown in figure 5.3 (see, for example, [3, 16, 19]). In this chapter, we consider the surface charge of the cell membrane formed by negative ions trapped in the potential wells formed by the dipole heads of the membrane phospholipids. These ions are strongly bound to the membrane surface: the ion binding energy U with the membrane surface is much greater than the thermal energy $k_B T$. This has allowed the construction of a self-consistent theory from the Gouy–Chapman–Stern theories and helped to determine the average charge density sitting on the membrane. We emphasize that this chapter does not discuss the passage of ions through transmembrane ion channels or pores. We limit ourselves to considering only the surface processes in the lipid membrane placed in the saline solution.

The main ions in the physiological solution are Na^+, K^+, Ca^{2+}, Mg^{2+}, and Cl^-. The total concentration of these ions is $n_i \approx 1.8 \cdot 10^{26}\,\mathrm{m}^{-3}$ (300 mmol l^{-1}) [20], but

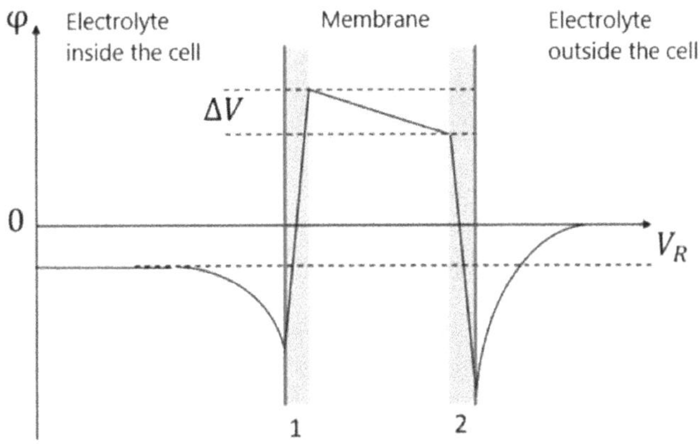

Figure 5.3. Potential distribution inside and outside the membrane when the inside and outside of the membrane have different surface charges: 1 and 2—dipole head regions on the inner and outer membrane surfaces. V_R is the resting membrane potential, equal to the potential difference between the electrolyte inside and outside the cell, and ΔV is the potential difference inside the membrane. Vertical red lines show the charges on the membrane surfaces (Stern layer).

for simplicity, we only consider the case where the bilayer phospholipid membrane is immersed in a water solution of NaCl.

5.2 An electrostatic model of the phospholipid membrane. Potential distribution near the membrane surface

Below, we mainly follow [21, 22].

It is known that the phospholipid molecules of the cell membrane form a mosaic (matrix) structure in which the dipole heads are directed toward the fluid (the positively charged head faces outward from the membrane) [16]. The average surface area per lipid molecule is ≈ 0.5 nm^2, the length of the polar head is ~ 0.5–1 nm, the radius of the head is $\sim 0.2 - 0.3$ nm, and the distance between the hydrophilic heads of the membrane is in the range of $5 - 7$ nm [23, 24]. The dipole moment of the phospholipid head is $18.5 - 25$ D [25] (1D $= 3.34 \cdot 10^{-30}$ C $\cdot$ m), which is more than ten times larger than the dipole moment of water molecules. Based on the geometric dimensions of the cell membrane and the size of water molecules, it can be concluded that the free spaces between phospholipid heads do not exceed the size of a water molecule (~ 0.275 nm). This means that the membrane interacting with the ions of the surrounding liquid cannot be considered a dielectric medium with an infinitesimal dipole size.

These facts allow us to consider the following simplified model of ion interaction with the membrane:

1. The membrane is a matrix (figure 5.4) with a mesh size of $a \times a$. The dipoles are located in the nodes of the cells; the charge of the dipole head is q; the distance between charges (the dipole length) is d; and the distance between dipoles along the axis z is l.

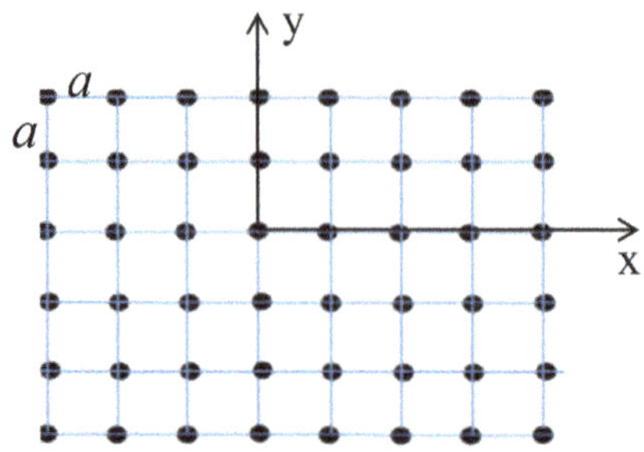

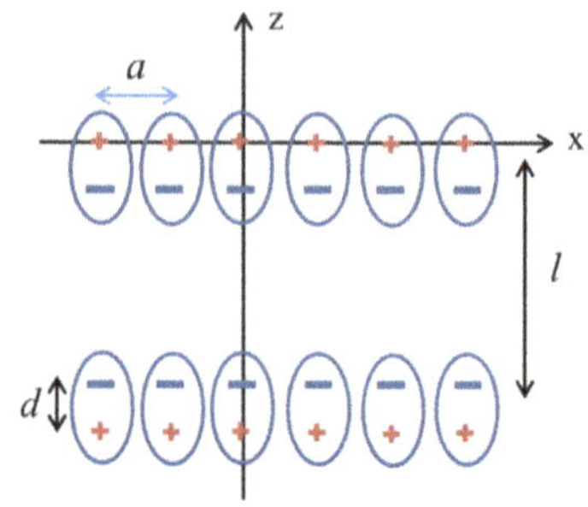

Figure 5.4. A simplified mosaic model of a membrane: the membrane is a matrix with dipoles in the nodes, a is the mesh size of the matrix, d is the distance between the charges of the dipole heads, and l is the distance between dipoles along the z-axis.

2. Ionic membrane permeability is a separate problem that is not considered in this work; for us, it is important to know how strongly ions are attached to the surface of the membrane.

The following expression gives the membrane potential in a cylindrical coordinate system (r, θ, z) at a point above the membrane surface (figure 5.5):

$$U(r, \theta, z) = \sum_{i=-N}^{N}\sum_{j=-N}^{N} U_{i,j}(r, \theta, z) =$$

$$\sum_{i=-N}^{N}\sum_{j=-N}^{N}\frac{q}{4\pi\varepsilon_0}\left(\frac{1}{\sqrt{r^2 + r_{i,j}^2 - 2rr_{i,j}\cos\left(\theta - \theta_{i,j}\right) + z^2}}\right.$$
$$-\frac{1}{\sqrt{r^2 + r_{i,j}^2 - 2rr_{i,j}\cos\left(\theta - \theta_{i,j}\right) + (z + d)^2}} \tag{5.1}$$
$$-\frac{1}{\sqrt{r^2 + r_{i,j}^2 - 2rr_{i,j}\cos\left(\theta - \theta_{i,j}\right) + (z + l)^2}}$$
$$\left.+\frac{1}{\sqrt{r^2 + r_{i,j}^2 - 2rr_{i,j}\cos\left(\theta - \theta_{i,j}\right) + (z + l + d)^2}}\right).$$

Here, the radial and angular coordinates $r_{i,j}$ and $\theta_{i,j}$ correspond to the position of the dipole at the node numbered (i, j), q is the dipole charge, and ε_0 is the permittivity of free space. The value of N in (5.1) is chosen so that the potential near the membrane does not depend on the size of the matrix n. The count goes from the node (dipole head) (figure 5.5): $r = (x^2 + y^2)^{1/2}$, $\theta = \operatorname{atan}(y/x)$.

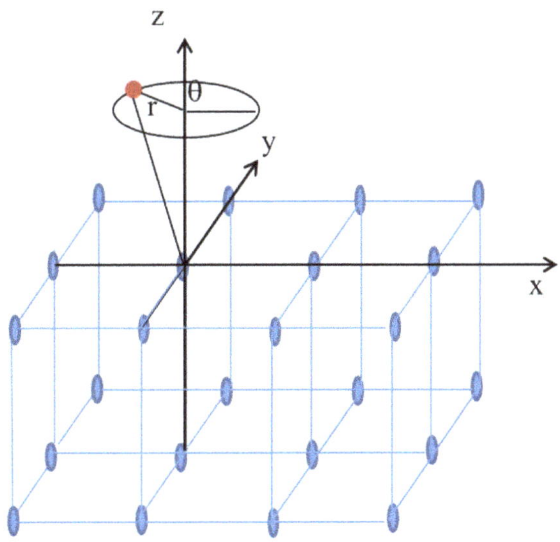

Figure 5.5. Spatial lattice of dipoles in a bilayer lipid membrane. The ellipsoids at the lattice sites correspond to the dipole heads of the phospholipid molecules.

We expand the potential U in a Fourier series by θ. Taking into account the rotational symmetry over $\pi/2$ rotations for the assumed square matrix of the dipole heads, we obtain:

$$U(r,\theta,z)=U_0(r,z)+\sum_{j=1}^{J}U_j(r,z)\cos(4j\theta)+\sum_{j=1}^{J}V_j(r,z)\sin(4j\theta), \tag{5.2}$$

where

$$U_0(r,z)=\frac{2}{\pi}\int_0^{\pi/2}U(r,\theta,z)\mathrm{d}\theta, \tag{5.3}$$

$$\begin{aligned} U_{j\neq0}(r,z)&=\frac{4}{\pi}\int_0^{\pi/2}U(r,\theta,z)\cos(4j\theta)\,\mathrm{d}\theta,\\ V_{j\neq0}(r,z)&=\frac{4}{\pi}\int_0^{\pi/2}U(r,\theta,z)\sin(4j\theta)\,\mathrm{d}\theta. \end{aligned} \tag{5.4}$$

In the framework of the model presented above, estimates show that the influence of the dipoles located on the bottom side of the membrane (figure 5.4) on the potential distribution φ at $z>0$ can be neglected. The same is true for the effect of the dipoles on the top of the membrane on the potential at $z<-(l+d)$.

For example, consider the case where the bilayer phospholipid membrane is immersed in an NaCl solution with the following set of parameters: $a=0.7$ nm, $d=0.5$ nm, $l=8$ nm, and $q=1.6\cdot10^{-19}$ C [14]. The dependencies of the zero harmonics of the potential U on r and z for this case are shown in figures 5.6(A) and

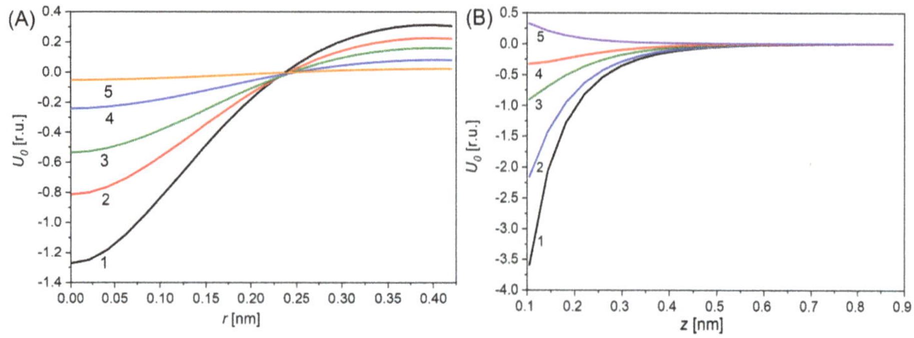

Figure 5.6. The dependencies of a zero harmonic of the potential U on r (A) and on z (B). In (A), curve 1 corresponds to $z = 0.182$ nm, 2—$z = 0.2205$ nm, 3—$z = 0.259$ nm, 4—$z = 0.336$ nm, and 5—$z = 0.49$ nm. In (B), curve 1 corresponds to $r = 0$, 2—$r = 0.084$ nm, 3—$r = 0.147$ nm, 4—$r = 0.189$ nm, 5—$r = 0.273$ nm, and 6—$r = 0.42$ nm $r = 0.42$ nm. The increasing potential at $r > 0.2$ nm in (A) is due to the influence of the dipoles at the points (0, 0.35 nm), (0, −0.35 nm), (0.35 nm, 0), and (−0.35 nm, 0).

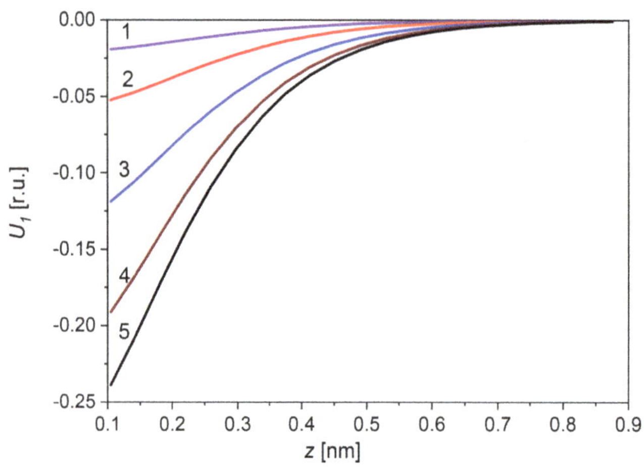

Figure 5.7. The dependencies of the first harmonic of the potential U on z. Curve 1 corresponds to $r = 0.231$ nm, 2—$r = 0.294$ nm, 3—$r = 0.342$ nm, 4—$r = 0.357$ nm, and 5—$r = 0.399$ nm.

(B), respectively. The dependencies of the first harmonic of the potential U on z are shown in figure 5.7. Regarding the dependence of U on θ, in the region $r \leqslant a/2 = 0.35$ nm, the contribution of the harmonics higher than zero order does not exceed 7%, so we neglect them hereafter.

As shown in figure 5.8, the value of $W_{\mathrm{ef}}/k_B T$ decreases exponentially with the distance from the membrane, and the ratio $W_{\mathrm{ef}}/k_B T$ is about ten at a distance of $z/a = 0.5$. Although this is still a fairly deep potential at $z/a = 1$, the effect of the membrane on the ions can be neglected.

Let us determine the energy of a negative ion of finite size. Consider the ion as a uniformly charged sphere with radius r_{ion} and the dipole heads as elongated ellipsoids with point charges inside. Let r_h be the minimum distance from which

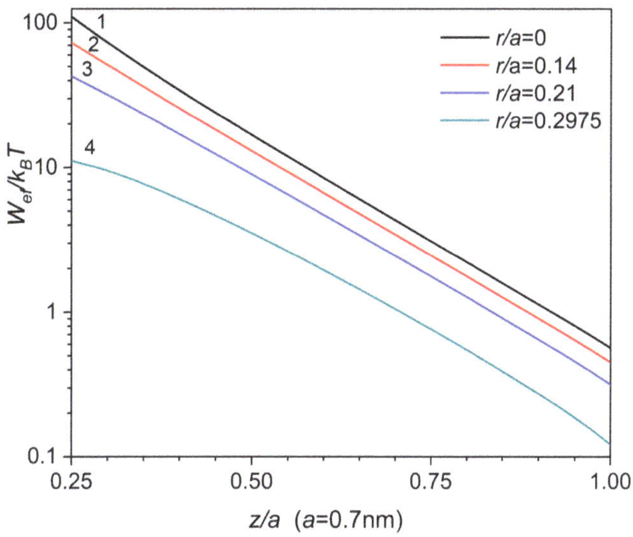

Figure 5.8. The dependence of the parameter $W_{\mathrm{ef}}/k_B T$ on z at $r = 0$. Curve 1 corresponds to $r/a = 0$, 2—$r/a = 0.14$, 3—$r/a = 0.21$, and 4—$r/a = 0.30$.

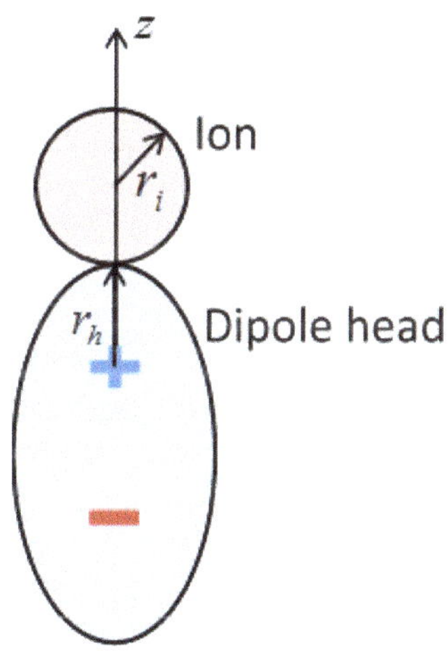

Figure 5.9. The negative ion is located near the head of the dipole of the phospholipid molecule. The ion is a uniformly charged sphere with radius r_{ion}, and r_h is the distance from the positive charge of the dipole to the head of the ion.

the ion can approach a positively charged charge, as shown in figure 5.9 In this case, the binding energy of the negative ion is W_{ef}.

$$\frac{W_{\mathrm{ef}}}{k_B T} = \frac{2\pi}{k_B T} \frac{3}{4\pi r_{\mathrm{ion}}^3} \int_{r_h}^{r_h + 2r_{\mathrm{ion}}} \mathrm{d}z \int_0^{\sqrt{r_{\mathrm{ion}}^2 - (r_h + r_{\mathrm{ion}} - z)^2}} U(r,\, z) r \mathrm{d}r. \tag{5.5}$$

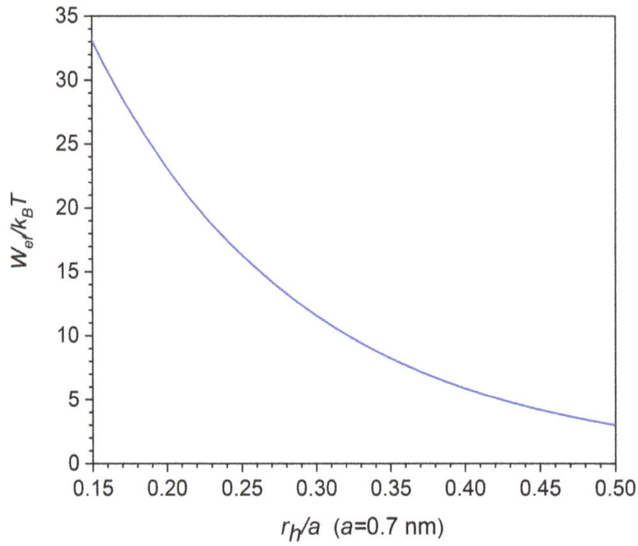

Figure 5.10. The dependence $W_{\text{ef}}/k_B T$ on the size of the head at the assumed radius of the ion $r_{\text{ion}} = 0.18$ nm (Cl^-).

Since we are considering the simplest electrolyte, an aqueous solution of NaCl salt, the negative ion of the electrolyte is the Cl^- ion. The dependence of the effective potential of the ion Cl^- in the potential well on the size of the head r_h is shown in figure 5.10. The chloride ion radius $r_{\text{ion}} = 0.18$ nm, and its atomic weight is $M_{\text{ion}} = 35.4$ AMU.

The typical size of the dipole head is $r_h = 0.2$ nm ($r_h/a \approx 0.3$), and the reduced potential depth is $W_{\text{ef}}/k_B T \approx 11$. Thus, the captured ion is quite tightly bound to the membrane. It should be noted that for electrolytes with a different composition of negative ions, for example, in the axon, where the major negative ions are anion groups of macromolecules and phosphates, estimates of the potential will differ from those shown in figure 5.10.

In the evaluation of (5.5), we considered the chloride ion to be dehydrated. Since the dipole moment of the phospholipid head is 18.5–25 D and that of water molecules is 1.84 D, it is energetically more advantageous for the ion to shed the water shell and 'attach' to the phospholipid head.

Obviously, the trapped Cl^- ions form a potential barrier to the entry of other chloride ions into the potential well region, so in general, the potential for chloride ions near the membrane should behave as shown in figure 5.11.

5.3 Phenomenological theory of surface charge (Stern layer) on the phospholipid membrane

For simplicity, we assume the ions to be point charges, but consider the finite size of the ion to be the minimal separation between the ion and the membrane. As

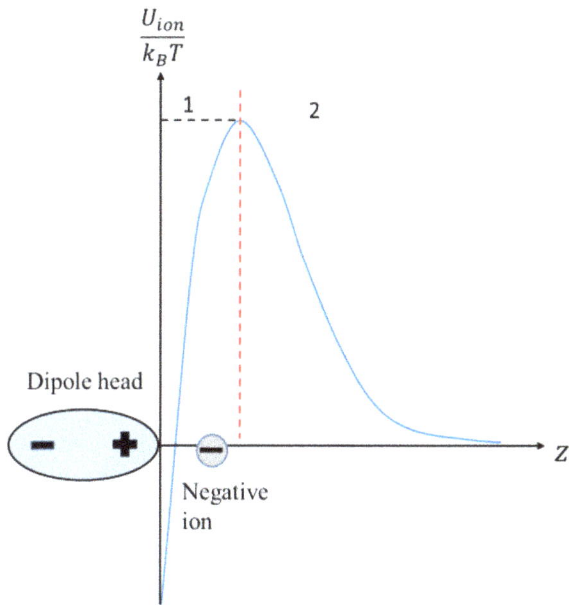

Figure 5.11. Potential energy of the chloride ion near the membrane: 1—potential wall associated with phospholipid dipole heads and 2—potential barrier associated with negative surface charge on the membrane. In the absence of surface charge on the membrane, phospholipid heads are positively charged on their exterior and attract negative ions, forming a potential well. Because ions have a finite size and phospholipid heads are dipolar, the depth of the potential well for negative ions is limited (figure 5.10). The surface charge on the membrane, on the other hand, repels the negative charge and forms a barrier to negative ions.

indicated above, this is a standard approach in models of ion interaction with dielectric surfaces.

We assume that the space charge on the membrane does not affect its structure (i.e. the dipole heads). Since the field of the membrane (without taking into account the ionic charge on it) is negligibly small at a distance on the order of the mesh size, and the distance between the free ions in the solution is larger than the mesh size, we can relate the charge on the membrane surface to the charges in solution by equating the flows at the membrane/liquid boundary (figure 5.12).

Following [26], the one-dimensional Poisson equation for ions in the field of the surface charge σ_{m} has the form:

$$\frac{\mathrm{d}^2\varphi}{\mathrm{d}z^2} = -\frac{qn_\infty}{\varepsilon\varepsilon_0}\left(e^{\frac{q\varphi}{k_B T}} - e^{-\frac{q\varphi}{k_B T}}\right) = -2\frac{qn_\infty}{\varepsilon\varepsilon_0}\mathrm{sh}\left(\frac{q\varphi}{k_B T}\right), \tag{5.6}$$

$$\left.\frac{d\varphi}{dz}\right|_{z=0} = -\frac{\sigma_{\mathrm{m}}}{2\varepsilon\varepsilon_0}, \tag{5.7}$$

$$\varphi|_{z\to\infty} = 0. \tag{5.8}$$

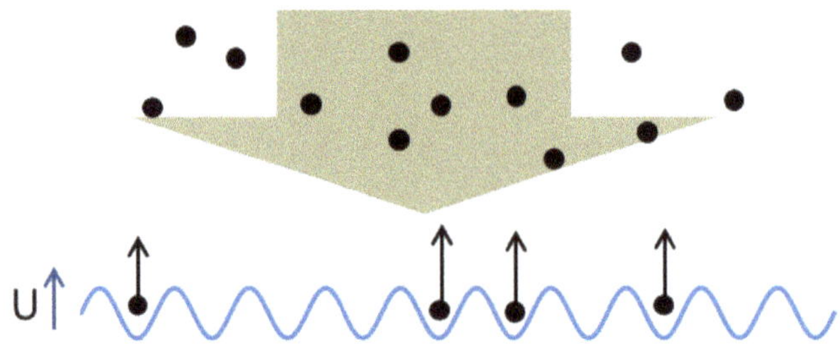

Figure 5.12. A scheme of the ion flows near the membrane: toward the membrane, and 'evaporation' from potential wells of depth W_{ef} outward from the membrane.

Multiplying the left and right parts of the equation by $\frac{d\varphi}{dz}$, we get:

$$\frac{1}{2}\frac{d}{dz}\left(\left(\frac{d\varphi}{dz}\right)^2\right) = -\frac{2n_\infty k_B T}{\varepsilon\varepsilon_0}\frac{d}{dz}\left(\cosh\left(\frac{q\varphi}{k_B T}\right)\right) \tag{5.9}$$

Integrating (5.9) and taking into account the boundary condition (5.8), we obtain:

$$\frac{\mathrm{d}\varphi}{\mathrm{d}z} = \left(\frac{4n_\infty k_B T}{\varepsilon\varepsilon_0}\right)^{1/2}\left(\cosh\left(\frac{q\varphi}{k_B T}\right) - 1\right)^{1/2}. \tag{5.10}$$

Since $(\cosh(\frac{q\varphi}{k_B T}) - 1)^{1/2} = \pm\sqrt{2}\sinh(\frac{q\varphi}{2k_B T})$, it is convenient to rewrite (5.10) in the form:

$$\frac{\mathrm{d}\varphi}{\mathrm{d}z} = -\left(\frac{8n_\infty k_B T}{\varepsilon\varepsilon_0}\right)^{\frac{1}{2}}\sinh\left(\frac{q\varphi}{2k_B T}\right), \tag{5.11}$$

given that:

$$\int\frac{\mathrm{d}u}{\sinh(u)} = \ln\left(\tanh\left(\frac{u}{2}\right)\right) + \text{const.} \tag{5.12}$$

Then, by integrating (5.11), we obtain:

$$\ln\frac{\tanh\left(\frac{q\varphi_0}{4k_B T}\right)}{\tanh\left(\frac{q\varphi}{4k_B T}\right)} = \left(\frac{2n_\infty q^2}{\varepsilon\varepsilon_0 k_B T}\right)^{\frac{1}{2}} z = \frac{z}{\lambda_D}. \tag{5.13}$$

From (5.13), it follows that:

$$\frac{q\varphi}{k_B T} = 4\text{artanh}\left(\tanh\left(\frac{q\varphi_0}{4k_B T}\right)e^{-\frac{z}{\lambda_D}}\right). \tag{5.14}$$

From equation (5.11), taking into account the boundary condition (5.7), we obtain the equation for determining φ_0:

$$\sinh\left(\frac{q\varphi_0}{2k_BT}\right) = \sigma_\mathrm{m}\left(\frac{1}{32n_\infty k_B T\varepsilon\varepsilon_0}\right)^{\frac{1}{2}} \tag{5.15}$$

Since $\tanh(u/2) = \frac{\sinh(u)}{\cosh(u)+1} = \frac{\sinh(u)}{(\sinh^2(u)+1)^{1/2}+1}$, then

$$\tanh\left(\frac{q\varphi_0}{4k_BT}\right) = \frac{\sigma_\mathrm{m}\left(\frac{1}{32n_\infty k_B T\varepsilon\varepsilon_0}\right)^{\frac{1}{2}}}{\left(\frac{\sigma_\mathrm{m}^2}{32n_\infty k_B T\varepsilon\varepsilon_0}+1\right)^{1/2}+1} \tag{5.16}$$

and, respectively,

$$\frac{q\varphi}{k_BT} = 4\operatorname{artanh}\left(\frac{\sigma_\mathrm{m}\left(\frac{1}{32n_\infty k_B T\varepsilon\varepsilon_0}\right)^{\frac{1}{2}}}{\left(\frac{\sigma_\mathrm{m}^2}{32n_\infty k_B T\varepsilon\varepsilon_0}+1\right)^{1/2}+1}e^{-\frac{z}{\lambda_D}}\right) \tag{5.17}$$

Since the left-hand side of (5.13) decreases in absolute value as z increases, the maximum value of $|\varphi|$ occurs at $z = 0$. If $\frac{q|\varphi_0|}{4k_BT} < 1$, then it follows from (5.17) and (5.13) that:

$$\varphi = \varphi_0 e^{-z/\lambda_D}, \tag{5.18}$$

where

$$\varphi_0 = \frac{4\sigma_\mathrm{m}k_BT}{q}\left(\frac{1}{32k_BTn_\infty\varepsilon\varepsilon_0}\right)^{\frac{1}{2}} = \sigma_\mathrm{m}\left(\frac{k_BT}{2n_\infty\varepsilon\varepsilon_0 q^2}\right)^{\frac{1}{2}}. \tag{5.19}$$

Let us estimate the flux of ions falling on the membrane. We assume the Boltzmann distribution of negative ions outside the membrane is:

$$n_\mathrm{ion}(z) = n_\infty e^{-\frac{q|\varphi|}{k_BT}} \tag{5.20}$$

where q is the ion charge, n_∞ is the ion density at infinity, and φ is the potential at a distance z from the membrane (figure 5.1).

Since the ions in the pits are dehydrated, it is correct to assume that within the ζ-potential (figure 5.1), the flow of negative ions from the electrolyte to the membrane and their 'evaporation' from the potential pits can be considered a gas of dehydrated ions.

Assuming that the ions are in thermal equilibrium with the water molecules, we obtain the following estimate for the ion flux on the surface of the membrane:

$$P_\mathrm{in} = n_\infty\overline{v}e^{-\frac{q|\varphi|}{k_BT}} = n_\infty\left(\frac{k_BT}{2\pi M_i}\right)e^{-\frac{q|\varphi|}{k_BT}}. \tag{5.21}$$

Here, $\bar{v}$ is the averaged ion velocity of dehydrated ions.

On the other hand, an estimate of the ion flux 'evaporation' from the surface of the membrane is as follows: the flow of ions from the surface of the membrane can be considered the evaporative process of a liquid with a work function equal to the potential well W_{ef}. Since the characteristic oscillation time of an ion in the potential well is on the order of $a/\bar{v}$, where a is the size of the phospholipid cell, an estimation of the ion lifetime takes the form:

$$\tau_i \approx \frac{a}{\bar{v}}(e^{W_{ef}/k_B T} - 1). \tag{5.22}$$

Accordingly, the flux of 'evaporating' ions equals:

$$P_{out} = \frac{1}{a^2}\frac{N_i}{\tau_i} = \frac{\bar{v}N_i}{a^3}\frac{1}{e^{W_{ef}/k_B T} - 1}. \tag{5.23}$$

Here, N_i is the relative population of the potential wells with ions. Equating the incident flux of the ions on the membrane to the flow 'evaporating' from it, we obtain the relative population of the potential wells:

$$\frac{N_i}{1 - N_i} = a^3 n_\infty e^{-\frac{q|\varphi_0|}{k_B T}}(e^{W_{ef}/k_B T} - 1) \tag{5.24}$$

where φ_0 is the potential on the membrane. In (5.24), we have considered that the probability of the incident ion being trapped in a potential well is proportional to $1 - N_i$.

For a known value of N_i, we can estimate the surface charge density on the membrane as follows:

$$\sigma_m = -N_i q/a^2. \tag{5.25}$$

The calculated dependencies of the surface charge values on the effective depth of the potential wells for different possible values of the ion concentrations of the NaCl solution under consideration are shown in figure 5.13.

The maximum absolute value of the surface charge density shown in figure 5.13, $\approx 0.32\ \mathrm{C\ m^{-2}}$, corresponds to the case where all of the cells (figure 5.4) are full, that is, one negative ion is in every cell. It can be seen that even for small values of $W_{ef}/k_B T$, the relative occupancy of the potential wells with charges is large enough, and the charge density of the charges, which are tightly bound to the membrane, can reach hundredths of coulombs per square meter. It should be noted that in this estimation, we did not consider the interaction between the ions bonded to the membrane, which can certainly play an important role in a more accurate calculation of the occupancy of the potential wells.

This section is reproduced with permission from [22].

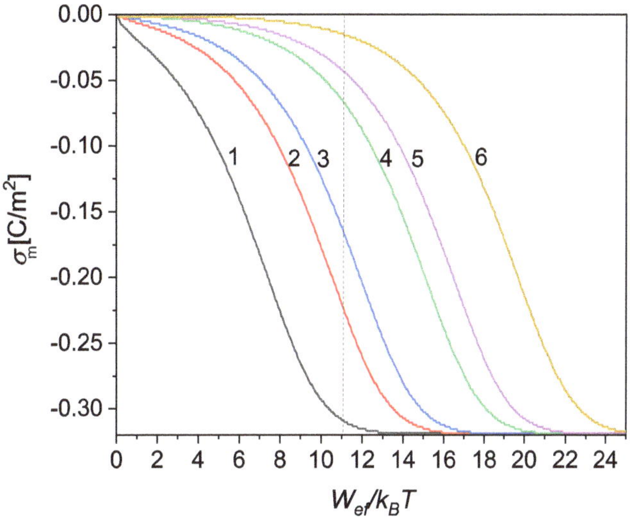

Figure 5.13. Dependencies of the surface charge density σ_m on the reduced potential W_{ef}/k_BT. Curve 1 corresponds to $n_\infty = 5 \cdot 10^{26}$, curve 2 to $n_\infty = 10^{26}$, curve 3 to $n_\infty = 5 \cdot 10^{25}$, curve 4 to $n_\infty = 10^{25}$, curve 5 to $n_\infty = 5 \cdot 10^{24}$, and curve 6 to $n_\infty = 10^{24}$ m^{-3}. The vertical dashed line corresponds to the potential $W_{ef}/k_BT = 11$ (figure 5.10).

5.4 Discussion

In this chapter, we examined the behavior of a membrane surface with dipole heads placed in an electrolyte solution. However, despite this very simple approach, the results are directly related to processes in biological lipid membranes, such as the membranes of the axon. Because the negative ions inside the axon differ from those located on the outside (on the inside, the main negative ions are anion groups of macromolecules and phosphates, but on the outside, the main group consists of chloride ions), it is expected that the surface charge density of ions sitting on the membrane is different. Figure 5.3 shows the potential distributions inside and outside the membrane, where the inner and outer sides of the membrane have different surface charges.

The methods of molecular dynamics were used in [27–31] to study the penetration of Na^+ and Cl^- ions into the phospholipid membrane. However, in those articles, the binding energy of the ions with phospholipid heads was not illustrated. Therefore, it would be of value to compare the results of our model with those of calculations performed using molecular dynamics.

This section is reproduced with permission from [22].

5.5 Conclusions

Based on the considerations presented in this chapter, the following conclusions can be drawn:

The effective energy binding the ion to the membrane is on the order of several $k_B T$; that is, the ions are firmly bound to the membrane surface. The value of the potential decays exponentially with distance from the membrane, so that at a distance greater than 0.7 nm, the influence of the membrane on the electrolyte ions can be neglected.

The ions forming the surface charge are located in relatively deep potential wells near the dipole heads of the phospholipid membrane, which prevents them from sliding along the membrane surface.

A qualitative, self-consistent theory of the potential distribution near the membrane indicates or suggests that the density of bound charges on the membrane can reach hundredths of $\mathrm{C\,m^{-2}}$. This chapter supports the assumption underlying the studies reported in [17, 18], namely that the ions on the excitable axon membrane are tightly bound to it. Therefore, the electric field component of a microwave field interacting with the ions transfers energy and momentum directly to the membrane. This interaction leads to a forced mechanical vibration of the membrane and, consequently, to a redistribution of transmembrane protein ion channels.

According to (5.11), the surface charge of the membrane increases as the density of dissolved salts in the solution increases. The redistribution time of ion channels in the microwave radiation field is inversely proportional to the square of the surface charge density (chapter 4). Therefore, by varying the salinity of the solution, we can change the redistribution time of ion channels in the initial segments of axons and thus affect the characteristic time for changes in the threshold of neuronal excitation.

References

[1] Craig J, Franklin J G, Cafiso D S, Flewelling R F and Hubbell W L 1993 Probes of membrane electrostatics: synthesis and voltage dependent partitioning of negative hydrophobic ion spin labels in lipid vesicles *Biophys. J.* **64** 642

[2] Khalid M A A 2013 *Membrane Electrochemistry: Electrochemical Processes in Bilayer Lipid Membrane* (London: IntechOpen)

[3] Cevc G 1990 Membrane electrostatics *Biochim. Biophys. Acta* **1031** 311

[4] McLaughlin S 1989 The electrostatic properties of membrane *Annu. Rev. Biophys. Biophys. Chern.* **18** 113

[5] Flewelling R F and Hubbell W L 1986 Hydrophobic ion interactions with membranes. Thermodynamic analysis of tetraphenylphosphonium binding to vesicles *Biophys. J.* **49** 531

[6] Pikov V, Arakaki X, Harrington M, Fraser S E and Siegel P H 2010 Modulation of neuronal activity and plasma membrane properties with low-power millimeter waves in organotypic cortical slices *J. Neural Eng.* **7** 1

[7] Krasil'nikov P M 1999 Resonance interactions of surface charged lipid vesicles with the microwave electromagnetic field *Biofizika* **44** 1078

[8] Krasil'nikov P M 2001 Effect of the surface charge on deformation dynamics in lipid membranes *Biofizika* **46** 460

[9] Lakshminarayanaiah N and Murayama K 1975 Estimation of surface charges in some biological membranes *J. Membr. Biol.* **23** 279

[10] Heimburg T 2009 Physical properties of biological membranes arXiv:0902.2454v2

[11] Gouy G 1909 Sur la Constitution de la Charge Electrique á la Surface d'un Electrolyte *Comt. Rend* **149** 654 https://gallica.bnf.fr/ark:/12148/bpt6k3103r/f654.item
[12] Chapman D L 1913 A contribution to the theory of electrocapillarity *Phil. Mag.* **6** 475
[13] Stern O Z 1924 Zur theorie der elektrolytischen doppelschicht *Z. Elektrochem Angew. Phys. Chem.* **30** 508
[14] Delgado A V, González-Caballero F, Hunter R J, Koopal L K and Lyklema J 2005 Measurement and interpretation of electrokinetic phenomena *J. Colloid Interface Sci.* **309** 194
[15] Korobeynikov S M, Melekhov A V, Furin G G, Charalambakos V P and Agoris D P 2002 Mechanism of surface charge creation due to image forces *J. Phys. D: Appl. Phys.* **35** 1193
[16] Alberts B, Johnson A, Lewis J, Raff M, Roberts K and Walter P 2002 *Molecular Biology of the Cell* 4th edn (New York: Garland Science)
[17] Shneider M N and Pekker M 2013 Non-thermal mechanism of weak microwave fields influence on nerve fiber *J. Appl. Phys.* **114** 1
[18] Shneider M N and Pekker M 2014 Non-thermal influence of a weak microwave on nerve fiber activity *J. Phys. Chem. Biophys.* **4** 164
[19] Ermakov Y A 2023 Electric fields at the lipid membrane interface *Membranes* **13** 883
[20] Herman I P 2007 *Physics of the Human Body* 1st edn (Berlin: Springer)
[21] Pekker M and Shneider M N 2014 The surface charge of a cell lipid membrane ArXiv:1401.4707v2 [physics.biof]
[22] Pekker M and Shneider M N 2015 Interaction between electrolyte ions and the surface of a cell lipid membrane *J. Phys. Chem. Biophys.* **5** 1000177
[23] Nagle J F and Tristram-Nagle S 2000 Structure of lipid bilayers *Biochim. Biophys. Acta* **1469** 159
[24] Saiz L and Klein M L 2001 Electrostatic interactions in a neutral model phospholipid bilayer by molecular dynamics simulations *J. Chem. Phys.* **116** 3052
[25] Mashaghi A, Partovi-Azar P, Jadidi T, Nafari N, Maass P, Tabar M R R, Bonn M and Bakker H J 2012 Hydration strongly affects the molecular and electronic structure of membrane phospholipids *J. Chem. Phys.* **136** 114709
[26] Electrical Double Layers in Biology 1985 *Electrochemical Society Symp. on Electrical Double Layers in Biology (Toronto, Canada)*
[27] Ben-Tal N, Honig B, Peitzsch R M, Denisov G and McLaughlin S 1996 Binding of small basic peptides to membranes containing acidic lipids: theoretical models and experimental results *Biophys. J.* **71** 561
[28] Gurtovenko A A 2005 Asymmetry of lipid bilayers induced by monovalent salt: atomistic molecular-dynamics study *J. Chem. Phys.* **122** 244902
[29] Bockmann R A, Hac A, Heimburg T and Grubmuller H 2003 Effect of sodium chloride on a lipid bilayer *Biophys. J.* **85** 1647
[30] Lopez Cascales J J, Garcia de la Torre J, Marrink S J and Berendsen H J C 1996 Molecular dynamics simulation of a charged biological membrane *J. Chem. Phys.* **104** 2713
[31] Vácha R, Berkowitz M L and Jungwirth P 2009 Molecular model of a cell plasma membrane with an asymmetric multicomponent composition: water permeation and ion effects *Biophys. J.* **11** 4493

Chapter 6

Bypassing damaged areas in neural tissues

This chapter discusses the fundamental possibility of bypassing damaged, demyelinated portions of neural tissue, thereby restoring its normal function for the passage of action potentials.

6.1 Introduction

Violations of nerve fiber integrity, such as partial demyelination or microrupture, lead to dysfunction of the nervous system and its components [1–5]. For example, damage or loss of the myelin coating of neurons, which can be caused by various diseases, slows down or even blocks action potentials. This results in a variety of disorders, including sensory impairment, multiple sclerosis, blurred vision, difficulty controlling movement, and problems with bodily functions and responses [1–6]. The problem of restoring damaged nerve tissue function has been the subject of numerous articles and patents [7–19].

Many of these have proposed a recovery scheme in which an electrical signal is read from one or more needle electrodes in contact with an individual neuron or group of neurons and then processed and transmitted to another group of neurons with additional needle electrodes (figure 6.1).

Based on calculations shown in [20], the theoretical possibility of restoring the normal work of a partially demyelinated neuron cell that remains alive and functional was demonstrated by appropriate stimulation of the axon away from the damaged area, which led to normal passage of the action potential while bypassing the demyelinated area. Such stimulation can be a local change in membrane potential induced by currents in saline, similar to the synchronization of neurons considered in chapter 2.

In this chapter, we discuss the possibility of bypassing damaged nerve fibers (or a bundle of damaged nerve fibers) using noncontact electrodes. In recent years, the creation of such electrodes has become technically feasible. In order to better

doi:10.1088/978-0-7503-6034-0ch6

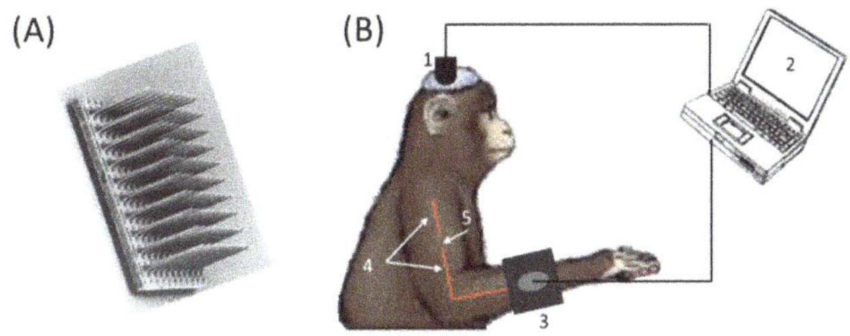

Figure 6.1. Schematic representation of an example of restoration of nerve tissue functions using a bypass of needle electrodes. (A) System of needle electrodes. Reprinted from [19], Copyright (1998), with permission from Elsevier. (B) Example of bypass: 1—system of needle electrodes for reading the signal from the motor areas of the brain, 2—system for processing the signal coming from the motor areas of the brain and for generating an output for control of the arm muscles, 3—system of needle electrodes for the stimulation of neurons in the muscle tissue, 4—nerve tissue connecting the motor areas of the brain with the muscles of the hand, and 5—ruptured (damaged) neural tissue.

understand the practicality of a bypass based on noncontact electrodes, comprehensive experimental studies are required.

6.2 Bypassing a damaged area of nerve tissue by transmitting an action potential

It is known (e.g. see [21, 22]) that the excitation of the action potential in a nerve fiber requires the application of a stimulating voltage pulse at the threshold of ~10 mV and a duration of about 0.1–1 ms to the non-myelinated section of the axon membrane (figures 1.24 and 1.33 in chapter 1). Moreover, to stimulate the action potential in the entire fiber, it is sufficient to apply the voltage pulse to a small area of the initial segment of the axon.

In particular, it was shown in [23, 24] that as the action potential propagates along a fiber, the change in potential at the outer surface of the membrane differs by only a few microvolts from the potential elsewhere on the outer surface of the membrane at rest. It appears that at such small variations in surface potential, the excitation conditions between neighboring neurons cannot be established, and thus, neuronal interaction is considered impossible for most mammalian neural tissues [25–27]. As shown in chapter 2, this statement is incorrect because the resistance of the membrane is many orders of magnitude greater than the resistance of the electrolytes inside and outside the axon (see chapter 1, section 4). Therefore, for the same values of current in the electrolyte and across the membrane, the potential difference across the membrane is ~0.1 V, while the potential difference across the electrolyte section separating the axons of neighboring neurons is several orders of magnitude smaller. However, the threshold for action potential excitation is not determined by the potential difference in the electrolyte but by the potential difference across the membrane. Currents flowing through non-myelinated regions of the active axon charge the unmyelinated axon surfaces of nearby neurons to above-threshold potential differences, which can initiate the excitation of an action potential in neighboring, initially inactive axons. This is the mechanism of ephaptic coupling that we discussed in detail in chapter 2.

We believe that if the properties of nervous tissue (an axon bundle or even a single axon) are disordered (for example, if the myelin sheath in a part of the nerve tissue is damaged in such a way that the passage of the action potential becomes impossible), then the normal functioning of the axons can be made possible by the transfer of the action potential over the damaged area. The principle of such a transfer is similar to the transfer of excitation from one neuron to another in the case of ephaptic coupling. All parameters of the myelinated fibers correspond to frog (*Xenopus*) axons and are given in chapter 1, section 6. To calculate the damaged section, we assumed that demyelination occurs between the 12th and 22nd nodes of Ranvier in the calculations for the damaged axon model. Following [20], we mimicked neuronal demyelination by assuming a myelin sheath of smaller thickness, $\delta_M = 0.125$ μm, such that the full diameter of the myelinated segment $d_M = 9.25$ μm, whereas in normal intact regions, the thickness of the myelin sheath and the diameter of the myelinated segment are $\delta_M = 3$ and $d_M = 15$ μm, respectively. That is, in demyelinated areas, the capacitance per unit length greatly increases, and the resistance decreases. Calculations of the action potential saltatory propagation in undamaged and damaged axons were performed based on the Goldman–Albus equation (2.2) within the framework of the approximations and data used in [28].

Calculated examples of action potential propagation along undamaged myelinated and damaged, partially demyelinated axons are shown in figures 6.2(A) and 6.2(B), respectively. Under the assumed conditions, demyelination causes a complete block of the action potential. However, as shown in [29], an increase in the resting potential of 38 mV (~31.6% of the maximum amplitude of the action potential) at the first node of Ranvier after the demyelinated area is sufficient to restore normal propagation of the action potential (figure 6.2(C)). In this case, the action potential propagates down the axon, skipping the demyelinated area.

In [30], it was shown that if a partially demyelinated neuron remains alive and functional, appropriate stimulation of the axon away from the damaged area can lead to the normal passage of the action potential by bypassing the demyelinated area. Such stimulation can be a local change in membrane potential induced by a

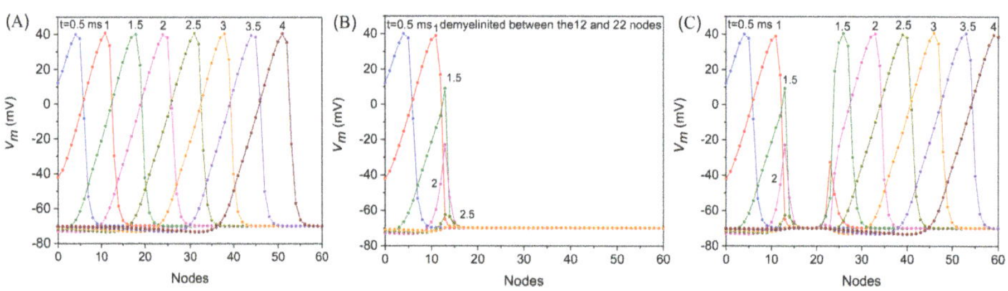

Figure 6.2. Results of model calculations of the myelinated axon [20]. (A) Saltatory action potential propagation in normal myelinated fibers. (B) Action potential blocking in a demyelinated area. (C) Bypass of the demyelinated area (between the 12th and 22nd nodes of Ranvier).

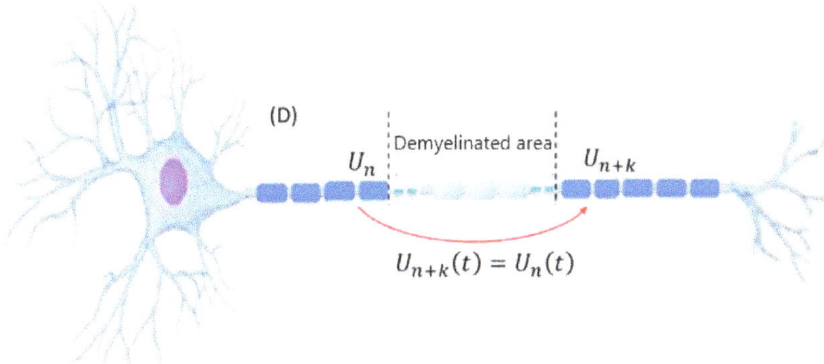

Figure 6.3. Schematic of a neuron with the characteristic elements of the myelinated axon. The demyelinated portions with damaged segments between the nth and $n + k$th nodes of Ranvier are also shown. The arrows indicate the bypass shunting of the demyelinated section.

current in saline, similar to that seen in the synchronization of neurons [30]. This can be done, for example, by changing the local probe potential, inducing a current in the saline, resulting in the membrane charging at a node of Ranvier until the potential difference across the membrane is sufficient to initiate an action potential outside the demyelinated area. The action potential can then propagate along the undamaged segments of the axon. As a result, the activity of the nerve is fully or partially restored. The principle of such shunting of the damaged part of the nerve is schematically shown in figure 6.3.

6.3 Discussion of the possibility of bypassing with noncontact electrodes

All the abovementioned axon damage associated with the demyelination and overgrowth of the nodes of Ranvier with an insulating coating is not accompanied by the death of neurons. Therefore, this question naturally arises: Is it possible to bypass a damaged area of nerve tissue and thus restore its normal function?

In chapter 2, we considered the mechanism of saltatory transition in detail and constructed a mathematical model that allowed us to estimate the scale at which ephaptic coupling between adjacent squid axons manifests [23, 24]. We showed that these currents can locally charge a region of the membrane of a neighboring neuron axon where a potential difference arises that is sufficient to excite the action potential. This approach allows one to estimate the range of synchronization (the correlation scale) of action potentials between non-myelinated fibers and the initial segments of myelinated fibers. As noted in chapter 2, these estimates of the correlation scales are in agreement with the experimental data. Thus, if we were to collect the currents coming from node n and 'transfer' them without loss to node $n + k$, we would be able to bypass the damaged (demyelinated) part of the axon.

Figure 6.4 shows the simplest scheme for implementing a bypass of the demyelinated region of an axon. During action potential propagation, the potentials

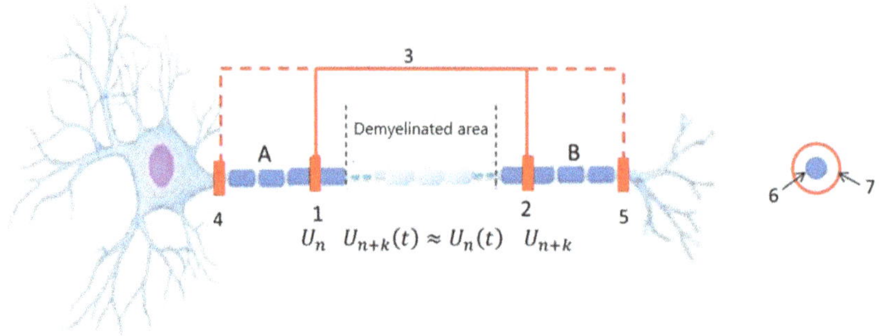

Figure 6.4. Schematic view of damaged myelin fibers, showing the presence of a demyelinated area in which the nodes of Ranvier are absent (overgrown). A and B are undamaged regions of the axon, and 1 and 2 are contactless electrodes: electrode 1 accumulates the charge induced by the propagating action potential, and electrode 2 is located beyond the damaged section of the myelinated fiber, while 3 is an insulated conductor that connects the two electrodes. Electrode 4 is a possible position for the electrode used for 'reading' the action potential; 5 is a possible position for the electrode used for propagating the action potential, bypassing the demyelinated section of the neuron; and 6 and 7 are the contactless electrode and the undamaged section of the myelinated fiber in a cross-sectional view, respectively.

of electrodes 1 and 2 are different; therefore, an electrical connection is established between areas A and B: part of the charge from area A flows into area B, which automatically leads to charging of the membrane of the axon in B. If the transferred charge is large enough that the local potential difference across the membrane of the nodes of Ranvier in area B exceeds the threshold value of $\sim$10–30 mV, an action potential is excited in B. Figure 6.4 also shows another way to bypass the demyelinated part of the axon. For example, one can take the signal from the initial segment of the neuron instead of from the node of Ranvier, or directly excite the peripheral region of the neuron. The possibility of identifying nodes of Ranvier and recording the current in their vicinity was demonstrated by Tasaki [31] and by Huxley and Stämpfli [32] (see chapter 1, section 6). It is also possible to take currents from several nodes of Ranvier in the intact area A, combine them, and send them to area B. Figure 6.4 shows a ring of noncontact electrodes, but the electrode structure may vary. The important thing is to induce a sufficiently large current to charge the membrane to a potential difference that exceeds the threshold for excitation of an action potential behind the damaged (demyelinated) region of the axon.

The use of non-needle, noncontact electrodes is not exotic today. For example, in [33], bipolar hook electrodes and a tripolar cuff electrode were used to stimulate, block, and record the action potential in the sciatic muscle of a frog placed in Ringer's solution,[1] as shown in figure 6.5. Note that this experiment with a frog was not performed to ensure the passage of the action potential by bypassing the

[1] Ringer's solution is a laboratory solution of salts dissolved in water used for a variety of medical conditions. It is an isotonic solution, which means it mimics the body fluids (blood) of animals. The solution typically contains sodium chloride, potassium chloride, calcium chloride, and sodium bicarbonate, which balance the pH.

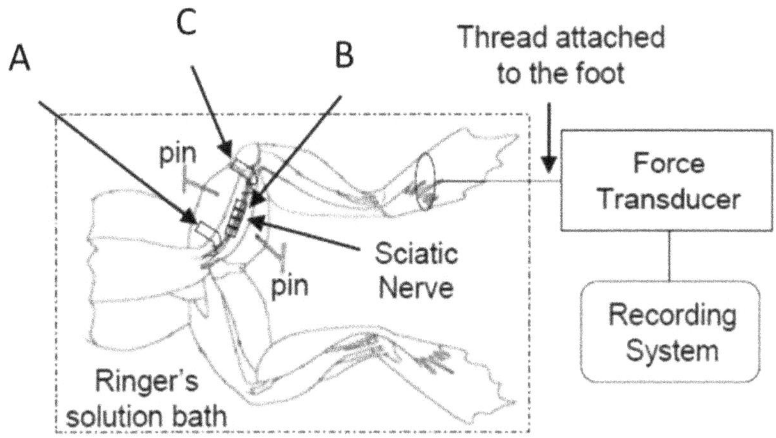

Figure 6.5. Experimental setup showing that the exposed sciatic nerve is stimulated by a bipolar hook electrode A and blocked by a tripolar cuff electrode B. A bipolar hook electrode C is used to confirm the nerve block. The frog legs are immersed in a Ringer's solution bath and fixed by multiple pins. Reprinted by permission from Springer Nature Customer Service Centre GmbH: [Springer], [Medical & Biological Engineering Computing] [33], Copyright (2017).

damaged area, but for the opposite task of blocking the action potential, that is, for anesthesia, which we will discuss in the next chapter. Here, we have presented this experiment only to illustrate the use of miniaturized noncontact electrodes to influence the activity of a single nerve.

We have considered the possibility of bypassing a damaged (e.g. demyelinated) axon section using noncontact electrodes. However, if the damaged axons are part of a nerve containing hundreds or thousands of axons, the use of needle electrodes, for example, makes it possible to isolate them and, using the scheme described above, bypass the damaged sections and thereby restore the activity of the entire nerve.

The possibility of bypassing demyelinated areas of nerve fibers requires experimental verification to assess the feasibility of its implementation in biomedical practice. To observe the propagation of the action potential, its bypass through damaged areas or a complete block may be possible by detecting the second harmonic generated by a laser pulse incident on a sample of nerve tissue, as suggested in [34, 35]. These results demonstrate that the second harmonic response can serve as a local probe of the state of the myelin sheath, providing high-contrast detection of neuronal demyelination.

6.4 Additional notes

It is not necessary for the noncontact electrodes considered in this work to have the shape of a ring. They can be made as half rings, small plates, or grids. The main requirement is that they effectively collect the current in the vicinity of an axon initiated by the action potential.

A positive feature of noncontact electrodes is that, in order to bypass the damaged part of nerve fibers, there is no need to use an external electronic device to amplify the signal from the active part of the fiber. However, if it is necessary to filter, amplify, delay, or suppress the signal from the active part of the nerve fiber or fiber bundle, the scheme proposed here allows this to be done using conventional electronic schemes designed for the system of needle electrodes [8–15].

Over the last 10–15 years, a completely new technology has been developed for the production of electrodes of submicron size (from 20 to 200 nm). These electrodes can take the form of needles, thin wires, or gratings. Therefore, the production of the required extended electrodes of the order of tens or hundreds of square micrometers and with a thickness of a few microns in the form of rings, small plates, or grids is not a technical problem today [19, 36–38].

References and further reading

[1] McDonald W 1963 The effects of experimental demyelination on conduction in peripheral nerve: a histological and electrophysiological study. II. Electrophysiological observations *Brain* **86** 501

[2] Waxman S G 1977 Conduction in myelinated, unmyelinated and demyelinated fibers *Arch. Neurol.* **34** 585

[3] Rasminsky M and Sears T A 1972 Internodal conduction in undissected demyelinated nerve fibers *J. Physiol. (Lond* **227** 323

[4] Waxman S G, Kocsis J D and Black J A 1995 Pathophysiology of demyelinated axons *The Axon* ed S G Waxman, J D Kocsis and P K Stys (Oxford: Oxford University Press) 438

[5] Stephanova D I and Chobanova M 1997 Action potentials and ionic currents through paranodally demyelinated human motor nerve fibers: computer simulations *Biol. Cybern.* **76** 311

[6] Love S 2006 Demyelinating diseases *J. Clin. Pathol.* **59** 1151

[7] Bouton C *et al* 2016 Restoring cortical control of functional movement in a human with quadriplegia *Nature* **533** 247

[8] Sharma G, Annetta N, Friedenberg D, Shaikhouni A, Blanco T, Rezai A and Bouton C 2015 Time stability and coherence analysis of multi-unit, single-unit and local field potential neuronal signals in chronically implanted brain electrodes *Bioelectron. Med.* **2** 63

[9] Opie N L, John S E, Rind G S, Ronayne S M, Grayden D B, Burkitt A N, May C N, O'Brien T J and Oxley T J 2016 Chronic impedance spectroscopy of an endovascular stent-electrode array *J. Neural Eng.* **13** 046020

[10] Wolpaw J R and McFarland D J 2004 Control of a two dimensional movement signal by a noninvasive brain computer interface in humans *Proc. Natl Acad. Sci. USA* **101** 17849

[11] Nunez P and Srinivasan R 2006 *Electric Fields of the Brain: The Neurophysics of EEG* 2nd edn (Oxford: Oxford University Press)

[12] Slutzky M W, Jordan L R, Krieg T, Chen M, Mogul D J and Miller L E 2010 Optimal spacing of surface electrode arrays for brain–machine interface applications *J. Neural Eng.* **7** 026004

[13] Velliste M, Perel S, Spalding M C, Whitford A S and Schwartz A B 2008 Cortical control of a prosthetic arm for self-feeding *Nature* **453** 1098

[14] Hochberg L R *et al* 2012 Reach and grasp by people with tetraplegia using a neurally controlled robotic arm *Nature* **485** 372

[15] Henderson P 2015 Implanted intracortical electrodes as chronic neural interfaces to the central nervous system *PeerJ PrePrints* **3** e1255v1

[16] Richardson-Burns S 2015 Co-electrodeposited hydrogel-conducting polymer electrodes for biomedical applications *US Patent* 20150369771 A1

[17] Abdelghani M, Jung R, Abbas J J and Horch K 2015 Neural interface activity simulator *US Patent* 20150213191

[18] Melosh N A, Verma P and Almquist B D 2014 Devices and methods for long-term intracellular access *US Patent* 20140353172

[19] Richardson-Burns S, Hendricks J L, Martin D C, Sereno A, King Z and Jan E 2015 Coelectrodeposited hydrogel-conducting polymer electrodes for biomedical applications *US Patent* 20150369771

[20] Shneider M N 2016 Bypassing damaged nervous tissue arXiv:1605.06469

[21] Debanne D, Campanac E, Bialowas A, Carlier E and Alcaraz G 2011 Axon physiology *Physiol. Rev.* **91** 555

[22] Colwell L J and Brenner M P 2009 Action potential initiation in the Hodgkin-Huxley model *PLoS Comput. Biol.* **5** e1000265

[23] Clark J and Plonsey R 1966 The mathematical evaluation of the core conductor model *Biophys. J.* **6** 95

[24] Clark J and Plonsey R 1968 The extracellular potential field of the single active nerve fiber in a volume *Biophys. J.* **8** 842

[25] Barr R C and Plonsey R 1992 Electrophysiological interaction through interstitial space between adjacent unmyelinated parallel fibers *Biophys. J.* **61** 1164

[26] Segundo J P 1986 What can neurons do to serve as integrating devices *J. Theor. Neurobiol.* **5** 1

[27] Esplin D W 1962 Independence of conduction velocity among myelinated fibers in cat nerve *J. Neurophysiol.* **25** 805

[28] Goldman L and Albus J S 1968 Computation of impulse conduction in myelinated fibers; theoretical basis of the velocity-diameter relation *Biophys. J.* **8** 596

[29] Platkiewicz J and Brette R A 2010 Threshold equation for action potential initiation *PLoS Comput. Biol.* **6** e1000850

[30] Shneider M N and Pekker M 2015 Correlation of action potentials in adjacent neurons *Phys. Biol.* **12** 066009

[31] Tasaki I 1959 *Conduction of nerve impulse Handbook of Physiology. Section I: Neurophysiology* **vol 1** ed J Field (Bethesda, MD: American Physiological Society) 75

[32] Huxley A F and Stämpfli R 1949 Evidence for saltatory conduction in peripheral myelinated nerve fibres *J. Physiol.* **108** 315

[33] Yang G, Wang J, Shen B, Roppolo J R, de Groat W C and Tai C 2017 Post-stimulation block of frog sciatic nerve by high-frequency (kHz) biphasic stimulation *Med. Biol. Eng. Comput.* **55** 585

[34] Shneider M N, Voronin A A and Zheltikov A M 2010 Modeling the action-potential-encoded second harmonic generation as an ultrafast local probe for nonintrusive membrane diagnostics *Phys. Rev.* E **81** 031926

[35] Shneider M N, Voronin A A and Zheltikov A M 2011 Modeling the action-potential-sensitive nonlinear-optical response of myelinated nerve fibers and short-term memory *J. Appl. Phys.* **110** 094702

[36] Almquist B D and Melosh N A 2011 Molecular structure influences the stability of membrane penetrating bio-interfaces *Nano Lett.* **11** 2066
[37] Zhang A, Zheng G and Lieber C 2016 *Nanowires: Building Blocks for Nanoscience and Nanotechnology* NanoScience and Technology (Cham: Springer International Publishing)
[38] Castleberry S A, Almquist B D, Li W, Reis T, Chow J, Mayner S and Hammond P T 2016 Self-assembled wound dressings silence mmp-9 and improve diabetic wound healing *in vivo* *Adv. Mater.* **28** 1809
[39] Swinney K R and Wikswo J J P 1980 A calculation of the magnetic field of a nerve action potential *Biophys. J.* **32** 719
[40] Roth B J and Wikswo J J P 1985 The magnetic field of a single axon *Biophys. J.* **48** 93

IOP Publishing

Low-Intensity Control of Nerve Tissue Activity

Mikhail N Shneider and Mikhail Pekker

Chapter 7

Theoretical model of external spinal cord stimulation

This chapter presents a theoretical model for the excitation of action potentials in multiple motor pools when stimulating current pulses are applied over the lumbosacral regions of the spinal cord. This model explains the known empirical data that have been obtained in medical experiments. It is shown that currents initiated in the intercellular conductive medium can non-synaptically excite neurons, analogous to ephaptic coupling, thereby facilitating the activation of spinal networks capable of generating motor-evoked potentials in different leg muscles. The selectivity of the effect of the stimulating current pulse on neurons of different types is discussed.

7.1 Introduction

Over the last decade, a significant number of experimental studies have demonstrated the effectiveness of restoring lower limb control by means of spinal cord stimulation in the lumbosacral regions of the spinal cord below the site of spinal cord injury. These effects have been observed with electrical stimulation using implanted epidural electrodes and with stimulation using non-invasive electrodes placed directly on the skin over the lower spinal cord [1–13].

The results obtained are surprising because they contradict the conventional opinion that recovery of motor function in the lower limbs is impossible after one year of complete motor paralysis. In fact, spontaneous regeneration of damaged axons or plastic remodeling of preserved fiber systems after spinal cord injury is very limited in mammals. The main reasons for this poor capacity for spontaneous regeneration appear to be an inadequate neuronal growth response to injury, components that inhibit neuronal tissue growth, and the formation of cysts and

doi:10.1088/978-0-7503-6034-0ch7

scar tissue at the site of injury. However, studies conducted in recent decades (see, for example, reviews [14–17]) provide hope that modern methods of medical treatment in combination with spinal stimulation of the lumbosacral regions of the spinal cord below the site of spinal cord injury will allow successful restoration of the activity of the damaged regions of the spinal cord and thus cure paralyzed people.

The spinal cord is a complex anatomical system. Thus, we will not go into details that are far beyond the scope of this book, but instead refer the reader to excellent reviews and books, for example, [18–21].

The human spinal cord is a tubular bundle of nerve tissue and supporting cells that extends from the brainstem to the lumbar vertebrae. Together, the spinal cord and brain form the central nervous system. The spinal cord carries nerve signals from the brain to the body and vice versa. These nerve signals help you feel sensations and move your body. Any damage to the spinal cord can affect the movement or function of the body. The structure of the spine and its cross-section with the spinal cord are shown in figure 7.1. In total, the human spinal cord contains 31 pairs of nerves and nerve roots. These include:

1. Eight cervical nerve pairs (nerves that start in your neck and run mostly to your face).
2. Twelve pairs of thoracic nerves (nerves in the upper body that run to the chest, upper back, and abdomen).
3. Five pairs of lumbar nerves (nerves in the lower back that go to the legs and feet).
4. Five sacral nerve pairs (pairs of nerves in the lower back that run to the pelvis).

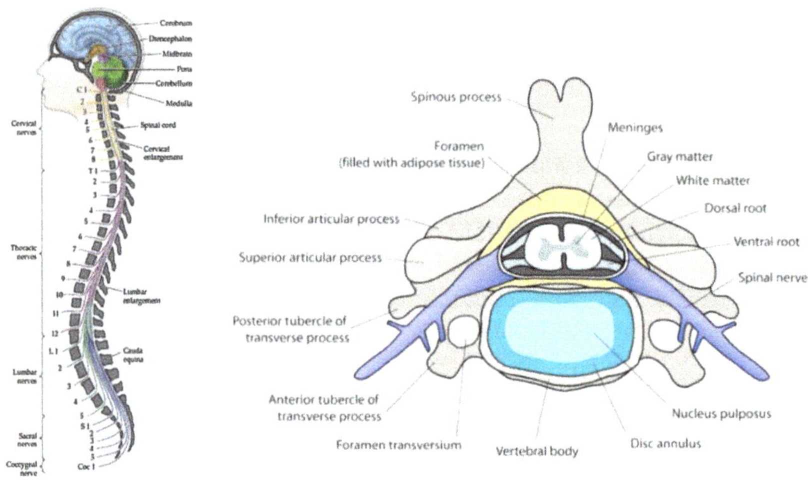

Figure 7.1. (Left) Anatomical structure of the spine. All 31 spinal nerves are shown. Reprinted from [21], Copyright (2014), with permission from Elsevier. (Right) Cross-section of a typical cervical vertebra with the spinal cord. Reproduced with permission from [22]. CC BY 3.0.

5. A nerve bundle at the base of the spinal cord, called the cauda equina. Cauda equina comes from the Latin word for 'horse's tail.' This name was used by early anatomists because they thought the nerve bundle looked like a horse's tail. The cauda equina contains nerves that provide sensation to your lower body.

For theoretical analysis, it is convenient to use simplified models of nerves. Figure 7.2 shows an example of such a simplified schematic view of the lumbar nerve, which is a bundle of isolated wires (fascicles) consisting of thin wires (axons) in a conducting medium. For nerves in and around the spinal cord, depending on their structure and location, the conducting medium may be cerebrospinal fluid (CSF), gray matter (GM), or white matter (WM), which have marked differences in conductance. Thus, according to [13], typical values of GM conductivity σ_g, longitudinal $\sigma_{w,\,\|}$ and transverse $\sigma_{w,\,\perp}$ WM conductivities, CSF σ_{cf}, and epidural fat σ_{ef} conductivities are $\sigma_g \approx 0.23$, $\sigma_{w,\,\|} \approx 0.6$, $\sigma_{w,\,\perp} \approx 0.083$, $\sigma_{\mathrm{cf}} \approx 1.7$, and $\sigma_{\mathrm{ef}} \approx 0.04\ \Omega^{-1}\,\mathrm{m}^{-1}$, respectively.

CSF is a fluid that constantly circulates in the brain ventricles, CSF tracts, subarachnoid space of the brain, and spinal cord. It protects the brain and spinal cord from mechanical influences and maintains constant intracranial pressure and water–electrolyte homeostasis. The GM and WM of the central nervous system (CNS) are conspicuous features that are attractive to quantify and compare across human and animal species. It should be noted that the GM of the spinal cord consists primarily of nerve cell bodies and their processes, which do not have myelin sheaths. In addition, the GM contains the processes of nerve cells located in other parts of the spinal cord and brain, neuroglia, blood vessels, and associated connective tissue. WM (white in color) consists mainly of myelinated axons of fibers, which distinguishes it from GM, and it is composed of bundles that connect different GM areas (the locations of nerve cell bodies) of the brain and carry nerve impulses between neurons. Recall that the role of the myelin sheath was discussed earlier in chapters 1 and 2, and it was shown that the myelin sheath acts as an

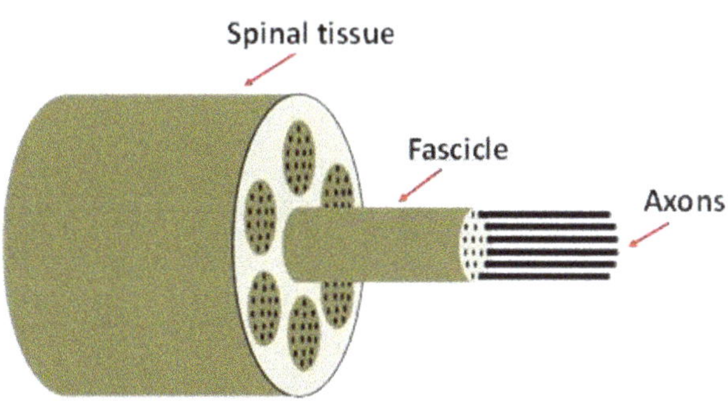

Figure 7.2. Schematic of one of the lumbar nerves, which is depicted as a bundle of isolated wires (fascicles) consisting of thin wires (axons).

insulator, allowing saltatory transmission of the action potential and thereby increasing the speed of transmission of nerve signals.

Before moving on to the model of electrical stimulation of spinal nerve activity, we should note that physiotherapy with electrical impulses has been successfully applied not only to patients paralyzed by spinal cord injury but also to those who have sustained injuries affecting other parts of the nervous system, for example, to restore normal function of the facial nerve [23].

7.2 Examples of electrical stimulation experiments on the spinal cord nerve

Electrode placement, geometry, and size may vary in different spinal cord electrical stimulation trials. Figure 7.3 shows an example of electrode placement for transcutaneous spinal cord stimulation.

In experiments [6, 8], slightly different electrodes and arrangements were used. A conductive rubber electrode with a radius of $R_{el} = 9$ mm was placed on the skin between the spinous processes T12–L1, T11–T12, and T10–T11 (figure 7.1) as a cathode, and two 5 × 9 cm self-adhesive electrodes (Pro-Patch) were placed symmetrically on the skin over the iliac crests as anodes. This electrode configuration provides a fairly uniform distribution of currents near the cathode. In these experiments, stimulation was delivered as a single square-wave pulse every 6 s, and the amplitudes of the stimulation current pulses, shown in figure 7.4, varied from $J_0 = 2$–100 mA [6, 8].

7.3 Computational models for epidural electrical stimulation of spinal nerves

The computer model for epidural electrical stimulation of the spinal nerve consists of two parts: a calculation model for the system of currents in the region of the spinal nerve and an excitation model for the action potential induced in the axon fiber by

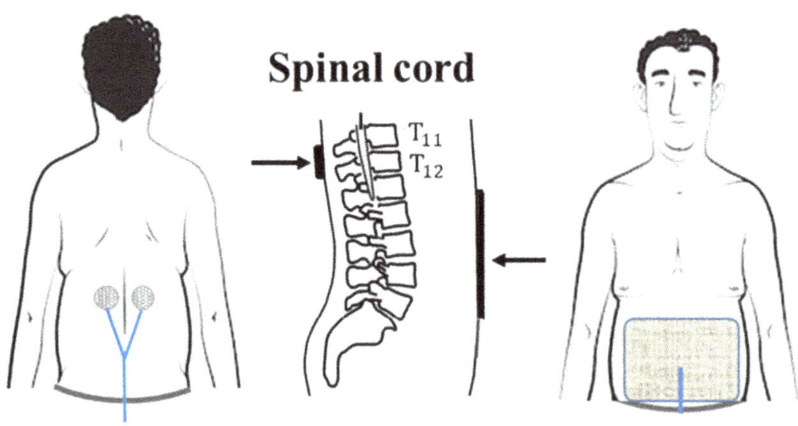

Figure 7.3. Example of electrode placement for transcutaneous spinal cord stimulation. Adapted from [24].

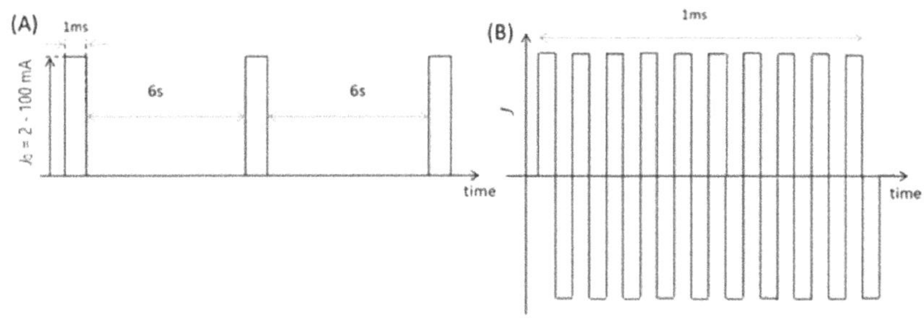

Figure 7.4. Periodic current pulses applied to the electrodes. (A) Time dependence of the current amplitude. (B) Current during the stimulation period.

these currents [25–32]. The calculation of currents in these works was carried out on the basis of solving the continuity equation for currents:

$$\nabla \cdot \vec{I} = \nabla \cdot \sigma \vec{E} = \nabla \cdot \sigma \nabla \varphi = 0, \tag{7.1}$$

with Dirichlet boundary conditions set at the outermost boundaries of the model:

$$\varphi(\mathrm{d}\Omega) = 0, \tag{7.2}$$

where φ, $\vec{I}$, and $\vec{E}$ are the distributions of potential, current density, and electric field in the electrolyte, respectively; σ is the conductivity; and $\mathrm{d}\Omega$ is the outermost surface of the model.

In fact, boundary condition (7.2) corresponds to an electrode and has nothing to do with the presence of a conductive fluid in which the spinal nerve is located. The correct numerical model for calculating the distribution of currents in the spinal nerve region (equation (7.1)) should include a second electrode.

The model of action potential initiation by currents flowing through the spinal cord in the axons of myelinated motoneurons described in [25, 31, 32] has the following form:

$$\frac{\mathrm{d}\varphi_n}{\mathrm{d}t} = \frac{1}{C_m}(G_a((\varphi_{i,\,n+1} - 2\varphi_{i,\,n} + \varphi_{i,\,n-1}) + (\varphi_{e,\,n+1} - 2\varphi_{e,\,n} + \varphi_{e,\,n-1})) - I_{i,\,n}) \tag{7.3}$$

$$\varphi_n = \varphi_{i,\,n} - \varphi_{e,\,n} + \varphi_r, \tag{7.4}$$

where $I_{i,\,n}$ is the ionic current density passing through the nth active part of the membrane with a capacitance of C_m, and G_a is the intra-axonal conductance between the centers of two adjacent segments. $I_{i,\,n}$ is a function of the voltage between the inner potential $\varphi_{i,\,n}$ and the outer potential $\varphi_{e,\,n}$ in the nth node of Ranvier, and φ_r is the inner resting potential. From (7.3), it follows that if the external potential at the membrane, determined by the currents flowing in the spinal cord, is constant, then the initiation of the action potential does not occur. This is not true, however, since the initiation of the action potential is due to the charging of the axon membrane by currents perpendicular to the surface of the neurons initiated by electrodes (the axon membrane is a cylindrical condenser filled with saline). An increase in the potential difference across the membrane lowers the excitation threshold of the action potential.

It should be noted that in all known numerical models of neuron excitation by external currents (see, for example, [24–35]), the potential $\varphi_{i,\,n}$ is calculated by considering the average conductivity of the medium in which the neurons are located. However, as shown in this chapter, the potential in the vicinity of a neuron depends on the radius of the neuron and can therefore differ significantly from the calculated potential.

Theoretical models discussed in [36] and [37] were developed to explain ephaptic coupling (chapter 2, section 2.3) and describe the bypass of a damaged section of myelinated axon (chapter 6), respectively. We consider the stimulation of nerves in a damaged but living spinal cord described by a similar model in [38]. The theoretical model proposed in [38] is based on a simple idea: the currents generated by external current sources charge the neuronal membranes to the potential at which the action potential is initiated. Since the potential at the nonconducting membrane φ_a is proportional to the radius of the axon a, given the same current density in the extracellular fluid and the same conductivity of the extracellular medium, the change in the potential difference across the membrane will be different for neurons with axons of different radii. Accordingly, for the same threshold potential difference, the excitation of neurons with axons of a larger radius should occur at a lower current density than that of neurons with axons of a smaller radius.

Since the radius of the spinal nerve does not exceed 2.4 mm [39] and the distance from the nerve fiber (spinal tissue) to the electrode (cathode) is less than the diameter of the electrode (e.g. ~18 mm for the experimental conditions given in [6, 8]), the distribution of currents in the region of the spinal cord can be considered perpendicular to the electrode and uniformly distributed over the area far from the fascia (or spinal root), as shown in figure 7.5.

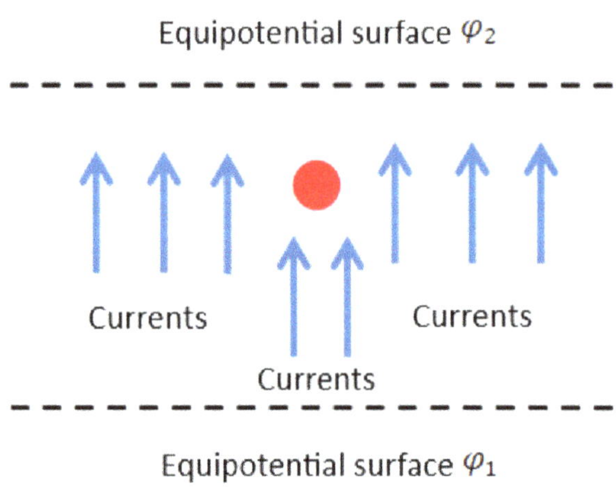

Figure 7.5. A sketch of the location of the fascia (or spinal root) in the area of current flow between the electrodes. The distance from the spinal nerve is much less than the diameter of the electrode. The dashed lines indicate equipotential surfaces away from the spinal tissue. The red disk represents a fascicle (or spinal root).

As proposed in [38], we consider the following model based on conditions corresponding to figure 7.5:

1. The axons of the fascicles are thin-walled cylinders that are far enough from each other that they can be viewed independently in the field of constant currents.
2. The conductivity of the medium in which the axon is located depends on its location. If the axon is in CSF, $\sigma = \sigma_{\mathrm{cf}}$; if in GM, $\sigma = \sigma_g$; if in WM, the conductivity of the medium depends on the direction of the current (orientation of the electric field). If the current is transverse to the spinal cord, then $\sigma = \sigma_{w,\perp}$; and if parallel, then $\sigma = \sigma_{w,\parallel}$. The corresponding quantitative values of the conductivities are given in section 7.1.
3. The membrane is impermeable to the ionic conduction currents that charge the capacitance. Instead, the current in the electrolyte completes its circuit path through the membrane's capacitance via the displacement current, $C_m \mathrm{d}V_m/\mathrm{d}t$, where c_m is the membrane capacitance per unit area and V_m is the voltage across the membrane. The axon (cylinder) membrane is charged by currents in the electrolyte until the additional surface charge accumulated on the membrane compensates for the radial field of the currents charging the membrane.

Without loss of generality, we assume that the currents that charge the membrane and change the potential difference across it are perpendicular to the axon surface (figure 7.6).

Consider the case where the time of the field change in the electrolyte is much longer than the charging time of the surface of the cylinder (the neuron membrane), as shown in figure 7.7. Equation (7.1) for the currents flowing in the external electrolyte has the following form:

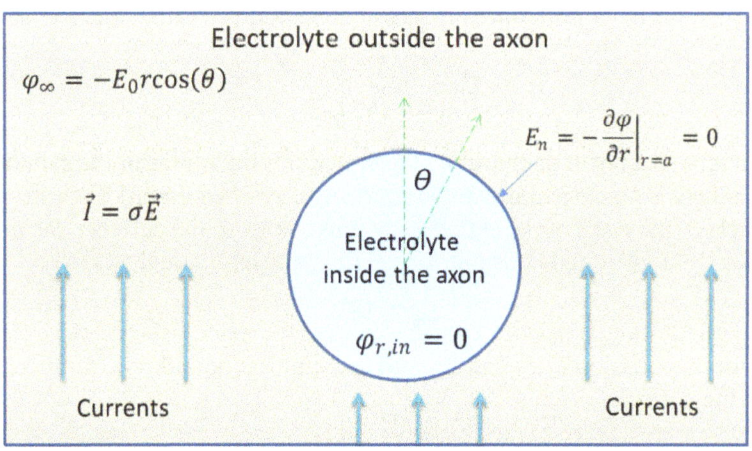

Figure 7.6. Schematic of a single axon cross-section in a field of currents uniformly distributed over the volume.

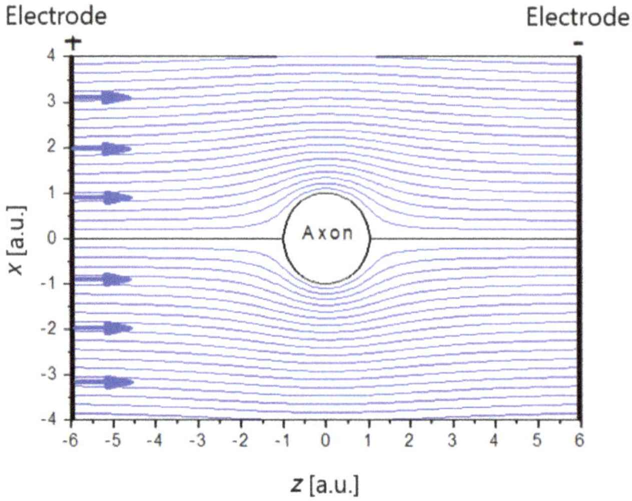

Figure 7.7. The current lines near the cylindrical axon, which is charged to a potential (7.15) corresponding to an electric field with components (7.13) and (7.14).

$$\mathrm{div}\vec{I} = -\sigma\left(\frac{1}{r}\frac{\partial}{\partial r}r\frac{\partial\varphi}{\partial r} + \frac{1}{r^2}\frac{\partial^2\varphi}{\partial\theta^2}\right) = 0, \tag{7.5}$$

where the conductivity σ of the electrolyte is assumed to be constant.

Far from the cylinder, the current density is constant, since the current is determined by the flat electrodes used in the experiments [6, 8], as shown schematically in figure 7.5. Accordingly, the current, the potential, and the electric field are represented by the relationship

$$\varphi_\infty = -E_0 r\cos(\theta) = -I_0 r\cos(\theta)/\sigma, \tag{7.6}$$

where $I_0 \approx J/\pi R_{\mathrm{el}}^2$ and J is the total current passing through the external electrodes. Since the membrane is impermeable to ion currents, the radial electric field

$$E_n = -\frac{\partial\varphi}{\partial r}\bigg|_{r=a} \tag{7.7}$$

must go to zero as a result of charging. Hereafter, a is the radius of the cylinder (axon).

Because there is no current inside the conductive cylinder (axon) when the stationary state is reached (the walls of the cylinder are impervious to the current), the potential of the cylinder is uniform and constant. For clarity, we set it equal to zero:

$$\varphi_{\mathrm{in}} = 0. \tag{7.8}$$

The solution of equation (7.5), taking into account the boundary condition (7.6), has the following form:

$$\varphi = -E_0 r\cos(\theta) + \sum_1^\infty B_n r^{-n}\cos(n\theta). \tag{7.9}$$

Since the radial field is zero at the boundary of the cylinder, from (7.9), we obtain:

$$E_n = -\frac{\partial \varphi}{\partial r}\bigg|_{r=a} = E_0 \cos(\theta) - \sum_1^{\infty} n B_n a^{-n-1} \cos(n\theta) = 0 \tag{7.10}$$

and

$$B_1 = -E_0 a^2,\ B_2 = B_3 = \ldots = B_n = 0 \tag{7.11}$$

$$\varphi = -E_0 \cos(\theta)\left(r + \frac{a^2}{r}\right). \tag{7.12}$$

Thus, the electric components are

$$E_r = E_0 \cos(\theta)\left(1 - \frac{a^2}{r^2}\right) = \frac{I_0}{\sigma} \cos(\theta)\left(1 - \frac{a^2}{r^2}\right), \tag{7.13}$$

$$E_\theta = E_0 \sin(\theta)\left(1 + \frac{a^2}{r^2}\right) = \frac{I_0}{\sigma} \sin(\theta)\left(1 + \frac{a^2}{r^2}\right). \tag{7.14}$$

In accordance with equations (7.12) and (7.9), the potential difference on the membrane is as follows:

$$\varphi_a = -2E_0 a \cdot \cos(\theta) = -\frac{2I_0}{\sigma} a \cdot \cos(\theta) = -\frac{2J}{\pi R_{\text{el}}^2 \sigma} a \cdot \cos(\theta). \tag{7.15}$$

It follows from (7.15) that the steady-state potential difference across the membrane depends only on the magnitude of the current and the radius of the cylinder. Figure 7.7 shows the current lines in the vicinity of the cylindrical axon charged to potential (7.15), corresponding to the electric field with components (7.13) and (7.14).

It can be seen that near the dielectric cylinder (axon membrane), the current lines (and the electric field) have only a tangential component. We now answer the question of how quickly the potential difference across the membrane is established when the current is applied. Obviously, this time is determined by the time required to charge the cylindrical capacitor to a potential equal to (7.15). For simplicity, we assume that the thin-walled dielectric cylinder does not disturb the electric field near its surface. In this case, the radial current is the one that charges the cylindrical capacitor:

$$I_n = -I_0 \cos(\theta). \tag{7.16}$$

Therefore, an estimate of the transition time (characteristic charging time of the capacitor) is given by:

$$\tau_{tr} \sim C_m \frac{\varphi_a}{I_n} = 2\frac{C_m a}{\sigma}, \tag{7.17}$$

Table 7.1. Transition times τ_{tr} (equation 7.17) of the axon surface charge of motoneurons of various types (differing in dimensions taken from [41]) at different ambient conductivities.

Type	Radius [μm]	Average [μm]	τ_{tr} [μs] CSF	τ_{tr} [μs] GM	τ_{tr} [μs] WM
α	6–10	8	0.094	0.695	1.92
β	2.5–6	4.25	0.050	0.370	1.02
γ	1.5–3	2.25	0.024	0.196	0.54
δ	1–2.5	1.75	0.021	0.152	0.42

where $C_m \approx 10^{-2}$ [m^{-2}] is the membrane capacitance per unit area [40]. It is important to note that in experiments [3, 5–8], this time is several orders of magnitude shorter than the duration of the current pulse in figure 7.4 (1 ms) and can therefore be neglected. The radius of motoneurons a is in the range of 6–10 μm for α motoneurons, 2.5–6 μm for β motoneurons, 1.5–3 μm for γ motoneurons, and 1–2.5 μm for δ motoneurons [34]. Table 7.1 presents estimates of the value of τ (7.17) for different types of neurons of various radius a located in CSF $\sigma = \sigma_{cf}$, in GM $\sigma = \sigma_g$, and in WM $\sigma = \sigma_{w,\perp}$.

7.4 Results and discussion

Since the duration of the current pulse in the experiments described in [3, 5–8] was 1 ms, which is almost four orders of magnitude longer than the charging time of the neuron membrane (see table 7.1), the potential difference across the membrane is constant over the duration of the current pulse and is given by formula (7.15).

In the experiments reported in [8], the amplitude of the current pulses shown in figure 7.4 varied in the range of $J = 2 - 100$ mA. Using formula (7.15), we can obtain an estimation formula for the critical current J_{cr} for the known critical perturbation value of the membrane potential δV_m:

$$J_{cr} \approx \frac{\pi R_{el}^2 \sigma}{2a} \delta V_m. \tag{7.18}$$

Since the ratio of the mean radii of the α, β, and γ neurons is 1.9:1:0.53, then for the same initiation voltage perturbation δV_m, the ratio of the critical currents should be 10.5:20:38. Let us assume that the critical perturbation of the membrane potential required for action potential excitation is the same for axons of all considered neuron types and is equal to $\delta V_m \approx 10$ mV. Then, by substituting the values $R_{el} = 9$ mm and $\sigma = \sigma_{w,\perp} = 0.083$ [Ω^{-1} m^{-1}] into (7.18), we can determine the values of the currents J_{cr} at which the excitation of action potentials occurs in axons of types α, β, γ, and δ located in the WM region. These critical current estimates are presented in table 7.2. Thus, the excitation of different types of neurons occurs at different critical currents. For example, if the current exceeds the critical value only by enough to excite the axons of the larger α neurons, the axons of other types of neurons within an axon fascicle will remain inactive. It should be noted, however, that the dynamic environment and the various cellular and synaptic components

Table 7.2. Estimates (7.18) of the excitation of the action potential threshold current in experiments [8] for different types of neurons in the WM area, where $\sigma = 0.083\ \Omega^{-1}\ \mathrm{m}^{-1}$ at $R_{el} = 9$ mm, and the voltage perturbation $\delta V_m = 10$ mV.

Neuron type	Radius [41] [μm]	Average Radius [μm]	J_{cr} [mA] WM
α	6–10	8	13.16
β	2.5–6	4.25	24.83
γ	1.5–3	2.25	46.83
δ	1–2.5	1.75	60.33

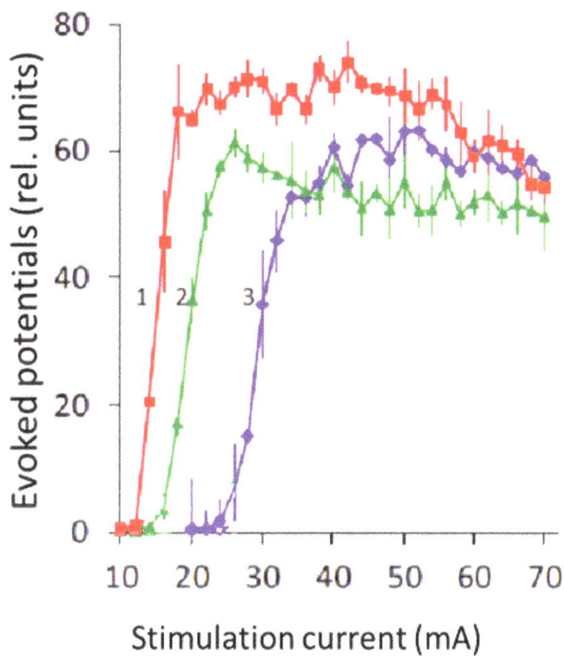

Figure 7.8. Evoked potentials in the medial gastrocnemius muscle of a human subject during transcutaneous electrical spinal stimulation delivered at different intensities at three spinal levels. Dependence of spinal nerve excitation in intervertebral regions [8]. Points 1, 2, and 3 represent thresholds of excitation in the areas T12–L1, T11–T12, and T10–T11 of the spinal nerve, respectively. Reproduced with permission from [8]. Copyright © 2015, The American Physiological Society.

within and between spinal networks functioning at different current levels under *in vivo* conditions are much more complex than those of a bundle of axons within a nerve fascicle. Intuitively, it would seem that this more complex environment under *in vivo* conditions would make the probability of excitation even higher than when modeling such a phenomenon based on the axonal diameter.

The data shown in figure 7.8 illustrate the effects of different currents applied transcutaneously at three different sites along the spinal axis. At each stimulation site, there is a clear threshold for action potential initiation, and the threshold is assumed to be largely determined by the size of the axons. The recruitment curves shown for each of the stimulation sites reflect monosynaptic responses recorded in the medial gastrocnemius muscle mediated by the activation of the largest axons within the dorsal roots. The estimates of critical currents and their dependence on axon type presented in table 7.2 are in qualitative and reasonable quantitative agreement with the experimental results presented in figure 7.8. One of the differences between the experimental data in figure 7.8 and the estimates in table 7.2 is most likely due to uncertainty in neuron size and action potential initiation voltage. In fact, after the action potential starts, the processes related to the opening of the ion channels are dominant, while the influence of external currents charging the membrane of the axons ceases to play a role. It should also be noted that the recovery time of the action potential is on the order of 0.01 s, which is much less than the time between the current pulses (figure 7.4).

According to (7.15), for a fixed current in the electrolyte, the potential difference across the membrane is directly proportional to the radius of the axon and inversely proportional to the conductivity of the electrolyte. In our opinion, the different excitation thresholds of action potentials in the lumbosacral regions of the spinal cord observed in [8] are largely due to differences in the radii of α, β, and γ motoneurons. This fact can explain the selectivity of the effect of the current pulse amplitude necessary to stimulate an action potential in neurons of different types.

Note that we have assumed that the spinal nerve axons are far enough apart that they can be treated independently. According to (7.13), the electric field from a charged cylinder falls as a^2/r^2, and the interaction of neurons with each other can be neglected if the distance between them is greater than the diameter of the axon. If the distance between neurons is on the order of or less than the diameter of the axon, then they can no longer be considered as single, i.e. unaffected by other neighboring neurons.

7.5 Concluding remarks

The considered mechanism of action potential excitation in motoneurons is inherently similar to the ephaptic coupling effect discussed in chapter 2. We have shown that action potential excitation by currents initiated by an external source in the intercellular conducting medium explains the experimental results for observed spontaneous limb movements. The proposed model can be effectively applied to predict and optimize the stimulation of nerve activity by external current sources.

References

[1] Angeli C A, Edgerton V R, Gerasimenko Y P and Harkema S J 2014 Altering spinal cord excitability enables voluntary movements after chronic complete paralysis in humans *Brain* **137** 1394

[2] Grahn P J *et al* 2017 Enabling task-specific volitional motor functions via spinal cord neuromodulation in a human with paraplegia *Mayo Clin. Proc.* **92** 544

[3] Gerasimenko Y P *et al* 2015 Noninvasive reactivation of motor descending control after paralysis *J. Neurotrauma* **32** 1968

[4] Gad P N, Gerasimenko Y P, Zdunowski S, Sayenko D, Haakana P, Turner A, Lu D, Roy R R and Edgerton V R 2015 Iron 'ElectriRx' man: overground stepping in an exoskeleton combined with noninvasive spinal cord stimulation after paralysis *2015 37th Annual International Conference of the IEEE Engineering in Medicine and Biology Society (EMBC)* (Piscataway, NJ: IEEE) 1124

[5] Gerasimenko Y *et al* 2016 Integration of sensory, spinal, and volitional descending inputs in regulation of human locomotion *J. Neurophysiol.* **116** 98

[6] Gerasimenko Y, Gorodnichev R, Moshonkina T, Sayenko D, Gad P and Edgerton V R 2015 Transcutaneous electrical spinal-cord stimulation in humans *Ann. Phys. Rehabil. Med.* **58** 225

[7] Gerasimenko Y, Gorodnichev R, Puhov A, Moshonkina T, Savochin A, Selionov V, Roy R R, Lu D C and Edgerton V R 2015 Initiation and modulation of locomotor circuitry output with multisite transcutaneous electrical stimulation of the spinal cord in noninjured humans *J. Neurophysiol.* **113** 834

[8] Gerasimenko Y P, Gorodnichev R, Puhov A, Moshonkina T, Savochin A, Selionov V, Roy R R, Lu D C and Edgerton V R 2015 Spinal segment-specific transcutaneous stimulation differentially shapes activation pattern among motor pools in humans *J. Appl. Physiol.* **118** 1364

[9] Possover M 2004 Laparoscopic exposure and electrostimulation of the somatic and autonomous pelvic nerves: a new method for implantation of neuroprosthesis in paralyzed patients? *J. Gynecol. Surg. Endosc. Imaging Allied Techniques* **1** 87

[10] Possover M, Baekelandt J, Flaskamp C, Dong L and Chiantera V 2007 Laparoscopic neurolysis of the sacral plexus and the sciatic nerve for extensive endometriosis of the pelvic wall *Minim. Invas. Neurosurg.* **12** 11

[11] Possover M, Baekelandt J and Chianteras V 2007 The Laparoscopic Implantation of Neuroprothesis (LION) Procedure to Control Intractable Abdomino-Pelvic Neuralgia *Neuromodulation* **10** 18

[12] Moraud E M, Capogrosso M, Formento E, Wenger N, DiGiovanna J, Courtine G and Micera S 2016 Mechanisms underlying the neuromodulation of spinal circuits for correcting gait and balance deficits after spinal cord injury *Neuron* **89** 814

[13] Schiff N D *et al* 2023 Thalamic deep brain stimulation in traumatic brain injury: a phase 1, randomized feasibility study *Nat. Med.* **29** 3162

[14] Fawcett J 2002 Repair of spinal cord injuries: where are we, where are we going? *Spinal Cord* **40** 615

[15] Nieuwenhuis B, Haenzi B, Andrews M R, Verhaagen J and Fawcett J W 2018 Integrins promote axonal regeneration afterinjury of the nervous system *Biol. Rev.* **93** 1339

[16] Tyzack G E *et al* 2014 Astrocyte response to motor neuron injury promotes structural synaptic plasticity via STAT3-regulated TSP-1 expression *Nature Commun.* **5** 4294

[17] Taylor C, McHugh C, Mockler D, Minogue C, Reilly R B and Fleming N 2021 Transcutaneous spinal cord stimulation and motor responses in individuals with spinal cord injury: a methodological review *PLoS One* **16** e0260166

[18] Bican O, Minagar A and Pruitt A A 2013 The spinal cord: a review of functional neuroanatomy *Neurol. Clin.* **31**

[19] Squire L, Berg D, Bloom F E, du Lac S, Ghosh A and Spitzer N C 2013 *Fundamental Neuroscience* 4th edn (Amsterdam: Elsevier/Academic Press)
[20] Siegel A and Sapru H N 2011 *Essential Neuroscience* 2nd edn (Philadelphia, PA: Wolters Kluwer)
[21] Silva N A, Sousa N, Reis R L and Salgado A J 2014 From basics to clinical: a comprehensive review on spinal cord injury *Prog. Neurobiol.* **114** 25
[22] Rehman M and El-Ost B 2011 *Relationships between AAA and cauda equina syndrome Diagnosis, Screening and Treatment of Abdominal, Thoracoabdominal and Thoracic Aortic Aneurysms* (Rijeka: InTech)
[23] Yoo M C, Kim J H, Kim Y J, Jung J, Kim S S, Kim S H and Yeo S G 2023 Effects of electrical stimulation on facial paralysis recovery after facial nerve injury: a review on preclinical and clinical studies *J. Clin. Med.* **12** 4133
[24] Ladenbauer J, Minassian K, Hofstoetter U S, Dimitrijevic M R and Rattay F 2010 Stimulation of the human lumbar spinal cord with implanted and surface electrodes: a computer simulation study *IEEE Trans. Neural Syst. Rehabil. Eng.* **18** 637
[25] McNeal D R 1976 Analysis of a model for excitation of myelinated nerve *IEEE Trans. Biomed. Eng.* **23 329** 1976
[26] Rattay F 1986 Analysis of models for external stimulation of axons *IEEE Trans. Biomed. Eng.* **33** 974
[27] Rattay F, Minassian K and Dimitrijevic M R 2000 Epidural electrical stimulation of posterior structures of the human lumbosacral cord: 2. quantitative analysis by computer modeling *Spinal Cord* **38** 473
[28] McIntyre c c, Richardson A G and Grill W M 2002 Modeling the excitability of mammalian nerve fibers: influence of afterpotentials on the recovery cycle *J. Neurophysiol.* **87** 995
[29] Capogrosso M, Wenger N, Raspopovic S, Musienko P, Beauparlant J, Luciani L B, Courtine G and Micera S 2013 A computational model for epidural electrical stimulation of spinal sensorimotor circuits *J. Neurosci.* **33** 19326
[30] Moraud E M, Capogrosso M, Formento E, Wenger N, DiGiovanna J, Courtine G and Micera S 2016 Mechanisms underlying the neuromodulation of spinal circuits for correcting gait and balance deficits after spinal cord injury *Neuron* **89** 814
[31] Struijk J J, Holsheimer J, van der Heide G G and Boom H B 1992 Recruitment of dorsal column fibers in spinal cord stimulation: influence of collateral branching *IEEE Trans. Biomed. Eng.* **39** 903
[32] Lempka S F, McIntyre c c, Kilgore K L and Machado A G 2015 Computational analysis of kilohertz frequency spinal cord stimulation for chronic pain management *Anesthesiology* **122** 1362
[33] Binder V E, Hofstoetter U S, Rienmüller A, Száva Z, Krenn M J, Minassian K and Danner S M 2021 Influence of spine curvature on the efficacy of transcutaneous lumbar spinal cord stimulation *J. Clin. Med.* **10** 554
[34] Danner S M, Hofstoetter U S, Ladenbauer J, Rattay F and Minassian K 2011 Can the human lumbar posterior columns be stimulated by transcutaneous spinal cord stimulation? A modeling study *Artif. Organs* **35** 257
[35] Danner S M, Hofstoetter U S and Minassian K 2015 Finite element models of transcutaneous spinal cord stimulation *Encyclopedia of Computational Neuroscience* ed D Jaeger and R Jung (New York: Springer) 1197

[36] Shneider M N and Pekker M 2015 Correlation of action potentials in adjacent neurons *Phys. Biol.* **12** 066009

[37] Shneider M N and Pekker M 2016 Bypassing damaged nervous tissue arXiv:1609.00739

[38] Shneider M N and Pekker M 2022 Theoretical model of external spinal cord stimulation *Phys. Biol.* **19** 044001

[39] Liu Y T, Zhou X J, Ma J, Ge Y B and Cao X 2015 The diameters and number of nerve fibers in spinal nerve roots *J. Spinal Cord Med.* **38** 532

[40] Glaser R 1996 *Biophysics* (Berlin: Springer)

[41] https://biologydiscussion.com/human-physiology/nerve-fiber-classification-and-properties-biology

Mikhail N Shneider and Mikhail Pekker

Chapter 8

Anesthesia stimulated by a train of electrical pulses

This chapter discusses electroacupuncture, local anesthesia, the reduction of postoperative and postamputation pain, and the stimulation of muscle activity using current pulses initiated by external sources in the electrolyte in which nerve tissue resides in the body. A theoretical model is proposed to determine the optimal parameters for the possible implementation of anesthesia; the model considers: (i) the required frequency of current pulse repetition, (ii) the electrical characteristics of the skin, (iii) the conductivity of the saline solution, and (iv) the characteristics of the myelinated nerve fibers. This model permits reversible blocking of action potential propagation.

8.1 Introduction

Acupuncture was originally an ancient Chinese practice of inserting fine needles through the skin at specific points to cure disease or relieve pain. This practice has existed since the third millennium BC and has remained virtually unchanged until today [1–6]. One of the modern innovations of the traditional acupuncture technique is the use of weak alternating current sources connected to needles (electroacupuncture). Experience has shown that this can significantly improve the effectiveness of acupuncture [7–9]. Figure 8.1 shows an example of the use of needles as electrodes to stimulate active points in the human body.

Currently, one of the 'nonstandard' methods of pain relief is electrical stimulation of certain parts of the human body with external electrodes placed on the body surface, as shown in figure 8.2. A review of the works devoted to these studies is far beyond the scope of our book, so we will focus only on a few implications that seem pertinent to us.

doi:10.1088/978-0-7503-6034-0ch8

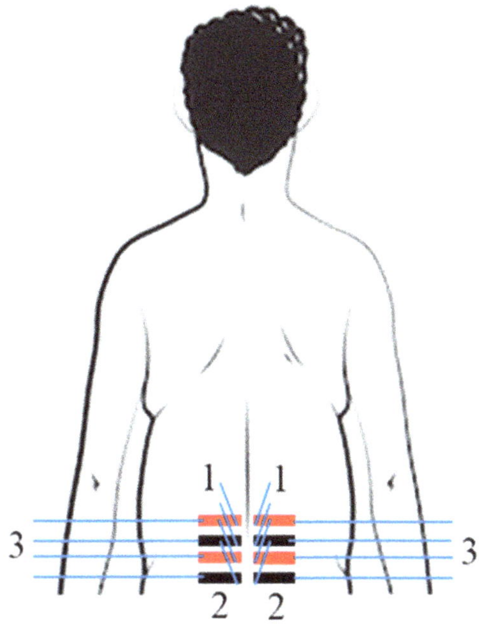

Figure 8.1. An example of how needle electrodes are used in electroacupuncture to target active points in the human body. 1–needles, 2–clamps, 3–wires.

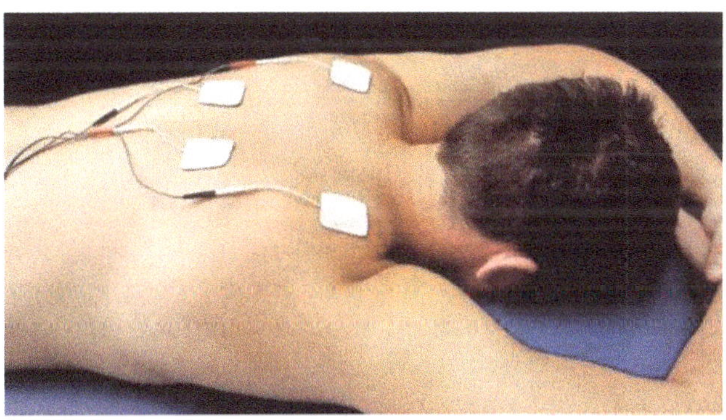

Figure 8.2. Schematic representation of external electrodes for pain relief or local activation of the nervous system in electrotherapy, as, for example, realized in [10]. 1—patches with electrodes, 2—wires. Adapted from [10].

The results reported in [11] show that the electrical stimulation of points near the ear (figure 8.3) reduces the amount of analgesic needed to relieve headache by 11%.

Postamputation pain is very common and difficult to treat. In the United States, more than one million people, including thousands of veterans who are amputees, suffer from postamputation pain. This represents a serious problem, as there are limited ways to treat this pain. It is often treated with strong narcotics, which are potentially dangerous because they can lead to addiction. The cause of postamputation pain is often the formation of a neuroma, a spherical tumor that grows at the end of severed nerves. Unregulated nerve regeneration occurs in the neuroma [12],

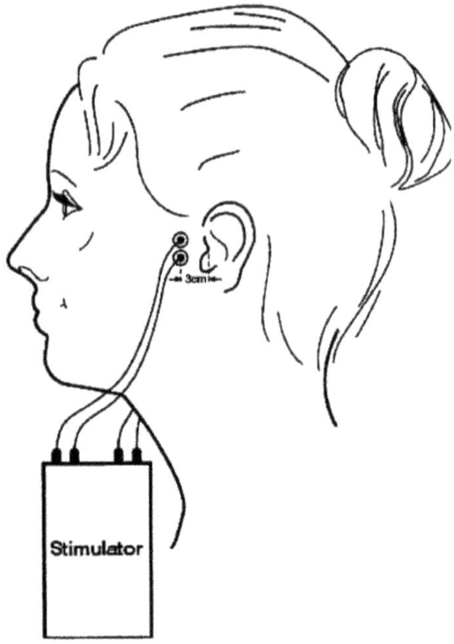

Figure 8.3. Schematic of the experiment. The active electrode was just above the acupuncture point, and the ground electrode was just below it. The current pulse had a rectangular shape and a pulse time of 0.2 ms. The time between pulses ranged from ~3 to 5 ms, and the current amplitude was 10 mA. Reproduced with permission from [11]. Copyright © 2002, American Society of Anesthesiologists.

with increased expression of sodium channels, which, as shown in chapter 1, results in a lower threshold for action potential excitability. Currently, it is believed that this abnormal hyperexcitability in the neuroma is the source of both stump pain and phantom pain [13, 14].

In [15], it was shown that the use of an electrical nerve block with high-frequency alternating current (the devices are shown in figure 8.4) applied to the peripheral nerve proximal to the neuroma reduced both residual limb pain and phantom pain in amputees suffering from chronic postamputation pain. As can be seen from the experimental data shown in figure 8.5, the pain relief was significant and sustained. In addition, the use of pain medication was significantly reduced, while daily functionality was significantly improved, as shown in figure 8.6.

Figure 8.7 shows a schematic diagram of an experiment that aimed to block the propagation of the action potential along a rat's sciatic nerve using an external electrode [16].

Most studies of nerve stimulation or anesthesia with low-amplitude electrical pulses have been empirical in nature. We have not found a convincing theoretical justification that explains how flat electrodes that are large enough and far enough away from the nerve fibers can relieve pain. In the following, we consider a simple theoretical model, recently proposed in [17], which enables us to qualitatively explain the experimentally observed anesthetic effect of current pulses and to obtain quantitative estimates that can be compared with experimental data.

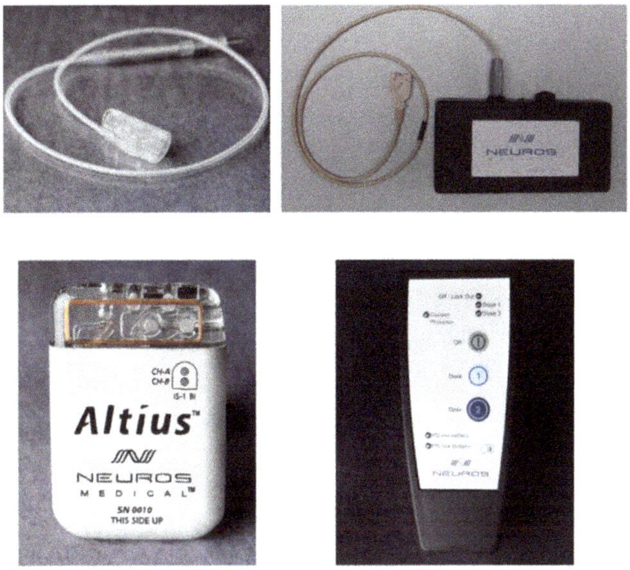

Figure 8.4. Electrical nerve block devices, including a nerve cuff electrode (top left), an external waveform generator (top right), an implantable waveform generator (bottom left), and an implantable generator controller (bottom right). Reprinted from [15], Copyright (2015), with permission from Elsevier.

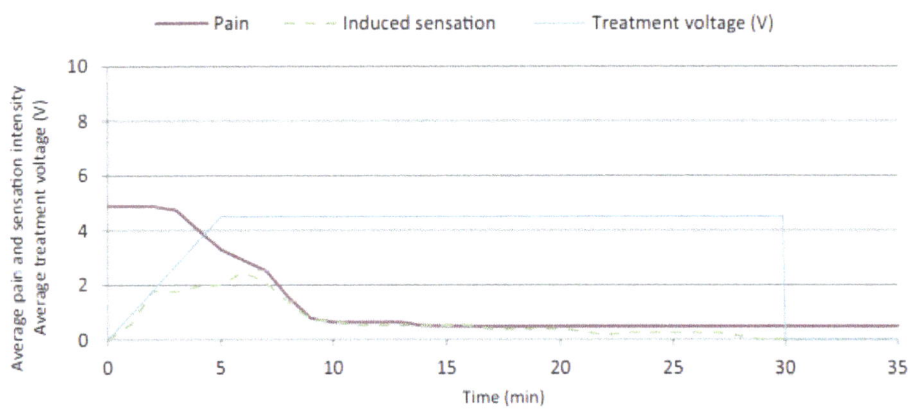

Figure 8.5. Pain intensity and therapy-related sensation during 30 min of electrical nerve block therapy. All patients were taking prescribed pain medication. Reprinted from [15], Copyright (2015), with permission from Elsevier.

For simplicity, consider finger anesthesia (figure 8.8(A)), where signals from receptors on the fingertips, such as thermal receptors, are blocked. Consider a model problem in which a nerve fiber (myelinated axon) of radius a is located on the axis of a hollow dielectric cylinder of radius R_0 ($a \ll R_0$), filled with a conductive liquid (saline) with specific conductivity σ (figure 8.8(B)). The currents inside the cylinder generated by ring electrodes fed with short unipolar current pulses are shown in figure 8.9.

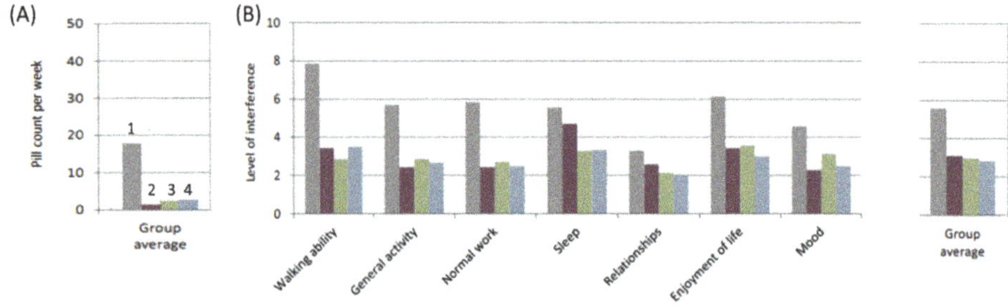

Figure 8.6. Results of the use of electrical nerve blocking. (A) Medication reduction at the three-month primary endpoint and follow-ups. (B) Pain interference reduction at the three-month primary endpoint and follow-up. Parts (A) and (B) reprinted from [15], Copyright (2015), with permission from Elsevier.

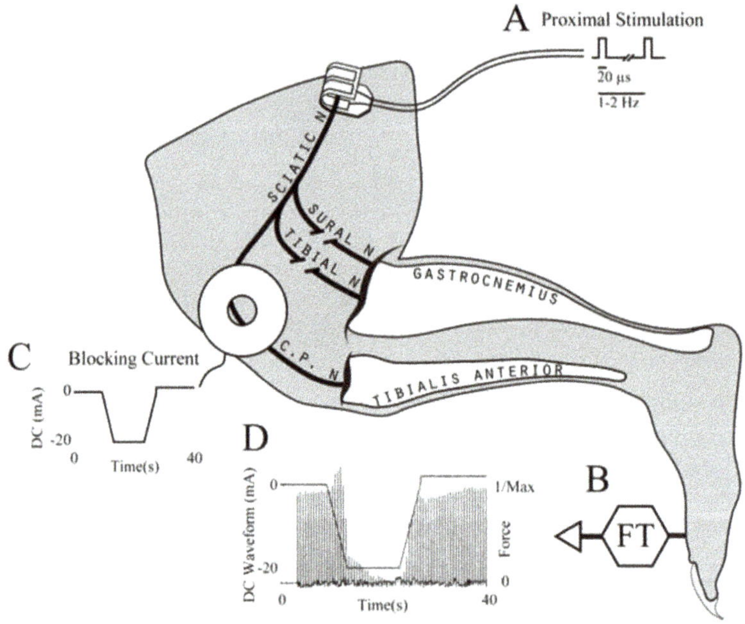

Figure 8.7. Schematic diagram of the experiment. (A) Stimulating electrode: half-ring covering 270° of the sciatic nerve. (B) A device for measuring the twitching force of the rat's leg. (C) Ring electrode with an inner diameter of 0.6 cm and an outer diameter of 1.2 cm. (D) Time dependence of the forces measured by device B (right vertical scale). The left vertical scale corresponds to the current pulse at electrode C [16] [2018], reprinted by permission of the publisher (Taylor & Francis Ltd, https://www.tandfonline.com).

8.2 Theoretical model

Let us consider the problem of generating currents in a saline solution inside a dielectric cylinder within the framework of a steady-state continuity equation, similar to that previously used in the theoretical model of stimulation of the injured spinal cord proposed in [18] (see chapter 7). For typical values of the conductivity of the physiological solution in which the nerve cells are located, $\sigma \sim 1 - 3\ \Omega^{-1}\,\mathrm{m}^{-1}$, and the Maxwell time is of the order of $\tau_M \sim 10^{-9}$ s (see chapter 2, section 2.3). This

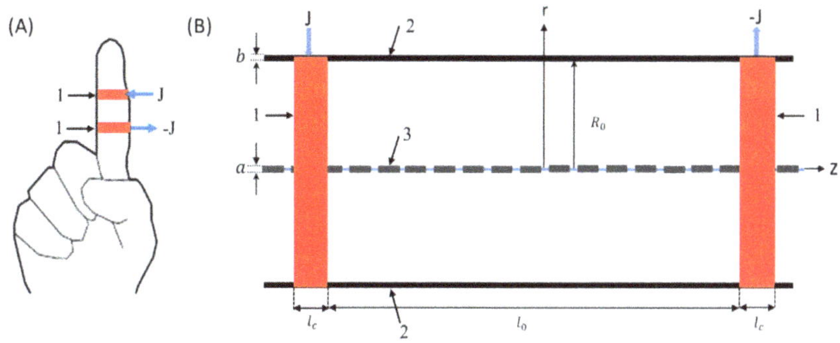

Figure 8.8. (A) Configuration of external ring electrodes and currents J in the considered example of finger anesthesia. (B) Corresponding model scheme: 1. Electrodes built into a dielectric cylinder. 2. The radius and thickness of the cylinder are R_0 and b, respectively, ($b \ll R_0$). The cylinder is filled with a physiological solution that has a conductivity of σ. 3. Myelinated nerve fiber (axon) of diameter a ($a \ll R_0$) located on the axis of the cylinder. Wide blue arrows show currents at electrodes 1. l_c and l_0 are the width of the electrodes and the distance between them, respectively.

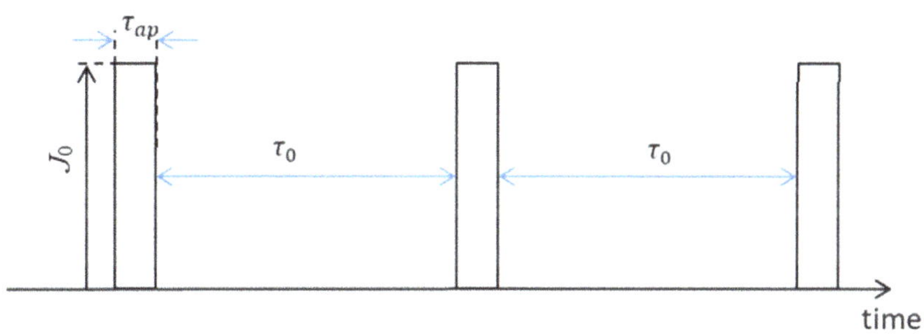

Figure 8.9. Periodic unipolar current pulses applied to the electrodes. τ_{ap}, τ_0, and J_0 are the current pulse duration, duty cycle, and normalized amplitude, respectively. Since the duration of the current pulse that blocks the propagation of the action potential must not be less than the action potential onset time $\tau_1 \sim 1$ ms [17], it is natural to assume that $\tau_{ap} \sim \tau_1$. Since the relaxation time of the action potential is $\tau_{rel} \sim 10-15$ ms, the duty cycle of the current pulses is $\tau_0 \sim \tau_{rel}$.

is five to six orders of magnitude shorter than the characteristic time of the excitation relaxation of the action potential in the axons, $\tau_1 \sim 1$ ms. In addition, the size of the non-quasi-neutral region near the membrane of axons is determined by the Debye length $\lambda_D \sim 0.5$ nm, which is at least three orders of magnitude smaller than the axon thickness a, so, as in previous chapters, we can use the continuity equation to calculate the currents inside the finger shown in figure 8.8:

$$\nabla \cdot \vec{I} = 0, \quad \vec{I} = \sigma \vec{E}. \tag{8.1}$$

Assuming the conductivity σ of the electrolyte inside the finger (figure 8.1) is uniform and constant in time, and that $\vec{E} = -\nabla \varphi$, the problem of determining the potential is reduced to the Laplace equation:

$$\Delta\varphi = 0, \quad \vec{E} = -\nabla\varphi. \tag{8.2}$$

Let us estimate the time required for the myelinated axon to be charged by the currents induced inside the dielectric cylinder (figure 8.1(B)). Since, in neurons with myelinated axons, the action potential is generated in unmyelinated areas, such as the initial segment and the nodes of Ranvier, we consider the charging of the membrane in the nodes of Ranvier, where the capacitance per unit area $C_m \approx 10^{-2}\,[\frac{\text{F}}{\text{m}^2}]$ [19] and the typical radius of the axon $a \sim 1.5$–8 μm [20].

Following [18], the estimation of the charging time of a cylindrical capacitor of radius a, capacitance per unit area C_m, and conductivity σ is:

$$\tau_m \sim 2\frac{C_m \cdot a}{\sigma}. \tag{8.3}$$

Substituting the above values of C_m, a, and $\sigma = 2\,\Omega^{-1}\,\text{m}^{-1}$ into (8.3), we determine that the charging time of the surfaces of the nodes of Ranvier of the myelinated axon is in the range of $\tau_m \sim 0.035$–0.1 μs.

Let us now estimate the charging time for the surface of the outer dielectric cylinder (skin) shown in figure 8.8(B), whose capacitance per unit area is:

$$C_{\text{skin}} = \frac{\varepsilon_0 \varepsilon_{\text{skin}}}{b_{\text{skin}}}, \tag{8.4}$$

where b_{skin} and $\varepsilon_{\text{skin}}$ are the thickness and relative permittivity of the skin, respectively (figure 8.8(B)). Let us assume that the permittivity of the outer cylinder and its thickness are each equal to the permittivity of the skin $\varepsilon_{\text{SKin}} = 12\ 000$ [21], and its thickness $b_{\text{skin}} \sim 0.5 - 4$ mm [22]. For estimates, we assume that $b_{\text{skin}} = 2$ mm. Substituting the values of ε_d and b into (8.4), we get $C_{\text{skin}} \approx 5.3 \cdot 10^{-5}\,[\frac{\text{F}}{\text{m}^2}]$. For clarity, we take the radius of the outer cylinder (finger) $R = R_0 = 0.01$ m. Substituting these values into (8.3), we determine that the charging time of the external cylindrical capacitor is $\tau_{\text{ec}} \sim 2\frac{C_{\text{skin}} \cdot R_0}{\sigma} \approx 0.5$ μs. That is, the membrane charging time in the nodes of Ranvier in the inner nerve fiber and the outer cylindrical capacitor formed by the skin of the finger is at least three orders of magnitude shorter than the duration of the current pulse τ_{ap} shown in figure 8.9. Therefore, during the action of the current pulse, the charge on the fiber membrane and on the surface of the cylinder can be considered constant. Note that the surface of the myelin fiber can be considered an impenetrable dielectric surface only until the potential on the membrane at the nodes of Ranvier reaches the threshold of excitation of the action potential. In the following, we assume that this condition is fulfilled.

8.3 Potential and current distribution inside the outer dielectric cylinder

Let us find the potential and current distributions in the electrolyte with the myelinated nerve fiber inside a dielectric cylinder with embedded ring electrodes.

Equation (8.2) in cylindrical coordinates has the form:

$$\frac{1}{r}\frac{\partial}{\partial r}r\frac{\partial \varphi}{\partial r} + \frac{\partial^2 \varphi}{\partial z^2} = 0. \tag{8.5}$$

As noted in the previous section of this chapter, the charge on the myelinated fiber membrane and on the dielectric surface of the outer cylinder can be considered constant during most of the stimulation current pulse. In this case, we can assume that the radial currents on them are zero:

$$I_r(z, r = a) = -\sigma\frac{\partial \varphi}{\partial r}\bigg|_{r=a} = 0, \tag{8.6}$$

$$I_r(z, r = R_0) = -\sigma\frac{\partial \varphi}{\partial r}\bigg|_{r=R_0} = 0. \tag{8.7}$$

Since $a \ll R_0$, the influence of the nerve fiber on the distribution of currents induced by external electrodes inside the dielectric cylinder is insignificant. Therefore, the presence of the myelinated fiber is neglected below.

From the symmetry of the problem of current distribution inside a dielectric cylinder with ring electrodes (figure 8.8(B)) (without the myelinated fibers on the axis), it follows that the radial current on the axis is:

$$I_r(z, r = 0) = -\sigma\frac{\partial \varphi}{\partial r}\bigg|_{r=0} = 0. \tag{8.8}$$

The boundary conditions for the potential φ on the inner surface of the dielectric cylinder have the form:

$$I_r = -\sigma\frac{\partial \varphi}{\partial r}\bigg|_{r=R_0,\, z} = 0,\ z < -\left(l_c + \frac{1}{2}l_0\right),\ -\frac{1}{2}l_0 < z < \frac{1}{2}l_0,\ l_c + \frac{1}{2}l_0 < z, \tag{8.9}$$

where l_c and l_0 are the width of the electrodes and the distance between them, respectively (see figure 8.8(B)).

On the ring electrodes, the current is given by:

$$I_r = -\sigma\frac{\partial \varphi}{\partial r}\bigg|_{r=R_0,\, z} = \tilde{I},\ -\left(l_c + \frac{1}{2}l_0\right) \leqslant z \leqslant -\frac{1}{2}l_0, \tag{8.10}$$

$$I_r = -\sigma\frac{\partial \varphi}{\partial r}\bigg|_{r=R_0,\, z} = -\tilde{I},\ \frac{1}{2}l_0 \leqslant z \leqslant \left(l_c + \frac{1}{2}l_0\right). \tag{8.11}$$

Without loss of generality, the stepwise longitudinal current distribution on the electrodes can be approximated by taking the sum of the exponents:

$$\tilde{I}(z) = \tilde{I}(t)\left(\sum_{k=1}^{N}\mu_k \exp(-s^2(z - z_k)^2) - \sum_{k=1}^{N}\mu_k \exp(-s^2(z + z_k)^2)\right), \tag{8.12}$$

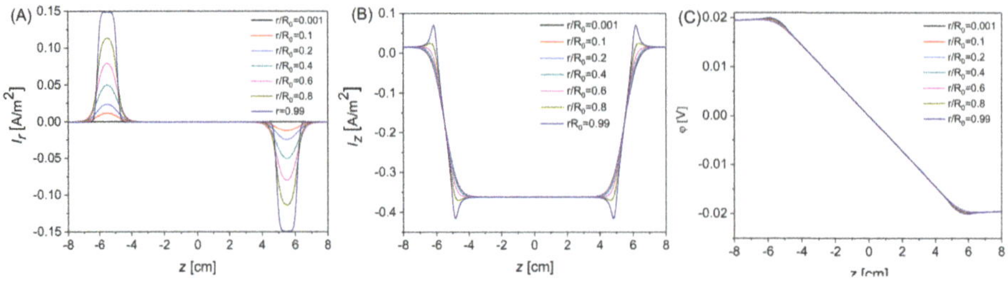

Figure 8.10. (A), (B) and (C) Dependencies of radial and longitudinal current densities and of potential distributions on z for different values of the distance from the axis. The calculations have been performed for selected parameters: $R_0 = 1$ cm, $l_0 = 10$ cm, $z_1 = 5$ cm, $z_2 = 5.25$ cm, $z_3 = 5$ cm, $z_4 = 5.75$ cm, $z_5 = 6$ cm, $s = 5\ \text{cm}^{-1}$, and $\tilde{I}_0 = 0.15\ \text{A m}^{-2}$.

where $\tilde{I}(t)$ is the current density, which is a step function corresponding to figure 8.9, and μ_k and z_k are constant values. Assuming that all $\mu_k = 1$, we obtain the distributions of current and potential inside the dielectric cylinder [23–25]:

$$\varphi(r, z, t) = \frac{\tilde{I}(t)}{\sqrt{\pi} s\sigma} \int_0^{\infty} \frac{I_0(\xi r/R_0)}{\xi I_1(\xi)} \exp\left(-\xi^2/(2sR_0)^2\right) \sum_{k=1}^{N} \left(\cos\left(\xi \frac{z - z_k}{R_0}\right) - \cos\left(\xi \frac{z + z_k}{R_0}\right)\right) d\xi, \quad (8.13)$$

$$I_r(r, z, t) = \frac{\tilde{I}(t)}{\sqrt{\pi} sR_0} \int_0^{\infty} \frac{I_1(\xi r/R_0)}{I_1(\xi)} \exp\left(-\xi^2/(2sR_0)^2\right) \sum_{k=1}^{N} \left(\cos\left(\xi \frac{z - z_k}{R_0}\right) - \cos\left(\xi \frac{z + z_k}{R_0}\right)\right) d\xi, \quad (8.14)$$

$$I_z(r, z, t) = -\frac{\tilde{I}(t)}{\sqrt{\pi} sR_0} \int_0^{\infty} \frac{I_0(\xi r/R_0)}{I_1(\xi)} \exp\left(-\xi^2/(2sR_0)^2\right) \sum_{k=1}^{N} \left(\sin\left(\xi \frac{z - z_k}{R_0}\right) - \sin\left(\xi \frac{z + z_k}{R_0}\right)\right) d\xi. \quad (8.15)$$

I_0 and I_1 in (8.13)–(8.15) are modified Bessel functions of the first kind.

Figure 8.10 shows an example of the calculation results for the selected maximum current density on the electrode, $\tilde{I}_0 = 0.15\ \text{A m}^{-2}$, and dimensions $R_0 = 1$ cm, $l_0 = 10$ cm, $z_1 = 5$ cm, $z_2 = 5.25$ cm, $z_3 = 5.5$ cm, $z_4 = 5.75$ cm, $z_5 = 6$ cm, and $s = 5\ \text{cm}^{-1}$.

8.4 Discussion

According to the calculated results for the considered example, the radial current (figure 8.10(A)) near the axis of the external dielectric cylinder tends to zero, and the potential (figure 8.10(B)) is practically independent of the radius. Thus, the variation of the potential across the membranes of the nodes of Ranvier (figure 8.8(B)) can be considered equal to the variation of the potential on the axis of the considered dielectric cylinder. Therefore, according to the results of the calculation, the potential on the membrane of the nodes of Ranvier in the vicinity of the longitudinal coordinate corresponding to the left electrode becomes about 20 mV higher than the rest potential, and on the right electrode, it becomes 20 mV lower.

Consider the case of action potential propagation along the fiber from right to left. It was shown in [22, 23] that when an action potential is excited in the nth node of Ranvier, the induced potential in adjacent (non-excited) nodes of Ranvier depends on the length of the myelinated segments. If the myelinated areas are

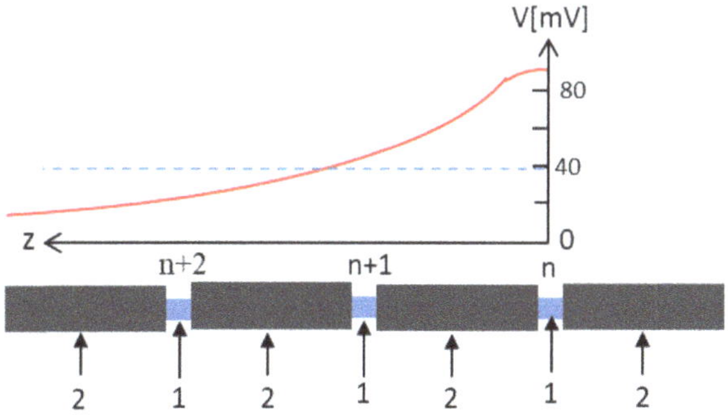

Figure 8.11. Schematic representation of an action potential propagating from right to left in a myelinated fiber. 1. Nodes of Ranvier. 2. Myelinated areas. The time is indicated when the action potential in the nth node of Ranvier reached its maximum; in the $(n + 1)$th node, when the potential reached the threshold value; and in the $(n + 2)$th node, when the potential did not reach the threshold excitation.

long enough, then the action potential excitation threshold of 40–45 mV is only reached at the $(n + 1)$th node of Ranvier in figure 8.11, where an action potential is definitely initiated. Recall that examples of calculations of the dependence of the voltage on time for different values of the myelinated coating lengths and the maximum voltage on the distance from the active node of Ranvier, based on the model given in [22], are shown in figures 2.5(A) and (B), respectively (see chapter 2, section 2.1).

According to the calculation results shown in figure 8.10(C), the potential in the nodes of Ranvier near the right electrode is lowered by ~20 mV relative to the resting potential, so the excitation threshold in them increased from 40–45 mV to 60–65 mV. Therefore, the propagation of the action potential near the right electrode is blocked. Obviously, an action potential propagating from left to right is also blocked at the right electrode.

Let us now consider the case where the myelinated fiber is not on the cylinder's axis. From the graphs shown in figure 8.10, it can be seen that when moving to the left from the right electrode at a distance equal to the electrode size $z > (2l_c + \frac{1}{2}l_0)$, the current components J_r and J_z are close to zero, regardless of r, while the potential φ remains practically constant and independent of r. Therefore, blocking of the action potential propagating from right to left can be expected to occur regardless of the radial position of the myelinated fiber. The same reasoning is also valid in the case of propagation of the action potential from left to right, and it is also blocked behind the right electrode, regardless of the radial position of the myelinated fiber.

Note that there is a significant difference between the initiation of the action potential during the stimulation of spinal nerves, considered in the previous chapter according to the model given in [18], and the opposite task—blocking the action potential—presented in this chapter corresponding to the model given in [17]. The stimulation of spinal cord nerves with axons perpendicular to the currents induced in a conducting fluid, as shown in [18], significantly changes the structure of the currents near the axons. In this chapter, the opposite case is considered, where mainly longitudinal currents are induced and radial currents are small and cannot significantly affect the membrane potential; they only cause the membrane potential to become equal to the electrolyte potential near the membrane. In the case of a fiber that is not on the axis of the dielectric cylinder with ring electrodes, all the above considerations remain valid.

8.5 Conclusions

We considered a possible approach to anesthesia without the use of anesthetics. We showed that this is possible using a sequence of current pulse excitations in the vicinity of the nerve fiber; thus, a reversible loss of sensitivity can be achieved without the use of anesthetics. However, it will be possible to draw final conclusions and discuss the application of the considered approach only after experimental verification of the theory.

References and further reading

[1] White A and Ernst E 2004 A brief history of acupuncture *Rheumatology* **43** 662
[2] Huang K C 1996 *Acupuncture: The Past and the Present* (New York: Vantage)
[3] Ma K W 1992 The roots and development of Chinese acupuncture: from prehistory to early 20th century *Acupunct. Med.* **10** 92
[4] Basser S 1999 Acupuncture: a history *Sci. Rev. Altern. Med.* **3** 34
[5] Chen Y 1997 Silk scrolls: earliest literature of meridian doctrine in ancient China *Acupunct. Electrother. Res.* **22** 175
[6] Dorfer L, Moser M, Bahr F, Spindler K, Egarter-Vigl E, Giullén S, Dohr G and Kenner T 1999 A medical report from the stone age? *Lancet* 1999 **354** 1023
[7] Li Y, Tougas G, Chiverton S G and Hunt R H 1992 The effect of acupuncture on gastrointestinal function and disorders *Am. J. Gastroenterol.* **87** 1372
[8] Lux G, Hagel J, Backer P, Backer G, Vogl R, Ruppin H, Domschke S and Domschke W 1994 Acupuncture inhibits vagal gastric acid secretion stimulated by sham feeding in healthy subjects *Gut* **35** 1026
[9] Zhou L and Chey W Y 1984 Electric acupuncture stimulates non parietal secretion of the stomach in dog *Life Sci.* **34** 2233
[10] https://aosm.in/electrotherapy/
[11] Greif R, Laciny S, Mokhtarani M, Doufas A G, Bakhshandeh M, Dorfer L and Sessler D I 2002 Transcutaneous electrical stimulation of an auricular acupuncture point decreases anesthetic requirement *Anesthesiology* **96** 306
[12] Hsu E and Cohen S P 2013 Postamputation pain: epidemiology, mechanisms, and treatment *J. Pain Res.* **6** 121
[13] Flor H, Nikolajsen L and Jensen S T 2006 Phantom limb pain: a case of maladaptive CNS plasticity? *Nat. Rev. Neurosci.* **7** 873
[14] Subedi B and Grossberg G T 2011 Phantom limb pain: mechanisms and treatment approaches *Pain Res. Treat.* **2011** 864605
[15] Soin A, Shah N S and Fang Z-P 2015 High-frequency electrical nerve block for post-amputation pain: a pilot study *Neuromodulation* **18** 197
[16] Van Acker G M, Vrabec T L, Bhadra N, Chae J, Kilgore K L and Bhadra N 2018 Block of motor nerve conduction via transcutaneous application of direct current *Bioelectronics Med.* **1** 107

[17] Shneider M N and Pekker M 2023 The possibility of anesthesia stimulated by a train of current pulses *Biomed. Phys. Eng. Express* **9** 035032

[18] Shneider M N and Pekker M 2022 Theoretical model of external spinal cord stimulation *Phys. Biol.* **19** 044001

[19] Glaser R 1996 *Biophysik* (Berlin, Heidelberg, New York: Springer)

[20] https://biologydiscussion.com/human-physiology/nerve-fiber-classification-and-properties-biology

[21] Gabriel S, Lau R W and Gabriel C 1996 The dielectric properties of biological tissues: II. Measurements in the frequency range 10 Hz to 20 GHz *Phys. Med. Biol.* **41** 2251

[22] Oltulu P, Ince B, Kokbudak N, Findik S and Kilinc F 2018 Measurement of epidermis, dermis, and total skin thicknesses from six different body regions with a new ethical histometric technique *Turk. J. Plast. Surg.* **26** 56

[23] Shneider M N and Pekker M 2015 Correlation of action potentials in adjacent neurons *Phys. Biol.* **12** 066009

[24] Shneider M N and Pekker M 2019 Stimulated activity in the neural tissue *J. Appl. Phys.* **125** 211101

[25] Shneider M N and Pekker M 2021 Physical model of electrical synapses in a neural network *bioRxiv preprint*

[26] https://drlorischneider.com/services/electro-acupuncture

Chapter 9

Effects of osmotic pressure variations on cell membranes

This chapter considers the physical basis of osmosis. It discusses the possible role of osmosis in experiments that have studied the interaction of low-temperature plasma with physiological solutions containing cell cultures. It has been shown that changes in the ionic composition of the intercellular medium can lead to changes in the water content of the lipid membrane and consequently to changes in the dielectric constant of cell membranes. As a result, the physiological consequences can be significant, such as altered resting potentials, reduced action potential excitation thresholds in neurons, and changes to the velocity of action potential propagation along axons.

9.1 Introduction to osmosis

Osmosis plays a very important role in the vital activity of cells, so we decided to include a brief overview of this phenomenon in this book and note its possible manifestations in the behavior of excitable nervous tissues.

Osmosis (/*dz*'moƱsɪs) is the spontaneous movement or diffusion of solute molecules across a selectively permeable membrane from a region of lower solute concentration to a region of higher solute concentration. The phenomenon of osmosis is well illustrated by a simple experiment with communicating vessels separated by a membrane impermeable to the solute, as shown in figure 9.1. The solvent flows across the membrane until the solute concentrations in the two vessels are equalized. As a result, a pressure difference $\Delta\pi$ develops between the two sides of the membrane, and the solvent flow stops.

A liquid with a low density of solute is called hypotonic, and one with a higher density of solute is called hypertonic. To avoid confusion, it should be noted that

doi:10.1088/978-0-7503-6034-0ch9

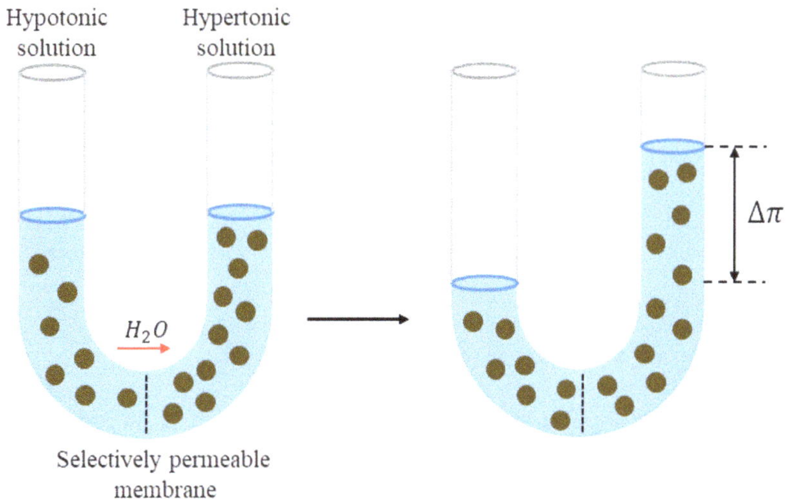

Figure 9.1. The osmotic pressure drop $\Delta\pi$ across a membrane that is permeable to a solvent but not to a solute. The red arrow indicates the direction of fluid flow from one vessel to another. Pumping a solvent (such as water) from the left half of a communicating vessel to the right half results in an increase in the amount of water in the right half and a corresponding pressure drop. This pressure difference is called the osmotic pressure.

when determining the osmotic pressure, it is assumed that there is no water flow through the membrane if there are no dissolved species in both vessels or if the concentrations of solutes are the same on both sides of the membrane.

Manifestations of osmosis in nature, both living and nonliving, have been observed for thousands of years, but the phenomenon was first documented in 1748 by Jean-Antoine Nollet (1700–70) [1]. Osmosis is an important process that largely determines the vital activity of cells and whole organisms. To date, the phenomenon of osmosis and its role in the biophysics of animal and plant cells and of whole organisms has been studied in great detail and is described in textbooks and monographs on biology, biophysics, and medicine (see, for example, [2–4]).

The contribution to the osmotic pressure difference of a component of the mixture is determined by a formula proposed by van't Hoff in 1886 [5], similar to the pressure drop formula for an ideal gas:

$$\Delta\pi_i = k_B T(n_{i,\,\text{in}} - n_{i,\,\text{out}}), \tag{9.1}$$

where $n_{i,\,\text{in}}$ and $n_{i,\,\text{out}}$ are the concentrations of solute components separated by the membrane. The total osmotic pressure drop is determined by the contribution of all components in solution:

$$\Delta\pi = \sum_i \Delta\pi_i = k_B T \sum_i (n_{i,\,\text{in}} - n_{i,\,\text{out}}). \tag{9.2}$$

Note that van't Hoff's equation (9.1) holds for sufficiently dilute solutions. There are several ways to indicate the effects caused by interactions between solute molecules at higher concentrations. For simplicity, we will consider only dilute solutions.

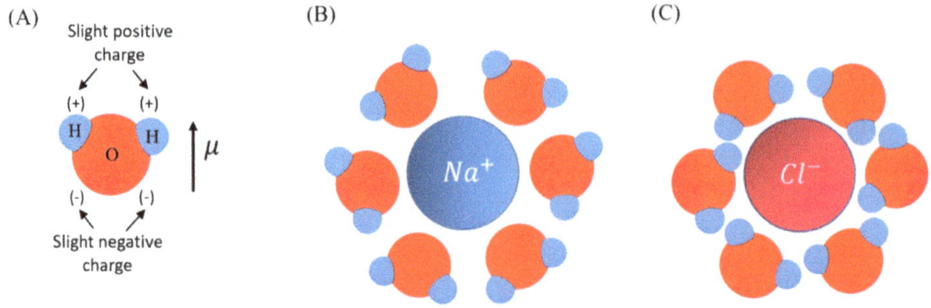

Figure 9.2. (A) A water molecule (H_2O), a polar molecule with a permanent dipole moment of $\mu = 1.84$ D. (B) Hydrated sodium (cations) and chloride (anions) ions in aqueous solution.

Water molecules are polar molecules with a constant dipole moment $\mu = 1.84$ D (figure 9.2(A)), so that ions dissolved in water are hydrated; that is, each ion is surrounded by several water molecules, which together with it form a single cluster (quasi-molecule). For an example, see [6]. Examples of hydrated positive sodium ions (cations) and negative chloride ions (anions) formed by the dissociation of table salt in an aqueous solution are shown in figure 9.2(B). Obviously, the charge of the hydrated ions is equal to the charge of the original 'bare' ion. It should be noted that in the physical chemistry literature, one may frequently encounter the concept of solvated ions. Solvation (from Latin 'solvo,' which means 'to dissolve') is an electrostatic interaction between the particles (ions, molecules) of a dissolved substance and a solvent. Solvation in aqueous solutions is called hydration.

The ions become hydrated, acquiring a shell of polar water molecules. This significantly increases their effective size and weight. This leads to a significant decrease in mobility and diffusion coefficient, a significant slowing down of recombination, and other consequences. Free water molecules pass through a water-permeable lipid membrane, but water molecules in a cluster with a hydrated ion cannot. In chapter 1, section 1.5, we describe how the passage of ions through ion channels embedded in cell membranes is accompanied by dehydration, which means release from their water shells (figure 1.30).

There are three main types of solutions in which cells are located, depending on the relationship between the osmotic pressures outside and inside the cell (for example, see [3]). A solution is called isotonic when the osmotic pressure in the solution is equal to the osmotic pressure in the cell. In such a solution, no water enters or leaves the cell, or, the water fluxes inside and outside the cell are equal, as shown in figure 9.3(A), because the concentrations of ions inside and outside the cell are the same.

A solution is called hypotonic when its osmotic pressure is less than the osmotic pressure inside the cell. In such a solution, water flows through the membrane into the cell, as shown in figure 9.3(B). The cell swells in such an environment and may burst.

If the osmotic pressure of a solution is greater than that inside the cell, the solution is hypertonic. Water leaves the cell through the membrane, as shown in figure 9.3(C), causing it to shrink.

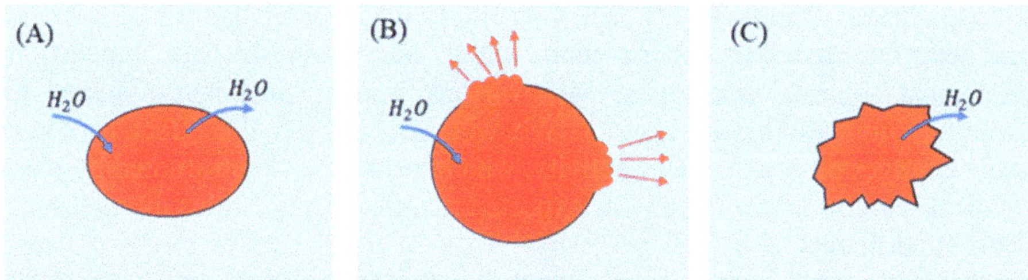

Figure 9.3. Water flows across the cell membrane in the major types of solutions in which cells are located. (A) Isotonic solution. (B) Hypotonic solution. (C) Hypertonic solution.

The effect of osmotic pressure on the vital activity of cells is well known in cell physiology [7]. For example, the phenomenon of erythrocyte osmotic fragility (osmotic hemolysis), which involves the destruction of erythrocyte cells, is relatively well studied. These cells have been subjected to osmotic stress by placing them in a hypotonic solution [8, 9].

9.2 Experiments on cells in physiological solution interacting with plasma

In recent decades, plasma medicine has developed significantly. A number of experimental studies have convincingly demonstrated that the action of a weakly ionized nonequilibrium plasma jet on a physiological solution can selectively affect the cells present in it [10–19]. Of particular interest are studies that have observed the selective stimulation of apoptosis in cancer cells [13–19]. However, the mechanism by which plasma affects cells in saline is still unclear (for example, see [10–12]). When considering the interaction of weakly ionized plasma jets with cellular structures, various physical and chemical processes caused by currents induced in the physiological solution and cells must be taken into account (for example, see [19]). A well-established experimental fact is that when plasma is exposed to a saline solution, long-lived (tens of minutes or even hours) hydrated ions and electrons appear in the solution [20].

Since phospholipid cell membranes are permeable to water molecules and poorly permeable to hydrated ions (see chapter 1, section 1.2), a change in the composition of ions in a physiological solution leads to a change in the osmotic pressure across the cell membrane and consequently to the stretching or shrinking of the membrane and changes in cell volume and shape. However, to the best of our knowledge, plasma medicine research has not addressed the role of the change in osmotic pressure in cells due to the exposure of physiological saline solutions to plasma sources.

In [21, 22], it was shown that the hydrated ions, electrons, and neutral molecules supplied by a plasma can cause a significant change in osmotic pressure and, consequently, a change in the pressure drop across the cell membrane. Since osmotic pressure depends on the permeability of the membrane to water molecules, the degree of osmosis varies depending on the membrane, for example, between healthy and diseased cells. Following [21, 22], we will briefly consider the role of osmosis in typical plasma medicine experiments, where cell ensembles are studied in a physiological solution interacting with various sources of weakly ionized low-temperature nonequilibrium plasma. We will also discuss the effect of osmotic pressure changes on neural tissue activity, which has not yet been studied by plasma medicine researchers, and review the expected manifestations of this interaction and possible experiments.

Figure 9.4 shows examples of hypotonic and hypertonic cell deformations observed in an experiment following an interaction between a physiological solution and a source of low-temperature nonequilibrium plasma produced by a dielectric barrier discharge (DBD) in air [23]. The corresponding measured changes in cell area are shown in figure 9.5.

In these experiments, changes in the shape and size of human thyroid epithelial cells were observed in a physiological solution in Petri dishes. Nanosecond DBD was used to treat cells in plastic Petri dishes. Briefly, short high-voltage (HV) pulses at 9 kV (pulse amplitude is doubled at the electrode) with a 30 ns duration were generated by a commercial pulser and transmitted to the discharge cell via a 25 m long coaxial cable. The total energy deposited in the plasma for one HV pulse was about 18 mJ. The plasma was generated in a 2 mm air gap between the open flat high-voltage electrode and the medium in the Petri dish. The ground electrode was placed under the Petri dish. For all plasma treatments, 10 000 pulses were applied at a frequency of 300 Hz. In the experiments, changes in the shape and size of cells in plasma-activated saline were observed for a long time after the discharge effect.

From the results of experiments performed with nonequilibrium DBD plasma, it can be concluded that ions entering the physiological solution with the cells led to the realization of a hypertonic scenario; that is, water flowed out of the cells to

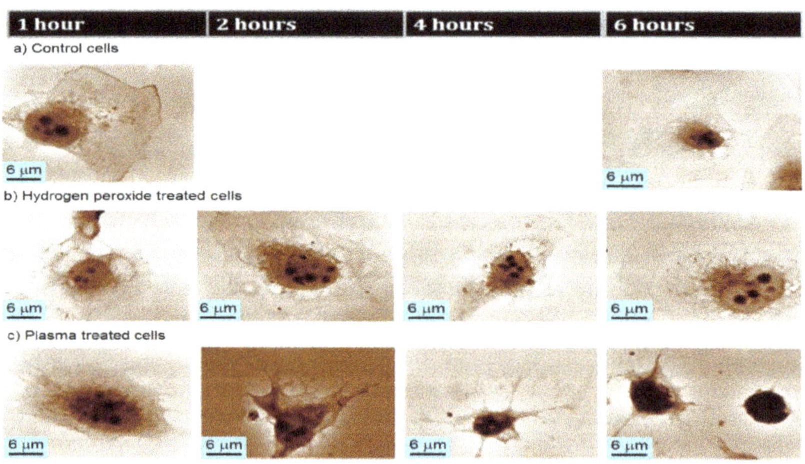

Figure 9.4. Images obtained using a numerical high-pass filter for detail enhancement at 150x, showing the cellular conditions at different times after treatment. Reprinted from [23], with the permission of AIP Publishing.

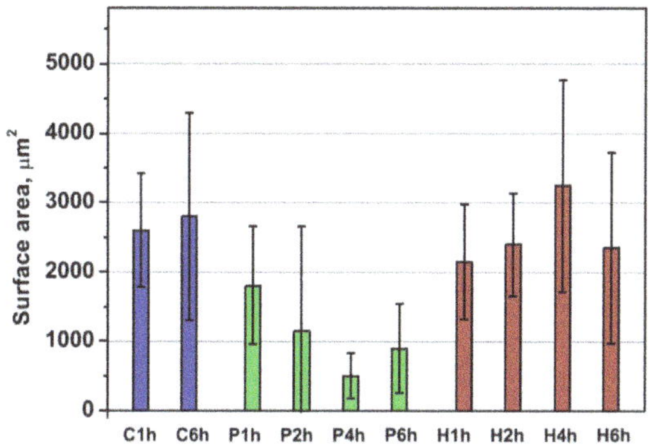

Figure 9.5. Average cell surface areas and their standard deviations measured at 40x magnification. Results are shown for each treatment condition (*C* for control cells, *P* for plasma treatment, and *H* for H_2O_2 treatment). Reprinted from [23], with the permission of AIP Publishing.

reduce the concentration of hydrated ions, to which the cell membranes were impermeable (see chapter 1, section 1.2); the cell thus shrank.

Hydrogen peroxide (H_2O_2) is a broad-range chemical catalyst with both reducing and oxidizing properties. It has been shown to be a reactive oxygen species (ROS) that has an active effect on cell viability [24], including the cells of the nervous system [25]. We will not focus here on the important biochemical processes in cells caused by the addition of hydrogen peroxide to the solution. We note, however, that according to experiments [23], as shown in figure 9.4(B), when H_2O_2 was added to a physiological solution, the cell swelled, i.e. the addition of hydrogen peroxide made the solution hypotonic. In the absence of catalysts in the solution, this appears to have been due to an exothermic disproportionation reaction [26]:

$$2H_2O_2 \rightarrow 2H_2O + O_2. \tag{9.3}$$

This means that adding hydrogen peroxide to a solution increases the concentration of water outside the cell and decreases the concentration of ions in the solution. Lipid cell membranes are known to allow the diffusive transport of H_2O_2 molecules [27, 28], resulting in changes in osmotic pressure. Therefore, water flows into the cell to equalize the concentration of ions in the solutions outside and inside the cell. A similar effect is observed when distilled water is added to blood: the isotonic solution that blood represents is transformed into a hypotonic physiological solution, with erythrocytes swelling due to the influx of water from outside the cell (see, e.g. [8, 9]).

Note that other, more complex reactions of hydrogen peroxide decomposition take place in physiological solutions that contain living cells, which, for example, are significantly accelerated by enzymes (see, e.g. [29]).

In our opinion, the results of experiments [23] shown in figures 9.4 and 9.5 confirm the osmotic nature of changes in cell morphology in a physiological solution interacting with plasma.

Figure 9.6 shows a schematic of a typical experimental setup for a plasma jet and cells in a physiological solution in a Petri dish (for example, see [13–18]). A weakly ionized plasma jet interacting with a physiological solution changes the local ionic

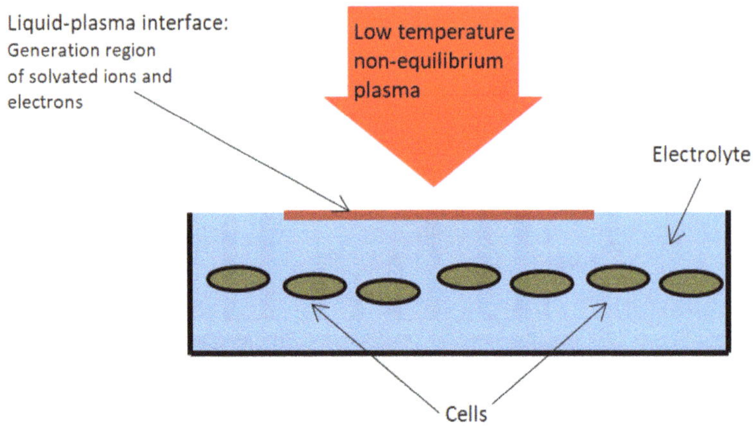

Figure 9.6. Schematic of the experimental setup for a plasma jet acting on cells in a Petri dish.

and molecular composition of the solution. Plasma-induced hydrated ions and neutral molecules then diffuse into the area where the cells are located. The density of charged particles in a saline electrolyte solution corresponding to a living organism is $n_i \approx 0.3\ \text{mol}^{-1} \approx 2 \cdot 10^{26}\ \text{m}^{-3}$ [30]. The characteristic Debye screening length corresponding to this ion density and temperature ~300 K does not exceed 1 nm. Due to the shielding of the electric field by electrolyte ions, the direct effect of plasma on the cells is insignificant. However, in principle, it is possible that additional charging of the cell membrane by currents induced in the electrolyte contributes to the critical voltage at which breakdown occurs in the membrane (its electroporation). This mechanism has been considered in many papers (for example, see [31–33]), so we do not dwell on it here.

9.3 Ions introduced by a plasma source at the interface and their deep diffusion into solution

Hydrated ions and neutral molecules introduced at the surface of a physiological solution by a plasma source (figure 9.6) propagate into the interior of the electrolyte by diffusion and turbulent mixing if turbulent macroscopic motion is initiated in a Petri dish. Let us show that for the characteristic operating time of the plasma source, the hydrated ions injected at the surface of the solution are likely to reach the cell surface. For simplicity, we consider only diffusion, which is the slowest process for transporting ions (and neutral molecules) from the plasma–liquid interface from the surface of the physiological solution to the depths where the cells are located.

The lifetime of hydrated ions and neutral molecules injected into saline is long enough to neglect decay and treat them as stable. For example, the lifetime of NO_3^- and NO_2^- ions and H_2O_2 molecules is on the order of several hours [34]. Therefore, to a first approximation, we can neglect the processes of ion recombination in a physiological solution. The radius of the region of plasma interaction with the surface of the liquid is greater than the distance from the surface to the cells, so the problem of diffusion of solvated charged particles (and neutral molecules) can be described by a one-dimensional diffusion equation:

$$\frac{\partial n}{\partial t} = D\frac{\partial^2 n}{\partial x^2}, \tag{9.4}$$

with boundary conditions in the injection region

$$D\frac{\partial n}{\partial x}\bigg|_{0,\, t>0} = J\theta\,(t_0 - t),\ \ \theta(t_0 - t) = \begin{cases} 1 \text{ at } t < t_0 \\ 0 \text{ at } t \geqslant t_0 \end{cases} \tag{9.5}$$

and at 'infinity'

$$n|_\infty = 0. \tag{9.6}$$

The right-hand side of (9.5) takes into account the time dependence of the flux of hydrated ions generated by the plasma source near the surface of the liquid. It is convenient to introduce the following dimensionless variables:

$$\tau = \frac{t}{t_0},\ \ \xi = \frac{x}{l_0} = \frac{x}{\sqrt{Dt_0}},\ \ \mu = \frac{n}{n_0} = \frac{n}{J}\sqrt{\frac{D}{t_0}}. \tag{9.7}$$

For boundary conditions (9.5) and (9.6), equation (9.4) has the following solution:

$$\mu = \int_0^\tau \frac{1}{\sqrt{\pi(\tau - \zeta)}} \exp\left(-\frac{\xi^2}{4(\tau - \zeta)}\right)\theta(1 - \zeta)\mathrm{d}\zeta. \tag{9.8}$$

Figure 9.7 shows the solution of (9.8) for different values of the dimensionless time τ.

In experiments [13–18], which studied the effect of plasma on cells in a Petri dish, the duration of the plasma source ranged from 0.5 to 2 min, and in [34], up to 60 min. For the vast majority of hydrated salt ions in water at a temperature of $\sim$25°C, the diffusion coefficient lies within the range of $D \sim 10^{-9} - 5 \cdot 10^{-9}\ \mathrm{m^2\,s^{-1}}$

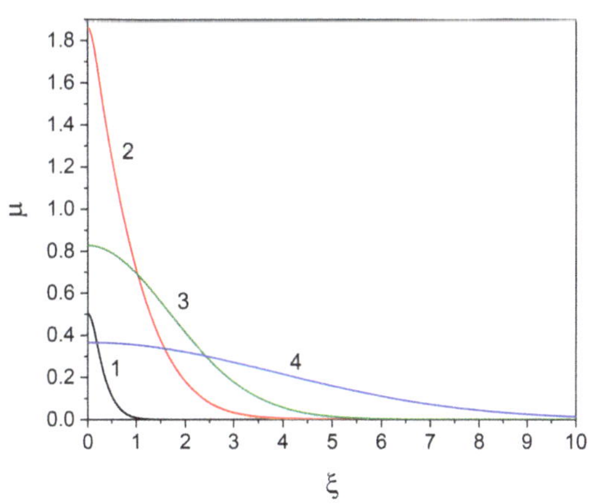

Figure 9.7. Solution of the diffusion equation for dimensionless variables. Line 1 corresponds to $\tau = 0.1$, line 2 to $\tau = 1$, line 3 to $\tau = 2$, and line 4 to $\tau = 4$.

(for example, see the data in [35, 36]). Thus, at $t_0 \sim 100$ s, $l_0 = \sqrt{Dt_0} \sim 0.3-1$ mm, that is, ions can diffuse to cells that are in the upper layers of a physiological solution in a Petri dish (with a typical depth of several millimeters). In this case, as in many experiments, when a plasma jet interacts with the surface of a physiological solution, the volume containing hydrated ions and neutral molecules is much larger because of the deformation of the surface of the liquid by the dynamic pressure of the plasma jet and the resulting hydrodynamic flows.

9.4 Estimation of cell size variation with changing ion concentration in solution

Suppose, for example, that a cell membrane is permeable only to water molecules but impermeable to hydrated ions. In such a case, the equilibrium radius of the cell is determined by the salinity of the solution inside and outside the cell. If the salinity of the solution inside is greater than the salinity outside, the cell absorbs water, and its volume grows until the salinity levels are equal. In the opposite case, the cell expels water, and its volume decreases until the salinity levels are equal.

Figure 9.8 shows a simplified scheme of water molecule transport across the cell membrane without and with solvated (hydrated) ions generated by a plasma source. In figure 9.8(A), the flux of water molecules out of the cell is equal to the flux of water into the cell. The osmotic pressure drop is zero because the ion densities outside and inside the cell are equal. In figure 9.8(B), the flux of water molecules out of the cell is greater than the flux into the cell, so the cell compresses due to mass loss. The compression continues until the flux of water molecules across the membrane is equalized; in other words, the degree of salinity of the water inside and outside the

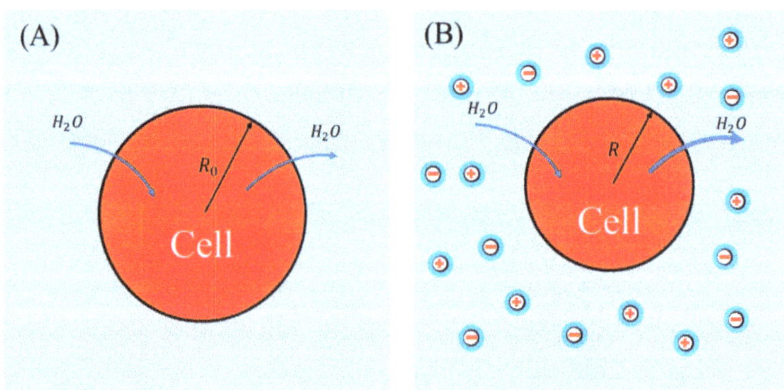

Figure 9.8. Diffusion of water molecules through a cell membrane. Arrows show the transport of water molecules through the membrane. (A) The flow of water molecules into and out of the cell is equal, and the osmotic pressure is zero. (B) The presence of additional solvated (hydrated) ions introduced by the plasma (denoted by smaller circles) reduces the number of free water molecules that can pass through the membrane. The flux of water molecules out of the cell exceeds the flux into the cell. Consequently, the pressure outside the membrane exceeds the pressure inside it, and osmotic pressure compresses the cell. Compression proceeds until the fluxes through the membrane equalize. Note that the densities of 'free' water molecules outside and inside the membrane are not equal, and, as a result, $R_0 > R$.

cell reaches the same level. The excess of ions outside the cell (figure 9.7(B)) leads to a decrease in osmotic pressure, which also contributes to cell compression.

Let $n_s = \sum_i n_i$ be the sum of the densities of all hydrated ions near the cell surface. The salinity of the solution is determined by the relative density of the hydrated ions:

$$\alpha_s = \frac{n_s}{n_w}, \tag{9.9}$$

where n_w is the local density of water molecules. Let the total density of ions near the cell increase by an amount δn_s due to ions injected by the plasma. In a hypertonic solution, under the simplest assumption of the sphericity of the cell shape, its radius decreases from the initial R_0 to R. The salinity of the solution inside the cell is determined by the ratio of the total number of ions in it, $N_s = \frac{4}{3}\pi R_0^3 n_s$, to the number of water molecules in it, $N_w = \frac{4}{3}\pi R_0^3 n_w$. Since the cell membrane is impermeable to ions and the density of water is constant, a change in the salinity of the cell associated with the outflow of water through the membrane only affects the radius of the cell as long as the salinities of the solution inside and outside the cell differ:

$$\alpha_s = \frac{N_s}{N_w} = \frac{\frac{4}{3}\pi R_0^3 n_s}{\frac{4}{3}\pi R^3 n_w} = \frac{\frac{4}{3}\pi R^3 (n_s + \delta n_s)}{\frac{4}{3}\pi R^3 n_w}, \tag{9.10}$$

where δn_s is the change in ion concentration in the cell associated with the change in the amount of water in the cell. Hence, taking into account that $\delta n_s \ll n_s$, the relative change in the radius of the cell is:

$$\frac{R - R_0}{R_0} = \frac{1}{(1 + \frac{\delta n_s}{n_s})^{1/3}} - 1 \approx -\frac{1}{3}\frac{\delta n_s}{n_s}. \tag{9.11}$$

Thus, for the same plasma source and exposure time but different initial salinities of the solution, the deformation of cells in solution is greater for lower initial salinities of the solution.

9.5 Estimation of the osmotic pressure drop across the cell membrane

Let us estimate the pressure drop across the cell membrane caused by the presence of hydrated ions injected by the plasma. The cells in the Petri dish are in equilibrium, so the solution can be considered isotonic before the plasma is exposed to the liquid. It is natural to assume that as a result of interaction with the plasma, additional ions appear in the solution outside the cells, since cell membranes are impermeable to them; in van't Hoff's formula (9.2), we can consider $\sum_i n_{i,\,\mathrm{in}} = 0$. As an example, we take the data given in [34], obtained by different researchers in experiments in which various air-discharge plasmas were studied in contact with water or saline solution. In these experiments, the densities of the NO_3^- and NO_2^- ions and the H_2O_2 molecules produced by the plasma in aqueous solutions were on the order of

0.1–2 $\text{mmol}\,\text{l}^{-1}$. Thus, at the solution temperature of T ~ 300 K, the resulting additional osmotic pressures $\Delta\pi$ were in the range of 0.5–10 kPa. It is known that the critical overpressure at which the phospholipid membrane is destroyed is on the order of 10–12 kPa [37], which is close in magnitude to the upper limit of our estimate. However, even small changes in pressure can disrupt the mechanical properties of membranes, thereby changing the transport into or out of the cell. In particular, changes in the mechanical properties of membranes could be one of the reasons for the selective effect of plasma on cells (for instance, the reason for the selective apoptosis observed in [13–19]).

It should be noted that estimate (9.2) is valid for weak solutions in which solutes can be considered an ideal gas that does not interact with the molecules of the solvent. In reality, the ions generated by the plasma interact with the water molecules (are hydrated), and therefore the pressure drop given by (9.2) is only a rough estimate.

We have shown that the selective effect of a plasma jet on living cells in a physiological solution can be related to a change in the osmotic pressure difference across the cell membrane as a result of the injection of additional long-lived solvated (hydrated) ions by the plasma. These ions result in an outflow of water from the cell volume; that is, the solution becomes hypertonic to the cells. This results in cell shrinkage and ultimately affects cell viability. We want to emphasize that the observed changes in cell morphology in the solution interacting with the plasma, an example of which is shown in figure 9.4, can be explained by the change in osmotic pressure in the solution interacting with the low-temperature plasma source. However, we are by no means claiming that osmotic changes are the only mechanism affecting cells in saline. We would like to point out a possible additional physical mechanism relevant to plasma-induced effects on living cells.

9.6 Selective effect of nonequilibrium low-temperature plasma interacting with healthy and cancerous cells in a Petri dish

Note that the considered effect of the dependence of potential difference across the membrane on water content at the same value of the surface charge can be directly related to the selective effect of nonequilibrium low-temperature plasma interacting with various cell cultures in a Petri dish (e.g. healthy and cancerous cells) observed in many experiments (for examples, see [13–16]). As discussed earlier in this chapter, the interaction of nonequilibrium plasma with a physiological solution changes the ionic composition of the solution and, consequently, the drop in osmotic pressure across the cell membranes. In [21, 22], it was supposed that the displacement of water from membranes and, consequently, the change in their dielectric constant were different between healthy cells and cancerous cells due to a noticeable difference in the mechanical properties of these cells. For example, the membrane properties of cancerous cells and healthy cells can be very different. The modulus of overall compression and the shear modulus for hepatocellular carcinoma cells (HCCs) in the measurements in [38] were $K_1 = 103.6\ \text{Nm}^{-2}$ and $K_2 = 42.5\ \text{Nm}^{-2}$, respectively, and for hepatocytes, they were $K_1 = 87.5\ \text{Nm}^{-2}$ and $K_2 = 33.3\ \text{Nm}^{-2}$, respectively. Resting potentials on the membranes of healthy and cancerous cells also differed markedly. For example, [39] showed that the transmembrane resting potentials in rat hepatocytes and hepatoma cells were −37.1 and −19.8 mV, respectively, and in mouse corneal fibroblasts and fibrosarcoma cells, the corresponding resting potentials were −42.5 and −14.3 mV. In other words, the resting potential in cancer cells was two times less than in healthy cells, indicating a difference in the transport properties of the membranes of healthy and cancerous cells.

It was shown in [40] that the compositions of phospholipids and their associated carboxyl and phosphate functional groups in the membranes of healthy and cancerous cells differ significantly. This, as well as the difference in the composition of ions in the cell [41, 42], apparently explains the difference in the resting potentials on the membranes [38, 39] of healthy and cancerous cells. It is possible that a small effect on the mechanical properties of the membranes or on the transmembrane potential difference might have a significant effect on the transport into and out of healthy and cancerous cells. We believe that the difference between the stiffnesses of healthy and diseased cells leads to differences in cell deformation and the displacement of water from cells for the same change in osmotic pressure as that caused by the interaction due to the appearance of hydrated ions (produced as a result of interaction with a source of low-temperature plasma with a physiological solution). Consequently, there were different changes of resting potential on the membranes of cells in this solution.

If, in addition, electric currents are induced in the solution, thus charging the membranes of these cells, then for the same additional charge on the membrane, the voltage on the membrane and the probability of its electroporation will be different for different cells. This, as was stated earlier in [21, 22], may be one of the reasons for the observed selective effect of nonequilibrium plasma on healthy and diseased cells in a physiological solution in a Petri dish.

9.7 Water flux across the lipid membrane induced by the change in osmotic pressure difference

As discussed above, ions and molecular clusters entering the physiological solution from the interface region of the interaction between the weakly ionized plasma and the surface of the solution change the osmotic pressure, leading to changes in the morphology of cells in the solution. When the ionic concentration of the solution is changed, a diffusive water flux occurs through the lipid bilayer membrane of the cell; that is, water molecules appear in its central hydrophobic part and diffuse through the membrane, changing the dielectric constant of the membrane. Note that we are talking about diffusive water flux through a bilayer lipid membrane without considering water flux through specific protein channels (aquaporins) or flux through pores in porous membranes. In general, however, the relationship between the concentration of water and that of a solute is not simple. The current state of the problem and possible solutions are discussed in many books and reviews, such as [4, 43, 44].

We will limit our discussion to water, but it applies to any other solvent. The volumetric water flux across a semipermeable membrane subjected to both a hydrostatic pressure difference and a difference in osmolarity (the total concentration of solutes in moles per unit volume) is determined by the water flux across the membrane [4, 43, 44], sometimes called the fundamental law of osmosis [43]:

$$J_v = -L_p(\Delta p - \Delta\pi), \tag{9.12}$$

where L_p is the hydraulic conductivity or the filtration coefficient and Δp and $\Delta\pi$ are the hydrostatic and osmotic pressure differences across the membrane. $\Delta\pi$ in (9.12) is determined by formula (9.2). The value of L_p depends on the specific composition and structure of the membrane that allows water to move across it. The hydraulic conductivity L_p is uniquely related to the osmotic water permeability coefficient, usually denoted by P_f and defined as $P_f = L_p\mathrm{RT}/v_w$, where R is the universal gas constant and v_w is the partial molar volume of water. The value of the permeability $P_f = 1\ \mathrm{cm}\cdot\mathrm{s}^{-1}$ at a solution temperature of $T = 298$ K corresponds to the hydraulic conductivity $L_p = 7.386\cdot 10^{-4}\ \mathrm{cm}\cdot\mathrm{s}^{-1}\cdot\mathrm{atm}^{-1}$ [45].

Note that it is possible for the hydraulic conductivity of the membrane to depend on the salinity of the electrolyte. For example, it has been demonstrated in experiments [46] that an increase in electrolyte salinity leads to an increase in membrane porosity, namely, an increase in the distance between the phospholipid heads. Therefore, with an increase in salinity, which is clearly associated with an increase in the density of ions in the electrolyte, it is expected that the amount of water in the membrane should also increase.

9.8 The dielectric constants of cell membranes and the excitation thresholds of the action potential

The water in the phospholipid membrane contributes to its effective permittivity. Therefore, an increase in the amount of water in the membrane should result in an increase in its dielectric constant.

Let us briefly describe the setting of the experiments and the results of [47], which showed that the addition of divalent chloride salts such as $CaCl_2$, $MgCl_2$, and $MnCl_2$ to a solution of NaCl reduces the voltage across the membrane's nerve fibers (resting potential). In [46], divalent chloride salts were added to a 112 $\mathrm{mmol\,l^{-1}}$ NaCl solution in a vessel containing frog myelinated nerve fibers, and a change in sodium transport activity across the membrane was observed as a function of the concentration of divalent ions. Figure 9.9 shows the required potential shifts at different concentrations of divalent ions, where sodium transport corresponds to a $[Ca^{2+}] \approx 2\ \mathrm{mmol\,l^{-1}}$ concentration, which was chosen as the reference point against which the measured shift in resting potential was determined when the concentration of dissolved divalent metal salt in the initial table salt solution was changed. For example, at a concentration of $[Ca^{2+}] \approx 0.1\ \mathrm{mmol\,l^{-1}}$, the potential between the inner electrolyte and the outer electrolyte should be increased by $\approx$16 mV so that the flux of sodium ions into the membrane corresponds to the flux at $Ca^{2+} \approx 2\ \mathrm{l^{-1}}$, and at $[Ca^{2+}] \approx 10\ \mathrm{mmol\,l^{-1}}$, the potential difference between the inner and outer

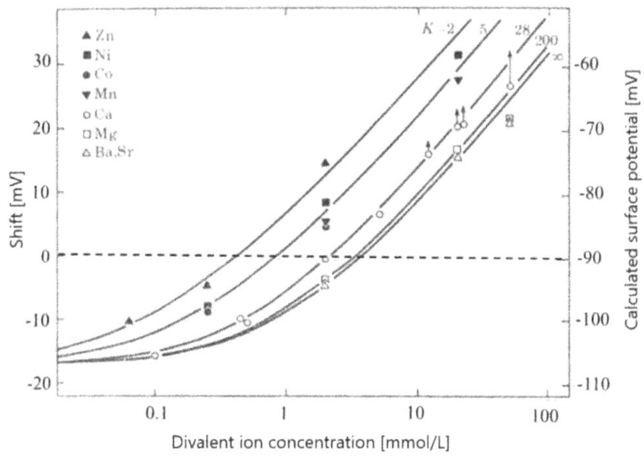

Figure 9.9. Voltage shifts due to different divalent ions. Shifts are plotted against the concentration of added divalent ions, with the horizontal line marking the control value for $Ca^{2+} \approx 2$ mmol l^{-1}. Each point is the mean of about four observations. Arrows on the points for $Ca^{2+} \approx$ 12, 20, 22, and 50 mmol l^{-1} show a correction attributable to the effect of the raised osmolality of those solutions explained in [47]. The right-hand scale shows the calculated surface (resting) potential (see [47] for details). Reproduced with permission from [47].

electrolytes should be decreased by $\delta V_m \approx 16$ mV. The corresponding resting potential, which corresponds to the right-hand axis in figure 9.9, was determined in [46] by empirical formulas, which we will not consider here.

Following [48, 49], considering the water contained in the lipid membrane as an impurity with a relative volume, in estimating the effective permittivity of the membrane ε_m, it is convenient to use the simplest approximate Rayleigh formula for the permittivity of two substances, one of which is continuous and the second of which is uniformly distributed small droplets of the impurity substance [49]:

$$\varepsilon_m \approx \varepsilon_e \left(1 + f \frac{3(\varepsilon_i - \varepsilon_e)}{\varepsilon_i + 2\varepsilon_e - f(\varepsilon_i - \varepsilon_e)} \right). \tag{9.13}$$

Here, ε_m, ε_e, and ε_i are the respective permittivities of the mixture, the main medium, and the impurity droplets, while f is the volume fraction of water. From (9.10), it follows that as $f \to 0$, $\varepsilon_m \to \varepsilon_e$, and as $f \to 1$, $\varepsilon_m \to \varepsilon_i$. Upon substituting the permittivity values $\varepsilon_e \approx 2$ for a dehydrated phospholipid membrane [50, 51] and $\varepsilon_i = \varepsilon_w = 81$ for water into (9.13), we obtain the dependence of the membrane permittivity ε_m on the volume fraction of water f, as shown in figure 9.10.

Since the capacitance of a unit area of a membrane is equal to $C_m = \varepsilon_m \varepsilon_0 / d_m$, then the potential difference across a membrane with a surface charge density of Σ_m is equal to:

$$U_m = \Sigma_m d_m / \varepsilon_m \varepsilon_0. \tag{9.14}$$

Recall that the resting potential at the membrane is determined by formula (1.10) and that it depends on the concentrations of sodium, potassium, and chloride ions

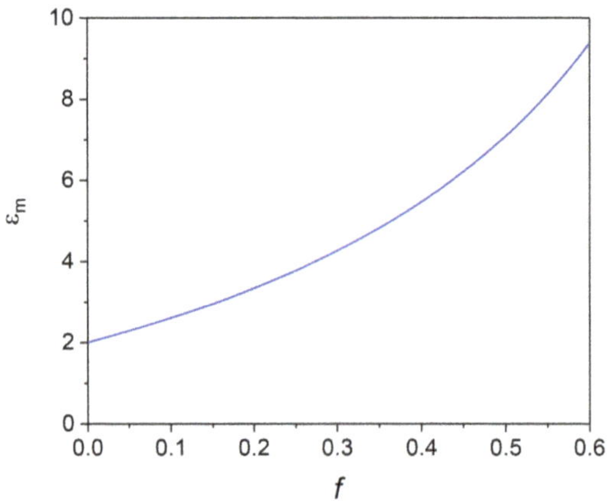

Figure 9.10. Dependence of the effective dielectric constant of the membrane ε_m on the water content f for $\varepsilon_e = 2$ and $\varepsilon_i = \varepsilon_w = 81$, calculated using formula (9.10).

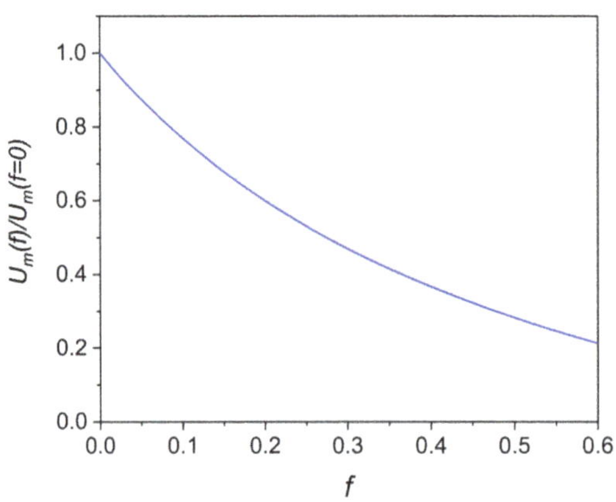

Figure 9.11. Dependence of the potential difference across the membrane on the water content f at a fixed value of the membrane surface charge Σ_m and thickness d_m.

on both sides of the membrane. Under equilibrium conditions, if no divalent metal salts are added to the physiological solution, as in experiments in [47], or if there is no interaction between the solution and a low-temperature plasma source, as in plasma medicine experiments, the solution can be considered isotonic. The appearance of additional ions in the solution, as a result of the dissociation of metal salts or coming from the area of plasma interaction, makes the solution hypertonic because the ions added to the physiological solution do not penetrate the membrane. The surface charge on the membrane is determined by the membrane capacitance and the resting potential $\Sigma_m = C_m U_m$. If we assume that when additional hydrated ions appear in the intercellular medium, making the solution hypertonic, the surface charge on the membrane and its thickness change little compared with the water content in the membrane, then $U_m \propto 1/\varepsilon_m$. In this case, the water content dependence of the ratio $U_m(f)/U_m(f=0)$ is shown in figure 9.11.

In our opinion, the saturation of the membrane with water explains the marked decrease in resting potential in the nervous tissue observed in [47]. A similar effect of resting potential reduction should be expected for nerve tissue in a physiological solution saturated with ions when the solution interacts with a low-temperature plasma source. On the other hand, a decrease in the resting potential leads to a decrease in the action potential excitation threshold, which is determined by voltage-gated protein channels for sodium ions. This effect could have medical applications, such as the stimulation of action potentials in the affected nerve tissue or, conversely, anesthesia, that is, blocking the action potential, based on the difference between the excitation thresholds of normal and plasma-activated physiological solutions. There is a certain analogy here to electrical stimulation with small-amplitude electrical pulses, which we discussed in chapter 7.

9.9 Changing the speed of action potential propagation

A change in the capacitance of a unit membrane area should lead not only to a change in the resting potential of the membrane, and hence in the excitation thresholds of the nerve tissue, but also to a change in the propagation velocity of the action potential. From our estimate of the action potential propagation velocity in the non-myelinated squid axon (1.47), we obtain:

$$v_{\text{ap}} \approx \frac{1}{C_m}\sqrt{\frac{aG_{Na}}{2r_{\|}}} \propto 1/\varepsilon_m. \tag{9.15}$$

In estimate (9.15), we have taken into account that the relative change in ion concentration inside and outside the axon is small, so that the change in resistance $r_{\|}$ can be neglected. Thus, if the axon membrane is saturated with water as a result of a change in osmotic pressure when the axon is in a physiological solution interacting with plasma, the rate of action potential propagation should decrease significantly. It would be very interesting to observe this phenomenon in an appropriate experiment using standard patch-clamp techniques or modern non-perturbative optical methods (for example, see [52]).

9.10 Concluding remarks

In this chapter, we showed the importance of considering osmosis when a physiological saline solution containing cells interacts with a low-temperature plasma source. This allowed us to explain the changes in cell morphology observed experimentally.

In addition, the resulting flow of water into or out of the cell causes a change in the water content of the lipid bilayer membranes, thereby increasing the dielectric constant of the membrane. In turn, the increase in the dielectric permittivity and, consequently, the capacitance of the cell membranes leads to an increase in the resting potential at the membrane (a decrease in absolute value), similar to the effect observed in experiments when divalent metal salts are dissolved in a physiological solution.

For nerve tissue in a physiological solution interacting with plasma, a significant decrease in excitation threshold and slower action potential propagation should be expected. However, a final conclusion about the possibility of these effects can only be reached after conducting appropriate experiments. Stimulating such experiments was the primary purpose of this chapter.

References

[1] L'Abbé Nollet 1748 Recherches sur les causes du bouillonnement des liquides (Researches on the causes of the boiling of liquids) *Histoire de l'Académie Royale des Sciences. Année MDCCXLVIII. Avec les Mémoires de Mathématique & de Physique, pour la même Anneé. Tirés des registres de cette Académie.* 57 https://gallica.bnf.fr/ark:/12148/bpt6k3546r/f203.item

[2] Glaser R 1996 *Biophysik* (Jena: Gustav Fischer Verlag)

[3] Sperelakis N 2011 *Cell Physiology Sourcebook: Essentials of Membrane Biophysics* 4th edn (New York: Academic Press)

[4] Kargol A 2019 *Introduction to Cellular Biophysics, Volume 1 Membrane transport mechanisms* (Bristol: IOP Publishing)

[5] Van't Hoff J H 1886 Une propriété général de la matière diluée *Kungliga Svenska Vetenskaps-Akademiens Handlingar* **21** 42–9

[6] Whittaker A G, Mount A R and Heal M R 2000 *Physical Chemistry* (Oxford: BIOS Scientific Publishers Limited)

[7] Lodish H, Berk A, Zipursky S L, Matsudaira P, Baltimore D and Darnell J 2000 *Molecular Cell Biology* 4th edn (New York: W H Freeman)

[8] Akeson S P and Mel H C 1982 Osmotic hemolysis and fragility. A new model based on membrane disruption, and a potential clinical test *Biochim. Biophys. Acta* **718** 201

[9] Goodhead L K and MacMillan F M 2017 Measuring osmosis and hemolysis of red blood cells *Adv. Physiol. Educ.* **41** 298

[10] Fridman A A and Friedman G D 2013 *Plasma Medicine* (New York: Wiley)

[11] Laroussi M, Richardson J P and Dobbs F C 2002 Effects of non-equilibrium atmospheric pressure plasmas on the heterotrophic pathways of bacteria and on their cell morphology *Appl. Phys. Lett.* **81** 772

[12] Lu X, Naidis G V, Laroussi M, Reuter S, Graves D B and Ostrikov K 2016 Reactive species in non-equilibrium atmospheric-pressure plasmas: generation, transport, and biological effects *Phys. Rep.* **630** 1

[13] Kim G J, Kim W, Kim K T and Lee J K 2010 DNA damage and mitochondria dysfunction in cell apoptosis induced by nonthermal air plasma *Appl. Phys. Lett.* **96** 021502

[14] Barekzi N and Laroussi M 2012 Dose-dependent killing of leukemia cells by low-temperature plasma *J. Phys. D: Appl. Phys.* **45** 422002

[15] Yan D, Sherman J H and Keidar M 2017 Cold atmospheric plasma, a novel promising anti-cancer treatment modality *Oncotarget* **8** 15977

[16] Yan D, Cui H, Zhu W, Nourmohammadi N, Milberg J, Zhang L G, Sherman J H and Keidar M 2017 The specific vulnerabilities of cancer cells to the cold atmospheric plasma-stimulated solutions *Sci. Rep.* **7** 4479

[17] Yan D, Talbot A, Nourmohammadi N, Sherman J, Cheng X and Keidar M 2015 Toward understanding the selective anti-cancer capacity of cold atmospheric plasma—a model based on aquaporins *Biointephases* **10** 040801

[18] Yan D, Xiao H, Zhu W, Nourmohammadi N, Zhang G, Bian K and Keidar M 2017 The role of aquaporins in the anti-glioblastoma capacity of the cold plasma-stimulated medium *J. Phys. D: Appl. Phys.* **50** 055401

[19] Stoffels E, Sakiyama Y and Graves D B 2008 Cold atmospheric plasma: charged species and their interactions with cells and tissues *IEEE Trans. Plas. Sci.* **36** 1441

[20] Bruggeman P and Leys C 2009 Non-thermal plasmas in and in contact with liquids *J. Phys. D: Appl. Phys.* **42** 053001

[21] Shneider M N and Pekker M 2018 Effect of weakly ionized plasma on osmotic pressure on cell membranes in a saline *J. Appl. Phys.* **123** 204701

[22] Shneider M N and Pekker M 2019 On the possible mechanisms of the selective effect of a non-equilibrium plasma on healthy and cancer cells in a physiological solution *Plasma Res. Express* **1** 045001

[23] Ohene Y, Marinov I, de Laulanié L, Dupuy C, Wattelier B and Starikovskaia S 2015 Phase imaging microscopy for the diagnostics of plasma-cell interaction *Appl. Phys. Lett.* **106** 233703

[24] Park W H 2013 The effects of exogenous H_2O_2 on cell death, reactive oxygen species and glutathione levels in calf pulmonary artery and human umbilical vein endothelial cells *Int. J. Mol. Med.* **31** 471

[25] Collin F 2019 Chemical basis of reactive oxygen species reactivity and involvement in neurodegenerative diseases *Int. J. Mol. Sci.* **20** 2407

[26] Petrucci R H 2007 *General Chemistry: Principles & Modern Applications* 9th edn (Hoboken, NJ: Prentice-Hall)

[27] Bienert G P, Schjoerring J K and Jahn T P 2006 Membrane transport of hydrogen peroxide *Biochim. Biophys. Acta* **1758** 994

[28] Branco M R, Marhino H, Cyrne L and Antunes F 2004 Decrease of H_2O_2 plasma membrane permeability during adaptation to H_2O_2 in *Saccharomyces cerevisiae J. Biol. Chem.* **279** 6501

[29] Pędziwiatr P, Mikołajczyk F, Zawadzki D, Mikołajczyk K and Bedka A 2018 Decomposition of hydrogen peroxide—kinetics and review of chosen catalysts *Acta Innovations* **N26** 45

[30] Aidly D J 1988 *The Physiology of Excitable Cells* 4th cdn (Cambridge: Cambridge University Press)

[31] Weaver J C and Chizmadzhev Y A 1996 Theory of electroporation: a review *Bioelectrochem. Bioenerg.* **41** 135

[32] Pavlin M, Kotnik T, Miklavčič D, Kramar P and Lebar A M 2008 Electroporation of planar lipid bilayers and membranes *Adv. Planar Lipid Bilayers Liposomes* **6** 165

[33] Debruin K A and Krassowska W 1998 Electroporation and shock-induced transmembrane potential in a cardiac fiber during defibrillation strength *Ann. Biomed. Eng.* **26** 584

[34] Lukes P, Dolezalova E, Sisrova I and Clupek M 2014 Aqueous-phase chemistry and bactericidal effects from an air discharge plasma in contact with water: evidence for the formation of peroxynitrite through a pseudo-second-order post-discharge reaction of H2O2 and HNO2 *Plasma Sources Sci. Technol.* **23** 015019

[35] Samson E, Marchand J and Snyder K A 2003 Calculation of ionic diffusion coefficients on the basis of migration test results *Mat. Struct. (MatÈriaux et Constructions)* **36** 156

[36] Li Y-H and Gregory S 1974 Diffusion of ions in sea water and in deep-sea sediments *Geochim. Gasmochim. Acta* **38** 703–14

[37] Gonzalez-Rodriguez D, Guillou L, Cornat F, Lafaurie-Janvore J, Babataheri A, de Langre E, Barakat A I and Husson J 2016 Mechanical criterion for the rupture of a cell membrane under compression *Biophys. J.* **111** 2711

[38] Zhang G, Long M, Wu Z-Z and Yu W-Q 2002 Mechanical properties of hepatocellular carcinoma cells *World J. Gastroenterol.* **8** 243

[39] Binggeli R and Cameron I L 1980 Cellular potentials of normal and cancerous fibroblasts and hepatocytes *Cancer Res.* **40** 1830–5

[40] Szachowicz-Petelska B, Dobrzyńska I, Sulkowski S and Figaszewski Z A 2012 Characterization of the cell membrane during cancer transformation *Colorectal Cancer Biology—from Genes to Tumor* ed R Ettarh (Rijeka: InTech) 241

[41] Dobrzyńska I, Szachowicz-Petelska B, Darewicz B and Figaszewski Z A 2015 Characterization of human bladder cell membrane during cancer transformation *J. Membr. Biol.* **248** 301

[42] Cameron I, Smith N K, Pool T B and Sparks R L 1980 Intracellular concentration of sodium and other elements as related to mitogenesis and oncogenesis *in vivo Cancer Res.* **40** 1493–500

[43] Manning G S and Kay A R 2023 The physical basis of osmosis *J. Gen. Physiol.* **155** e202313332 https://rupress.org/jgp/article/155/10/e202313332/276211/The-physical-basis-of-osmosisThe-physical-basis-of

[44] Fredrik K 1982 Mechanism of osmosis *Kidney Int.* **21** 303

[45] Fettiplace R and Haydon D A 1980 Water permeability of lipid membranes *Physiol. Rev.* **60** 510

[46] Petrache H I, Tristram-Nagle S, Harries D and Kučerka N 2006 Swelling of phospholipids by monovalent salt *J. Lipid Res.* **47** 302

[47] Hille B, Woodhull A M and Shapiro B I 1975 Negative surface charge near sodium channels of nerve: divalent ions, monovalent ions, and pH *Phil. Trans. R. Soc. London* **B 270** 301

[48] Shneider M N and Pekker M 2023 *The effect of intercellular medium salinity on the dielectric constant of cell membranes and the excitation thresholds of the action potential* (bioRxiv preprint

[49] Sihvola A 2000 Mixing rules with complex dielectric coefficients *Subsurface Sensing Tech. Appl.* **1** 393

[50] Huang W and Levitt D G 1977 Theoretical calculation of dielectric constant of a bilayer membrane *Biophys. J.* **17** 111

[51] Vitkova V, Mitkova D, Antonova K, Popkirov G and Dimova R 2018 Sucrose solutions alter the electric capacitance and dielectric permittivity of lipid bilayers *Colloids Surf. Physicochem. Eng. Asp.* **557** 51

[52] Emmenegger V, Obien M E J, Franke F and Hierlemann A 2019 Technologies to study action potential propagation with a focus on HD-MEAs *Front. Cell. Neurosci.* **13** 159

www.ingramcontent.com/pod-product-compliance
Ingram Content Group UK Ltd.
Pitfield, Milton Keynes, MK11 3LW, UK
UKHW051854100926
8556IPUK00005B/624

9 780750 360326